Rheumatoid Arthritis: From Pathophysiology to Management

Rheumatoid Arthritis: From Pathophysiology to Management

Editor: Travis Reagan

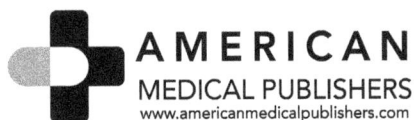

AMERICAN
MEDICAL PUBLISHERS
www.americanmedicalpublishers.com

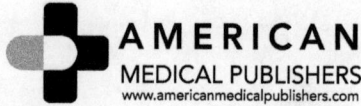

AMERICAN
MEDICAL PUBLISHERS
www.americanmedicalpublishers.com

Cataloging-in-Publication Data

Rheumatoid arthritis : from pathophysiology to management / edited by Travis Reagan.
   p. cm.
Includes bibliographical references and index.
ISBN 978-1-63927-476-5
1. Rheumatoid arthritis. 2. Rheumatoid arthritis--Pathophysiology. 3. Rheumatoid arthritis--Treatment.
4. Rheumatism. 5. Arthritis. I. Reagan, Travis.
RC933 .R443 2022

616.72--dc23

American Medical Publishers,
41 Flatbush Avenue,
1st Floor, New York,
NY 11217, USA

ISBN 978-1-63927-476-5 (Hardback)

This book contains information obtained from authentic and highly regarded sources. Copyright for all individual chapters remain with the respective authors as indicated. All chapters are published with permission under the Creative Commons Attribution License or equivalent. A wide variety of references are listed. Permission and sources are indicated; for detailed attributions, please refer to the permissions page and list of contributors. Reasonable efforts have been made to publish reliable data and information, but the authors, editors and publisher cannot assume any responsibility for the validity of all materials or the consequences of their use.

Trademark Notice: Registered trademark of products or corporate names are used only for explanation and identification without intent to infringe.

Contents

Preface

Rheumatoid arthritis (RA) is an autoimmune condition which affects the joints of the wrists, hands, elbows, feet, ankles and knees. It primarily causes the joints to swell. It may also affect other parts of the body. Symptoms tend to appear gradually over a period of weeks to months, as the disease progresses. The development of RA occurs with the activation of autoimmunity in joints and organs where it manifests. The disease starts with a phase of initiation due to non-specific inflammation, followed by a phase of amplification owing to T cell activation, and finally it enters a chronic inflammatory phase in which tissue injury starts to occur. The goal of treatment in RA is the reduction of pain and inflammation, and improvement in the overall functioning of the individual. Steroids, pain medications and NSAIDs are prescribed for the management of symptoms. This book contains some path-breaking studies in the pathophysiology and management of rheumatoid arthritis. It consists of contributions made by international experts. This book is an essential guide for both academicians and those who wish to pursue orthopedics further.

This book is a comprehensive compilation of works of different researchers from varied parts of the world. It includes valuable experiences of the researchers with the sole objective of providing the readers (learners) with a proper knowledge of the concerned field. This book will be beneficial in evoking inspiration and enhancing the knowledge of the interested readers.

In the end, I would like to extend my heartiest thanks to the authors who worked with great determination on their chapters. I also appreciate the publisher's support in the course of the book. I would also like to deeply acknowledge my family who stood by me as a source of inspiration during the project.

Editor

Glutaminase 1 plays a key role in the cell growth of fibroblast-like synoviocytes in rheumatoid arthritis

Soshi Takahashi[1], Jun Saegusa[1,2*], Sho Sendo[1], Takaichi Okano[1], Kengo Akashi[1], Yasuhiro Irino[3] and Akio Morinobu[1]

Abstract

Background: The recent findings of cancer-specific metabolic changes, including increased glucose and glutamine consumption, have provided new therapeutic targets for consideration. Fibroblast-like synoviocytes (FLS) from rheumatoid arthritis (RA) patients exhibit several tumor cell-like characteristics; however, the role of glucose and glutamine metabolism in the aberrant proliferation of these cells is unclear. Here, we evaluated the role of these metabolic pathways in RA-FLS proliferation and in autoimmune arthritis in SKG mice.

Methods: The expression of glycolysis- or glutaminolysis-related enzymes was evaluated by real-time polymerase chain reaction (PCR) and Western blotting, and the intracellular metabolites were evaluated by metabolomic analyses. The effects of glucose or glutamine on RA-FLS cell growth were investigated using glucose- or glutamine-free medium. Glutaminase (GLS)1 small interfering RNA (siRNA) and the GLS1 inhibitor compound 968 were used to inhibit GLS1 in RA-FLS, and compound 968 was used to study the effect of GLS1 inhibition in zymosan A-injected SKG mice.

Results: GLS1 expression was increased in RA-FLS, and metabolomic analyses revealed that glutamine metabolism was increased in RA-FLS. RA-FLS proliferation was reduced under glutamine-deprived, but not glucose-deprived, conditions. Cell growth of RA-FLS was inhibited by GLS1 siRNA transfection or GLS1 inhibitor treatment. Treating RA-FLS with either interleukin-17 or platelet-derived growth factor resulted in increased GLS1 levels. Compound 968 ameliorated the autoimmune arthritis and decreased the number of Ki-67-positive synovial cells in SKG mice.

Conclusions: Our results suggested that glutamine metabolism is involved in the pathogenesis of RA and that GLS1 plays an important role in regulating RA-FLS proliferation, and may be a novel therapeutic target for RA.

Keywords: Fibroblasts, Glutaminolysis, Glutamine, Metabolomics, Rheumatoid arthritis

Background

Rheumatoid arthritis (RA) is a systemic autoimmune disease characterized by immune cell infiltration and proliferation in the synovium, leading to progressive joint destruction. Although the etiology of RA is not fully understood, recent evidence indicates that resident fibroblast-like synoviocytes (FLS) play a major role in initiating and driving RA [1]. RA-FLS exhibit anchorage-independent proliferation, lack contact inhibition in vitro, and can attach to and invade articular cartilage [1, 2]. Furthermore, RA-FLS survive autonomously in a tumor-like environment that is enriched with oxygen radicals, nitric oxide, and cytokines [3, 4]. In recent years, the development of biologic therapies that target pro-inflammatory cytokines and immune cells have greatly improved the treatment of RA; however, some patients remain resistant to these therapies. Thus, new therapies designed to suppress RA-FLS proliferation could replace or complement existing RA treatments, increasing the therapeutic efficacy for the nonresponding population.

Many inflammation and hypoxia-induced signaling pathways have profound effects on intracellular metabolism,

* Correspondence: jsaegusa@med.kobe-u.ac.jp
[1]Department of Rheumatology and Clinical Immunology, Kobe University Graduate School of Medicine, 7-5-1, Kusunoki-Cho, Chuo-Ku, Kobe 650-0017, Japan
[2]Department of Clinical Laboratory, Kobe University Hospital, 7-5-1, Kusunoki-Cho, Chuo-Ku, Kobe 650-0017, Japan
Full list of author information is available at the end of the article

leading to effects on cell growth and survival. Recent studies of cancer cell metabolism have revealed cancer-specific metabolic changes that have led to the identification of new therapeutic targets. Most cancer cells consume glucose at higher rates than normal cells, a phenomenon known as the Warburg effect [5]. Many studies have shown that glycolytic enzyme inhibitors efficiently inhibit tumor growth, both in vitro and in vivo, by shifting glucose metabolism from glycolysis to glucose oxidation. This shift results in the release of proapoptotic mediators and reduces malignant cell proliferation, thus eliminating actively growing tumor cells while leaving normal cells unaffected [6]. Glutamine is another carbon source that is important in cell growth and energy metabolism [7, 8]. Glutamine provides a major energy source for respiration and serves as a precursor for the synthesis of macromolecules such as nucleotides and proteins [9, 10]. In tumor cells, pyruvate generated from the glycolytic pathway is converted to lactate, rather than being used in the tricarboxylic acid (TCA) cycle. Although the requirement for mitochondrial ATP production is reduced in tumor cells, the demand for biosynthetic precursors and NADPH is increased [11]. To compensate for these changes and to maintain a functional TCA cycle, cancer cells often rely on elevated glutaminolysis [12–15]. Several cancer cells, such as HeLa and basal-type breast cancer cells [12, 16, 17], even favor glutamine over glucose as an energy source.

RA-FLS exhibit several tumor cell-like characteristics, but the role of glycolysis in RA-FLS proliferation is unclear. The microenvironment in RA inflamed joints is characterized by hypoxia and low nutrient concentrations [18–20]. A few reports have addressed the metabolic changes in RA-FLS. For example, metabolome analysis showed the different metabolomic profiling between RA-FLS and osteoarthritis (OA)-FLS [21]. In addition, the inhibition of glucose transporter 1, choline kinase, monocarboxylate transporter (MCT4), and 6-phosphofructo-2-kinase, or the activation of pyruvate dehydrogenase or administration of fructose 1,6-bisphosphate, have each been shown to inhibit RA-FLS proliferation and/or ameliorate inflammatory arthritis in mice [22–27]. The metabolic changes identified in RA-FLS represent novel mechanisms that contribute to the pathogenesis of rheumatic diseases, and the targeting of metabolic dysfunction may provide a new therapeutic approach for RA.

Since the roles of glycolysis and glutaminolysis in RA have not been thoroughly investigated, here we examined the role of these pathways in RA-FLS proliferation and the development of arthritis in SKG mice. The glutamine catabolism pathway is initiated by the conversion of glutamine to glutamate by glutaminase (GLS)1, and several studies have shown that GLS1 inhibition significantly suppresses cancer cell proliferation [28–31]. Here,

we found that GLS1 expression was upregulated in RA-FLS, and that RA-FLS cell growth was decreased under glutamine-deprived, but not glucose-deprived, conditions. We also found that GLS1 inhibition suppressed RA-FLS proliferation and ameliorated inflammatory arthritis in SKG mice.

Methods

Mice

Female SKG mice were obtained from CLEA Japan (Tokyo, Japan). The mice were housed in the Kobe University animal facility at a constant temperature, with laboratory chow and water provided ad libitum. All animal protocols received prior approval by the institutional review board and all procedures were performed in accordance with the recommendations of the Institutional Animal Care Committee of Kobe University.

Reagents and antibodies

Zymosan A (ZyA) was obtained from Sigma-Aldrich (St. Louis, MO, USA). Cytokines and platelet-derived growth factor (PDGF) were from R&D Systems (Minneapolis, MN, USA). Compound 968, 5-(3-bromo-4-(dimethylamino)phenyl)-2,2-dimethyl-2,3,5,6-tetrahydrobenzo[a]phenanthridin-4(1H)-one, was obtained from Calbiochem (La Jolla, CA, USA). Anti-glutaminase and anti-Ki-67 antibodies were obtained from Abcam (Cambridge, UK).

Fibroblast-like synoviocytes and cell culture

Human studies were approved by the ethics committees of the Kobe University Hospital and conducted in accordance with the Declaration of Helsinki. Synovial tissue samples were obtained from RA and OA patients undergoing joint replacement surgery or synovectomy. The RA patients fulfilled the American College of Rheumatology 1987 criteria [32]. Collected synovial tissue samples were minced and incubated first with 4 mg/ml collagenase, and then with 0.05% trypsin (Difco, Detroit, MI, USA), as described previously [33]. The isolated cells were cultured in Dulbecco's modified Eagle's medium (DMEM) supplemented with 10% fetal bovine serum (FBS; GIBCO BRL, Palo Alto, CA, USA), 1% penicillin-streptomycin (Lonza Walkersville Inc., Walkersville, MD, USA), and 2 mM L-glutamine (GIBCO BRL). FLS cultures (used between passages 3–6) were maintained as previously described [33]. To determine the effects of glutamine or glucose deprivation, the FLS were cultured in DMEM with both L-glutamine and D-glucose (Wako, Osaka, Japan 044-29765), DMEM without L-glutamine (Wako 045-30285), or DMEM without D-glucose (Wako 042-32255), each of which was supplemented with 10% dialyzed FBS (Biowest, Nuaillé, France) and 1% penicillin-streptomycin.

Metabolomic analyses

FLS intracellular metabolites (0.2–1.0×10^6 cells) were analyzed by gas chromatography-mass spectrometry (GC/MS) and capillary electrophoresis-mass spectrometry (CE-MS; C-SCOPE, Human Metabolome Technologies Inc., Tsuruoka, Japan). GC/MS analysis was performed using a GC/MSQP2010 Ultra (Shimadzu Co., Kyoto, Japan) with a fused silica capillary column (CP-SIL 8 CB low bleed/MS; 30 m × 0.25 mm inner diameter, 0.25 μm film thickness; Agilent Technologies, Waldbronn, Germany), as described previously [34, 35]. 2-Isopropylmalic acid solution (Sigma-Aldrich) was added as an internal standard. The C-SCOPE analysis was performed as described previously [36]. 5-Hydroxy-N-methyl-tryptamine (Human Metabolome Technologies Inc.) was added as an internal standard.

Real-time polymerase chain reaction

Total RNA was isolated using RNeasy (Qiagen, Hilden, Germany), and 1 μg of total RNA was reverse-transcribed with a QuantiTect reverse transcription kit (Qiagen). Quantitative real-time polymerase chain reaction (PCR) was performed using a QuantiTect SYBR Green PCR Kit (Qiagen) with an ABI Prism 9900 instrument (Applied Biosystems, Foster City, CA, USA), according to the manufacturer's instructions. The primer pairs were from Qiagen and are shown in Additional file 1: Table S1. The mRNA levels were normalized to that of glyceraldehyde-3-phosphate dehydrogenase (GAPDH; QT01192646, Qiagen).

Western blotting

Cell lysates were analyzed by Western blotting with anti-GLS and anti-β-actin antibodies (Sigma-Aldrich). The bound antibodies were visualized using a chemiluminescence reagent (Super Signal West Dura Extended Duration Substrate, Thermo Fisher Scientific, Waltham, MA, USA) following the manufacturer's instructions. Immunoblot signals were quantified by densitometric scanning of the films, using ImageJ software.

Cell viability assays

Cell viability was determined using a WST-8 Cell Proliferation Cytotoxicity Assay Kit (Dojindo Laboratories, Kumamoto, Japan). Cells were seeded into 96-well plates (1×10^4 cells/well). After the culture period, the wells were pulsed with WST-8 for 3 h, and the optical density at 450 nm was measured with a microplate reader (Bio-Rad, Hercules, CA, USA).

Cell proliferation assays

Cells were seeded into 96-well plates (1×10^4 cells/well). After the culture period, cell proliferation was determined using a cell proliferation enzyme-linked immunosorbent assay (ELISA; BrdU; Roche, Basel, Switzerland) following the manufacturer's instructions, and by measuring optical densities at 450 nm with a microplate reader (Bio-Rad).

Arthritis induction and evaluation

Eight-week-old SKG mice were treated with 2 mg ZyA as previously described [37]. Briefly, ZyA suspended in saline was intraperitoneally injected on day 0, and arthritis developed 14 to 21 days later. Arthritis severity was assessed using a previously described scoring system (0 = no joint swelling, 0.1 = swelling of one digit joint, 0.5 = mild swelling of the wrist or ankle, and 1.0 = severe swelling of the wrist or ankle [38, 39]). The individual joint scores were totaled for each mouse.

Histology and immunohistochemistry

The hind paws of the mice were removed, fixed in 4% paraformaldehyde, decalcified in EDTA, embedded in paraffin, and sectioned. The samples were then stained with hematoxylin and eosin, and histological evaluation was performed. Histological evaluation was performed using a previously described scoring system (0 = no inflammation, 1 = slight thickening of the synovial cell layer and/or the presence of some inflammatory cells in the sublining, 2 = thickening of the synovial lining, infiltration of the sublining, and localized cartilage erosions, and 3 = infiltration in the synovial space, pannus formation, cartilage destruction, and bone erosion [39]). Paraffin-embedded tissue sections (5 μm) were deparaffinized and hydrated with xylene and graded alcohols using a standard protocol, and incubated overnight with primary antibodies at 4 °C in a humidified chamber, and then rinsed and incubated with biotinylated secondary antibodies for 30 min at room temperature. The slides were developed using the ImmunoCruz™ ABC Staining System (Santa Cruz Biotechnology, Santa Cruz, CA, USA) and were counterstained with Mayer's hematoxylin solution (Wako). Immunohistochemical staining of proliferating cells was performed with an anti-Ki-67 antibody. The Ki-67-positive cells in the lining of the synovium were quantified using ImageJ software.

Treatment of SKG mice with compound 968

Compound 968 was dissolved in dimethyl sulfoxide (DMSO; Sigma-Aldrich) and administered intraperitoneally to SKG mice at 25 mg/kg three times per week from day 14 (before the onset of arthritis) to day 42 after ZyA injection. DMSO was used as a negative control.

Statistical analysis

Results are expressed as the mean ± SEM. Statistical comparisons were performed using the Student's t test, Mann-Whitney U test, and Welch's t test, and two-way analysis of variance (ANOVA) using GraphPad Prism software as appropriate. *P* values less than 0.05 were considered statistically significant.

Results

Increased expression of mRNAs encoding HK2, MCT4, PDK1, and GLS1 in RA-FLS

To determine which metabolic pathways are upregulated in RA-FLS, we compared the expression of 14 glycolysis- or glutaminolysis-related genes in RA-FLS to that in OA-FLS by real-time PCR. We found that the mRNA levels of hexokinase (HK)2, MCT4, pyruvate dehydrogenase kinase (PDK)1, and GLS1 were significantly higher in RA-FLS than in OA-FLS. mRNA levels of glucose transporter (G6PD), pyruvate kinase isozyme (PKM)2, MCT3, and GLS2 were significantly higher in OA-FLS than in RA-FLS (Fig. 1). The expression level of GLS2 was extremely low compared to GLS1, suggesting that GLS1 plays a major role in glutamine metabolism (Additional file 2: Figure S1).

Upregulation of the glycolytic and glutaminolytic pathways in RA-FLS

To further elucidate the altered metabolic regulation in RA-FLS, we assessed the intracellular metabolomic profiles of RA-FLS and OA-FLS using GC/MS and CE-MS.

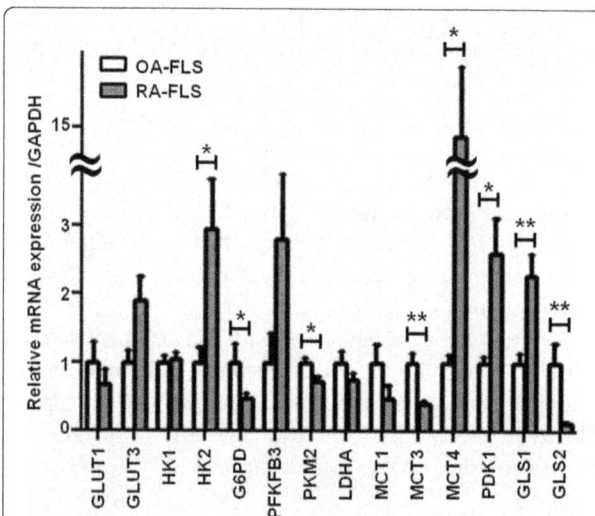

Fig. 1 RA-FLS exhibit higher HK2, MCT4, PDK1, and GLS1 mRNA levels than OA-FLS. Glycolysis- and glutaminolysis-related mRNAs were examined in 12 OA-FLS and 19 RA-FLS by real-time PCR, and their levels were normalized to that of GAPDH mRNA. Each experiment was performed in triplicate. Bars indicate mean ± SEM. *P < 0.05, **P < 0.01, versus OA-FLS by Student's *t* test. *G6PD* glucose-6-phosphate dehydrogenase, *GAPDH* glyceraldehyde-3-phosphate dehydrogenase, *GLS* glutaminase, *GLUT* glucose transporter, *HK* hexokinase, *LDHA* lactate dehydrogenase, *MCT* monocarboxylate transporter, *OA-FLS* fibroblast-like synoviocytes from osteoarthritis patients, *PDK* pyruvate dehydrogenase kinase; *PFK* 6-phosphofructo-2-kinase/fructose-2,6-bisphosphatase, *PKM* pyruvate kinase isozyme, *RA-FLS* fibroblast-like synoviocytes from rheumatoid arthritis patients

Both methods showed that the levels of glucose, glutamine, and glutamate tended to be lower in RA-FLS than in OA-FLS, suggesting that the glucose, glutamine, and glutamate consumptions were higher in RA-FLS (Fig. 2), although we did not find significant differences in the glutamine/glutamate ratio between OA-FLS and RA-FLS (Additional file 3: Figure S2). These results, together with the mRNA expression profiles (Fig. 1), indicated that both the glycolytic and glutaminolytic pathways are upregulated in RA-FLS.

Importance of glutamine for RA-FLS proliferation

We next examined the roles of HK2, MCT4, PDK1, and GLS1 in RA-FLS proliferation. Smaill interfering RNA (siRNA) efficiency is shown in Additional file 4: Figure S3. The knockdown of MCT4, PDK1, or GLS1, but not HK2, significantly inhibited RA-FLS proliferation (Fig. 3a). Silencing of MCT4, PDK1, or GLS1 did not significantly increase or decrease interleukin (IL)-6 or matrix metalloproteinase (MMP)-3 production (Additional file 5: Figure S4). We then studied the requirement of glucose or glutamine for RA-FLS proliferation and found that the RA-FLS cell growth was significantly reduced under glutamine-deprived, but not glucose-deprived, medium conditions (Fig. 3b). Under the glutamine-containing medium condition, we found that RA-FLS proliferation was increased after PGDF stimulation, whereas under the glutamine-deprived medium condition we found that RA-FLS proliferation was not increased even after PDGF stimulation (Additional file 6: Figure S5). These results suggested that glutamine plays a more important role than glucose in RA-FLS proliferation.

Upregulation of GLS1 in RA-FLS

Next, we evaluated the expression of GLS1, a key rate-limiting enzyme in glutaminolysis, in FLS. Western blot analysis revealed that the GLS1 expression was significantly higher in RA-FLS than in OA-FLS (Fig. 4a and b). We did not find upregulation of HK2, MCT4, or PDK1 in RA-FLS at a protein level. We then examined the effect of pro-inflammatory cytokines and growth factors implicated in the pathogenesis of RA on the GLS1 expression in RA-FLS. We found that IL-17 and PDGF significantly increased the GLS1 mRNA expression in RA-FLS, while lipopolysaccharide (LPS), tumor necrosis factor (TNF)-α, IL-1β, or IL-6 and soluble IL-6 receptor (sIL-6R) did not (Fig. 4c). We did not demonstrate upregulation of GLS1 in RA-FLS after IL-17 or PDGF stimulation at the protein level. IL-17 or PDGF stimulation did not significantly change the intracellular glutamine and glutamate levels in RA-FLS (Additional file 7: Figure S6).

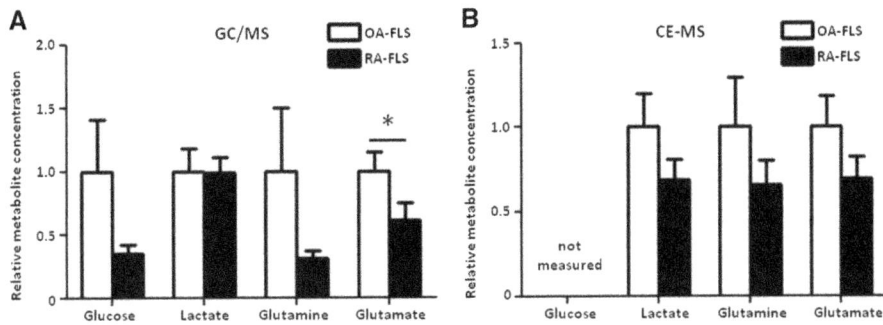

Fig. 2 Glucose, glutamine, and glutamate are more highly consumed in RA-FLS than in OA-FLS. **a** Relative levels of intracellular metabolites in 7 OA-FLS and 11 RA-FLS were analyzed by GC/MS. **b** Relative levels of intracellular metabolites in 3 OA-FLS and 3 RA-FLS were analyzed by CE-MS. Bars indicate mean ± SEM. *$P < 0.05$ by Mann-Whitney U test. *CE-MS* capillary electrophoresis-mass spectrometry, *GC/MS* gas chromatography-mass spectrometry, *OA-FLS* fibroblast-like synoviocytes from osteoarthritis patients, *RA-FLS* fibroblast-like synoviocytes from rheumatoid arthritis patients

GLS1 inhibition suppresses RA-FLS proliferation

We next investigated the effect of compound 968, a GLS1 inhibitor, on RA-FLS cell growth. We demonstrated that 10 μM compound 968 significantly inhibited RA-FLS proliferation (Fig. 5a) in a dose-dependent fashion (Fig. 5b). These results further supported the notion that GLS1 plays an important role in synovial hyperplasia in RA.

GLS1 inhibition ameliorates autoimmune arthritis in SKG mice

Next, we investigated the therapeutic effect of compound 968 on autoimmune arthritis in the SKG mice, an animal model of RA. We injected compound 968 (25 mg/kg) three times per week from day 14 to 42 after ZyA injection. We showed that the arthritis severity in the compound 968-treated group was significantly decreased compared to the DMSO-treated group (Fig. 6a). We also examined the compound 968-treated and DMSO-treated

SKG mice histologically. Arthritis histological scores were significantly lower in the compound 968-treated mice compared to DMSO-treated mice (Fig. 6b and c). Furthermore, immunohistochemical analysis revealed that compound 968 treatment significantly reduced the number of proliferative Ki-67-positive synovial cells (Fig. 6d and e), suggesting that GLS1 inhibition directly affects the cell-cycle progression of RA-FLS. We also measured the number of RORγt-expressing CD4[+] Th17 cells and FoxP3-expressing CD4[+] regulatory T (Treg) cells in the spleens from compound 968-treated and DMSO-treated SKG mice. There was no difference in the number of Th17 cells between the two groups, and the number of Treg cells was decreased in the compound 968-treated group, probably due to the amelioration of arthritis (Additional file 8: Figure S7). These results suggested that the influence of GLS1 inhibition on immune cells was minimal.

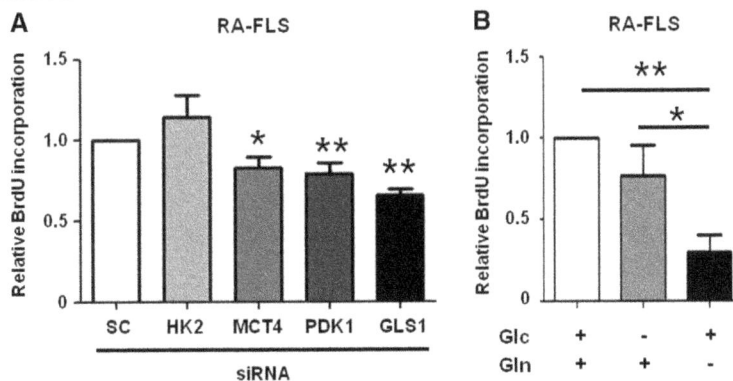

Fig. 3 Glutamine is required for the proliferation of RA-FLS. **a** RA-FLS proliferation was determined using the BrdU assay 96 h after transfection with HK2, MCT4, PDK1, GLS1, or SC siRNA ($n = 5$). Each experiment was performed in quintuplicate. Bars indicate the mean ± SEM. *$P < 0.05$, **$P < 0.01$ versus SC by Student's t test. **b** RA-FLS proliferation was determined using the BrdU assay 96 h after culturing in medium with both Glc and Gln, or in medium without Glc or Gln ($n = 7$). Each experiment was performed in quintuplicate. Bars indicate mean ± SEM. *$P < 0.05$, **$P < 0.01$. *Glc* glucose, *Gln* glutamine, *GLS* glutaminase, *HK* hexokinase, *MCT* monocarboxylate transporter, *PDK* pyruvate dehydrogenase kinase, *RA-FLS* fibroblast-like synoviocytes from rheumatoid arthritis patients, *SC* control scrambled, *siRNA* small interfering RNA

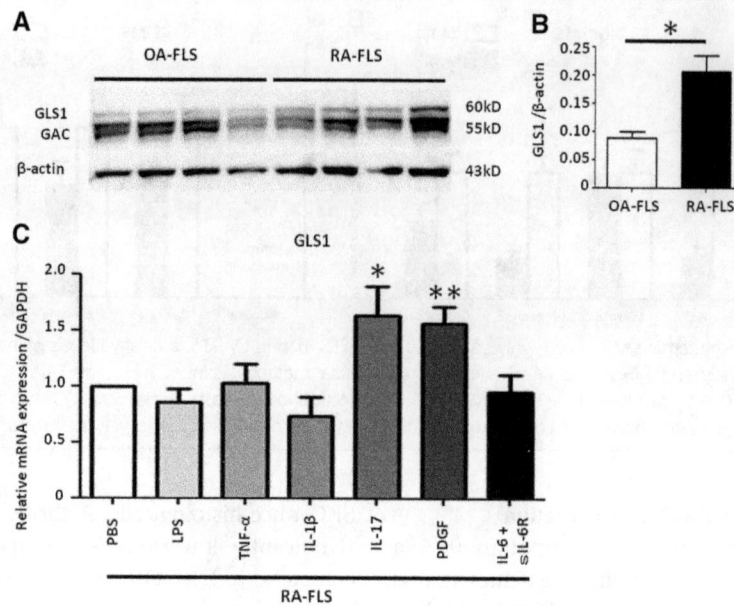

Fig. 4 GLS1 is upregulated in RA-FLS. **a** GLS1 protein levels in 4 OA-FLS and 4 RA-FLS were determined by immunoblotting. GAC is a splicing variant of GLS1. **b** Protein levels were calculated by phosphorimager analysis. Bars indicate mean ± SEM. *$P < 0.05$ by Mann-Whitney U test. **c** RA-FLS were stimulated with LPS (1 μg/ml), TNF-α (10 ng/ml), IL-1β (2 ng/ml), IL-17 (20 ng/ml), PDGF (10 ng/ml), and IL-6 (100 ng/ml) and sIL-6R (100 ng/ml), or PBS for 24 h, and the GLS1 mRNA levels were analyzed by real-time PCR ($n = 8$). Each experiment was performed in triplicate. Bars indicate mean ± SEM. *$P < 0.05$, **$P < 0.01$, versus PBS. *GAC* Glutaminase C, *GAPDH* glyceraldehyde-3-phosphate dehydrogenase, *GLS* glutaminase, *IL* interleukin, *LPS* lipopolysaccharide, *OA-FLS* fibroblast-like synoviocytes from osteoarthritis patients, *PBS* phosphate-buffered saline, *PDGF* platelet-derived growth factor, *RA-FLS* fibroblast-like synoviocytes from rheumatoid arthritis patients, *sIL-6R* soluble IL-6 receptor, *TNF* tumor necrosis factor

Discussion

In this study, we showed that GLS1 expression and glutamine and glutamate consumption were higher in RA-FLS than in OA-FLS. We also showed that glutamine deprivation or GLS1 inhibition suppressed RA-FLS proliferation. Finally, we showed that the administration of a GLS1 inhibitor ameliorated inflammatory arthritis in a mouse model of RA by suppressing FLS proliferation. Taken together, this is the first report to show the importance of glutaminolysis in the pathogenesis of RA.

We found that mRNAs encoding HK2, MCT4, and PDK1 were more highly expressed in RA-FLS than in OA-FLS, although we could not find demonstrate the upregulation of these enzymes at the protein level. We also showed that levels of glucose, glutamine, glutamate, and lactate tended to be lower in RA-FLS than in OA-FLS. The reduction of the lactate level seen in CE-MS may be due to the elevation of the MCT4, which exports intracellular lactate to the extracellular space. These results, together with the mRNA expression profile and the intracellular metabolomic profiles, indicate that both the glycolytic and glutaminolytic pathways are upregulated in RA-FLS, and are consistent with previous reports showing that the inhibition of HK2, MCT4, or PDK1 suppresses RA-FLS proliferation and arthritis in a mouse model [22, 24, 26]. In addition, we found that silencing of MCT4, PDK1, or GLS1 did not significantly

affect IL-6 or MMP-3 production from RA-FLS, suggesting that silencing of glycolytic or glutaminolytic enzymes may have little impact on cytokine production of these cells. Our findings that GLS1 plays key roles in RA-FLS proliferation and in a mouse model of arthritis further confirm that metabolic enzymes are involved in the pathogenesis of RA.

Cancer cells or highly proliferative cells exhibit a "glutamine addiction" phenotype [12]. To determine whether RA-FLS exhibit a similar phenotype, we investigated the effect of glucose or glutamine deprivation on RA-FLS proliferation. We found that RA-FLS proliferation was more dependent on glutamine than on glucose (Fig. 3b), and that GLS1 knockdown, but not HK2 knockdown, inhibited RA-FLS proliferation (Fig. 3a), consistent with a "glutamine addiction" phenotype of RA-FLS. Furthermore, we found that PDGF stimulation did not enhance the proliferation of RA-FLS under the glutamine-deprived condition. Notably, Colombo et al. [40] showed that HeLa cells, which strongly depend on glutamine for proliferation [14], transit through the S and enter the G2/M phase in the absence of glucose, but fail to enter G2/M in the absence of glutamine, suggesting that glutamine is critical for the entrance of highly proliferative cells into G2/M. They also showed that GLS1 is a substrate for the ubiquitin ligase anaphase promoting complex/cyclosome (APC/C)-Cdh1 in some cells [40, 41]. APC/C-Cdh1 inactivation is necessary

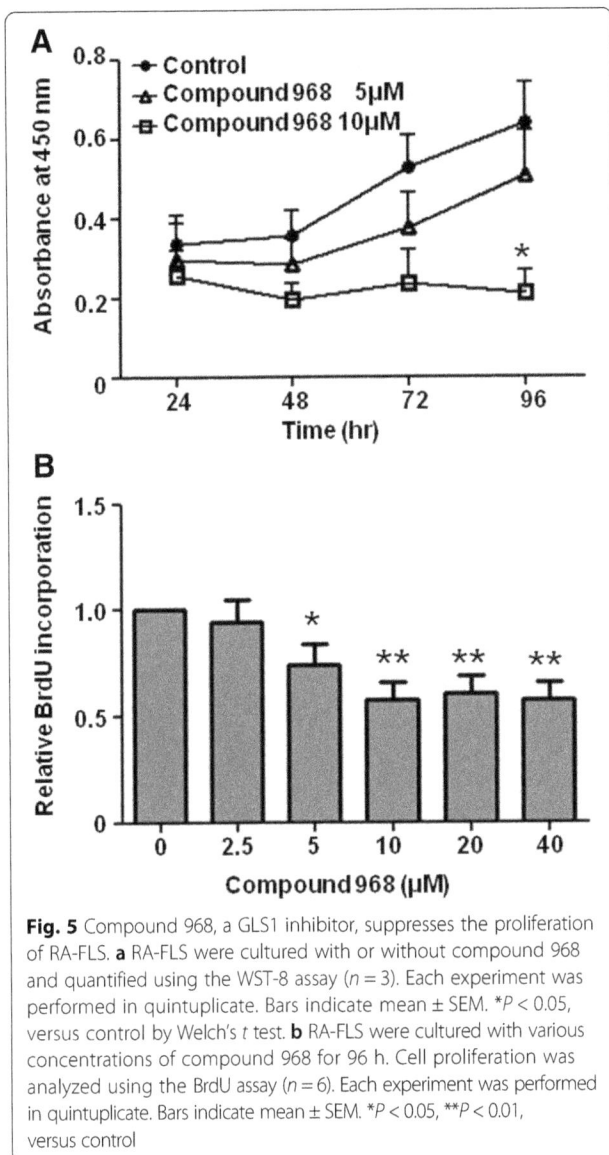

Fig. 5 Compound 968, a GLS1 inhibitor, suppresses the proliferation of RA-FLS. **a** RA-FLS were cultured with or without compound 968 and quantified using the WST-8 assay (n = 3). Each experiment was performed in quintuplicate. Bars indicate mean ± SEM. *P < 0.05, versus control by Welch's t test. **b** RA-FLS were cultured with various concentrations of compound 968 for 96 h. Cell proliferation was analyzed using the BrdU assay (n = 6). Each experiment was performed in quintuplicate. Bars indicate mean ± SEM. *P < 0.05, **P < 0.01, versus control

for S phase initiation, and APC/C-Cdh1 substrates are targeted for degradation through specific recognition motifs such as the KEN box. These previous findings are consistent with our result that compound 968 treatment of SKG mice significantly decreased the number of Ki-67-positive synovial cells.

Although the regulation of GLS1 in cancer cells is not well understood, several studies indicate a functional link between the oncogene *MYC* and glutamine metabolism. Bush et al. showed that three of the five enzymes involved in glutamine metabolism are directly regulated by MYC at the transcriptional level [42]. c-MYC, which is known to stimulate cell proliferation, transcriptionally represses miR-23a and miR-23b, which are repressors of GLS1 expression. In addition, Gao et al. reported that GLS1 levels are closely correlated with MYC expression

levels [16]. Studies also showed that the MYC expression is elevated in RA-FLS [43–45], raising the possibility that GLS1 expression is upregulated by MYC in these cells.

Our finding that PDGF or IL-17 augmented the GLS1 expression in RA-FLS at a mRNA level further supported the notion that glutaminolysis is important in RA-FLS metabolism, although we did not confirm the upregulation of GLS1 at the protein level nor the change in the intracellular glutamine and glutamate levels after IL-17 or PDGF stimulation. PDGF is a well-known growth factor for RA-FLS, and induces MYC expression [46]. IL-17 is also abundant in the rheumatoid synovium and contributes to RA pathogenicity by inducing RANKL expression. Interestingly, IL-17 is reported to upregulate MYC in some cancer cells [47, 48]. IL-1β, TNF-α, and LPS are known to have potent effects on the invasiveness of RA-FLS. In human neurons, GLS1 expression was upregulated by IL-1β or TNF-α treatment, and in a rat hepatoma model IL-6 or TNF-α treatment indirectly upregulated c-MYC expression [49, 50]. However, we did not observe upregulation of GLS1 by IL-1β, TNF-α, or LPS. Although the mechanism is unclear, IL-17-specific upregulation of GLS1 might be a cellular characteristic of RA-FLS, and suggests a novel role for IL-17 in RA-FLS and the pathogenesis of RA.

Since both glycolysis and glutaminolysis are associated with T-cell activation [51], GLS1 inhibition may also affect the immune system. Th17 cells and Treg cells show contrasting characteristics in terms of cellular metabolism; Th17 cells rely mainly on glycolysis [52], whereas Treg cells depend on glycolysis and fatty acid oxidation (FAO), and oxidative phosphorylation [53]. As Th17 cells and Treg cells are known to be two key players in the onset and maintenance of autoimmune arthritis in SKG mice [54], we studied the effect of GLS1 inhibition on Th17 and Treg cells. However, we found no difference in the number of Th17 cells and a decrease in the number of Treg cells in the spleens from compound 968- versus DMSO-treated SKG mice, suggesting that GLS1 inhibition minimally affected immune cells in our experimental system.

Several limitations of this study should be acknowledged. First, although we have revealed the critical role of GLS1 on cell proliferation of RA-FLS, we did not demonstrate the role of GLS1 on the invasive phenotype of RA-FLS. Second, we found that GLS1 mRNA was upregulated after cytokine stimulation, but we could not confirm the upregulation of GLS1 at the protein level. Third, we did not illustrate a precise molecular mechanism that is regulated by glutaminolysis in RA-FLS. To address this point, we examined the expression of c-MYC by immunoblotting (Additional file 9: Figure S8). Although there was no significant difference in c-MYC expression between RA-FLS and OA-FLS, we found that c-MYC expression tended to

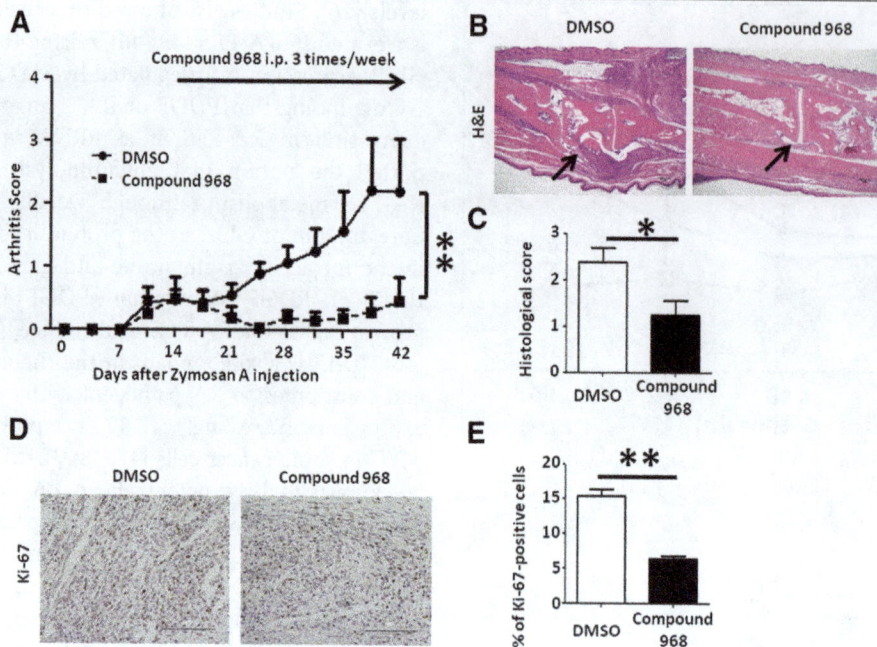

Fig. 6 GLS1 inhibition ameliorates autoimmune arthritis in SKG mice. Fourteen days after ZyA injection, compound 968 or DMSO was injected intraperitoneally into SKG mice three times per week (compound 968, $n = 4$; DMSO, $n = 5$). **a** Clinical arthritis scores were determined up to 42 days after ZyA injection. **$P < 0.01$ by two-way ANOVA using GraphPad Prism software. **b** Hind paws of compound 968- or DMSO-treated SKG mice were assessed for histopathological changes 42 days after ZyA injection. *Arrows* indicate the lining of the synovium. H&E original magnification × 40. **c** Histological arthritis scores were determined in the hind paws of compound 968- or DMSO-treated SKG mice. *$P < 0.05$ by Student's *t* test. **d** Immunohistochemical analysis of Ki-67 expression in the right hind paws of compound 968- or DMSO-treated SKG mice on day 42; original magnification × 400. **e** Quantification of Ki-67 staining from (**d**). Bars indicate mean ± SEM. **$P < 0.01$ by Student's *t* test. *DMSO* dimethyl sulfoxide, *H&E* hematoxylin and eosin, *i.p.* intraperitoneally

be higher in RA-FLS than in OA-FLS. Taken together, our in vitro and in vivo experiments suggest that glutaminolysis is activated in RA-FLS and that blocking glutaminolysis may be a novel therapeutic strategy for RA.

Conclusions

In this study, we found that GLS1 expression was upregulated in RA-FLS, and that RA-FLS cell growth was decreased under glutamine-deprived, but not glucose-deprived, conditions. We also found that GLS1 inhibition suppressed RA-FLS proliferation and ameliorated inflammatory arthritis in SKG mice. These results suggest that glutamine metabolism is involved in the pathogenesis of RA and that GLS1 plays an important role in regulating RA-FLS proliferation, and may be a novel therapeutic target for RA.

Additional files

Additional file 1: Table S1. Primer sequences used in this study. All primer sets were used for measuring gene expression by real-time PCR using SYBR® green chemistry. (DOCX 29 kb)

Additional file 2: Figure S1. GLS1 plays a major role in glutamine metabolism in FLS. GLS1 and GLS2 mRNAs were examined in 12 OA-FLS and 19 RA-FLS by real-time PCR, and the levels were normalized to that

of GAPDH mRNA. Each experiment was performed in triplicate. Bars indicate mean ± SEM. (TIF 2028 kb)

Additional file 3: Figure S2. Glutamine/glutamate ratio was not significantly different between OA-FLS and RA-FLS. Intracellular glutamine/glutamate ratio in 7 OA-FLS and 11 RA-FLS were analyzed by GC/MS, and in 3 OA-FLS and 3 RA-FLS were analyzed by CE-MS. Bars indicate mean ± SEM. (TIF 2028 kb)

Additional file 4: Figure S3. siRNA efficiency of HK2, MCT4, GLS1, and PDK1 in RA-FLS. After transfection with HK2, MCT4, PDK1, GLS1, or control siRNA, mRNA levels were examined by real-time PCR in RA-FLS ($n = 3$ for HK2, MCT4, and GLS1, $n = 4$ for PDK1). Each experiment was performed in triplicate. Bars indicate mean ± SEM. *$P < 0.05$, **$P < 0.01$. (TIF 2028 kb)

Additional file 5: Figure S4. Silencing of MCT4, PDK1, or GLS1 did not significantly affect IL-6 or MMP-3 production in supernatants. After silencing of MCT4, PDK1, or GLS1, IL-6 and MMP-3 levels in culture supernatants of RA-FLS were examined by ELISA ($n = 4$). Each experiment was performed in duplicated. Bars indicate mean ± SEM. *$P < 0.05$. (TIF 2028 kb)

Additional file 6: Figure S5. PDGF stimulation did not enhance the proliferation of RA-FLS under the glutamine-deprived medium condition. RA-FLS, culturing in medium with or without glutamine (Gln), were stimulated with or without PDGF (10 ng/ml). RA-FLS proliferation was determined using BrdU assay 48 h after stimulation ($n = 4$). Each experiment was performed in quintuplicate. Bars indicate mean ± SEM. **$P < 0.01$. (TIF 2028 kb)

Additional file 7: Figure S6. IL-17 or PDGF stimulation did not significantly change the intracellular glutamine and glutamate levels in RA-FLS. Relative levels of intracellular glutamine and glutamate in 3 RA-FLS after IL-17 or PDGF stimulation were analyzed by GC/MS. Bars indicate mean ± SEM. (TIF 677 kb)

Additional file 8: Figure S7. Influence of GLS1 inhibition on immune cells was minimal in arthritic SKG mice. The number of RORγt-expressing CD4+ Th17 cells and FoxP3-expressing CD4+ regulatory T (Treg) cells in the spleens from compound 968-treated and DMSO-treated SKG mice at day 42 after ZyA injection were analyzed by flow cytometry ($n = 5$ for Th17 cells in DMSO group, $n = 4$ for Treg cells in DMSO group, and $n = 4$ for Th17 cells and Treg cells in compound 968 group). (TIF 2028 kb)

Additional file 9: Figure S8. c-MYC expression in RA-FLS. c-MYC protein levels in 5 OA-FLS and 5 RA-FLS were determined by immunoblotting. Protein levels were calculated by phosphorimager analysis. Bars indicate mean ± SEM. (TIF 677 kb)

Abbreviations
APC/C: Anaphase promoting complex/cyclosome; CE-MS: Capillary electrophoresis-mass spectrometry; DMEM: Dulbecco's modified Eagle's medium; DMSO: Dimethyl sulfoxide; ELISA: Enzyme-linked immunosorbent assay; FAO: Fatty acid oxidation; FBS: Fetal bovine serum; FLS: Fibroblast-like synoviocytes; GAPDH: Glyceraldehyde-3-phosphate dehydrogenase; GC/MS: Gas chromatography-mass spectrometry; GLS: Glutaminase; HK: Hexokinase; IL: Interleukin; LPS: Lipopolysaccharide; MCT4: Monocarboxylate transporter; MMP: Matrix metalloproteinase; OA: Osteoarthritis; PCR: Polymerase chain reaction; PDGF: Platelet-derived growth factor; PDK: Pyruvate dehydrogenase kinase; RA: Rheumatoid arthritis; sIL-6R: Soluble interleukin-6 receptor; siRNA: Small interfering RNA; TCA: Tricarboxylic acid; TNF: Tumor necrosis factor; Treg: Regulatory T; ZyA: Zymosan A

Acknowledgements
The authors thank Shino Tanaka for providing technical assistance.

Funding
Not applicable.

Authors' contributions
ST designed the study, performed the experiments, analyzed the data, and drafted the manuscript. AM and JS made substantial contributions to study conception and design, as well as analysis and interpretation of data, drafting the article, and revising the manuscript. YI performed GC/MS analysis of metabolites and helped to revise the manuscript. SS, TO, and KA performed the experiments and helped to revise the manuscript. All authors read and approved the final manuscript.

Competing interests
The authors declare that they have no competing interests.

Author details
[1]Department of Rheumatology and Clinical Immunology, Kobe University Graduate School of Medicine, 7-5-1, Kusunoki-Cho, Chuo-Ku, Kobe 650-0017, Japan. [2]Department of Clinical Laboratory, Kobe University Hospital, 7-5-1, Kusunoki-Cho, Chuo-Ku, Kobe 650-0017, Japan. [3]Division of Evidence-Based Laboratory Medicine, Kobe University Graduate School of Medicine, 7-5-1, Kusunoki-Cho, Chuo-Ku, Kobe 650-0017, Japan.

References
1. Pap T, Muller-Ladner U, Gay RE, Gay S. Fibroblast biology. Role of synovial fibroblasts in the pathogenesis of rheumatoid arthritis. Arthritis Res. 2000;2:361–7.
2. Lafyatis R, Remmers EF, Roberts AB, Yocum DE, Sporn MB, Wilder RL. Anchorage-independent growth of synoviocytes from arthritic and normal joints. Stimulation by exogenous platelet-derived growth factor and inhibition by transforming growth factor-beta and retinoids. J Clin Invest. 1989;83:1267–76.
3. Bartok B, Firestein GS. Fibroblast-like synoviocytes: key effector cells in rheumatoid arthritis. Immunol Rev. 2010;233:233–55.
4. Bottini N, Firestein GS. Duality of fibroblast-like synoviocytes in RA: passive responders and imprinted aggressors. Nat Rev Rheumatol. 2013;9:24–33.
5. Vander Heiden MG, Cantley LC, Thompson CB. Understanding the Warburg effect: the metabolic requirements of cell proliferation. Science. 2009;324:1029–33.
6. Bonnet S, Archer SL, Allalunis-Turner J, Haromy A, Beaulieu C, Thompson R, et al. A mitochondria-K+ channel axis is suppressed in cancer and its normalization promotes apoptosis and inhibits cancer growth. Cancer Cell. 2007;11:37–51.
7. Buchakjian MR, Kornbluth S. The engine driving the ship: metabolic steering of cell proliferation and death. Nat Rev Mol Cell Biol. 2010;11:715–27.
8. Lunt SY, Vander Heiden MG. Aerobic glycolysis: meeting the metabolic requirements of cell proliferation. Annu Rev Cell Dev Biol. 2011;27:441–64.
9. DeBerardinis RJ, Mancuso A, Daikhin E, Nissim I, Yudkoff M, Wehrli S, et al. Beyond aerobic glycolysis: transformed cells can engage in glutamine metabolism that exceeds the requirement for protein and nucleotide synthesis. Proc Natl Acad Sci U S A. 2007;104:19345–50.
10. Wellen KE, Lu C, Mancuso A, Lemons JM, Ryczko M, Dennis JW, et al. The hexosamine biosynthetic pathway couples growth factor-induced glutamine uptake to glucose metabolism. Genes Dev. 2010;24:2784–99.
11. Frezza C, Gottlieb E. Mitochondria in cancer: not just innocent bystanders. Semin Cancer Biol. 2009;19:4–11.
12. Wise DR, Thompson CB. Glutamine addiction: a new therapeutic target in cancer. Trends Biochem Sci. 2010;35:427–33.
13. Medina MA. Glutamine and cancer. J Nutr. 2001;131:2539–42S.
14. Reitzer LJ, Wice BM, Kennell D. Evidence that glutamine, not sugar, is the major energy source for cultured HeLa cells. J Biol Chem. 1979;254:2669–76.
15. Lu W, Pelicano H, Huang P. Cancer metabolism: is glutamine sweeter than glucose? Cancer Cell. 2010;18:199–200.
16. Gao P, Tchernyshyov I, Chang TC, Lee YS, Kita K, Ochi T, et al. c-Myc suppression of miR-23a/b enhances mitochondrial glutaminase expression and glutamine metabolism. Nature. 2009;458:762–5.
17. Kung HN, Marks JR, Chi JT. Glutamine synthetase is a genetic determinant of cell type-specific glutamine independence in breast epithelia. PLoS Genet. 2011;7:e1002229.
18. Gaber T, Dziurla R, Tripmacher R, Burmester G, Buttgereit F. Hypoxia inducible factor (HIF) in rheumatology: low O2! See what HIF can do! Ann Rheum Dis. 2005;64:971–80.
19. Kennedy A, Ng CT, Chang CT, Biniecka M, O'Sullivan JN, Heffernan E, et al. Tumor necrosis factor blocking therapy alters joint inflammation and hypoxia. Arthritis Rheumatol. 2011;63:923–32.
20. Fisher BA, Donatien P, Filer A, Winlove CP, McInnes IB, Buckley CD, et al. Decrease in articular hypoxia and synovial blood flow at early time points following infliximab and etanercept treatment in rheumatoid arthritis. Clin Exp Rheumatol. 2016;34:1072–6.
21. Ahn JK, Kim S, Hwang J, Kim J, Kim KH, Cha H, et al. GC/TOF-MS-based metabolomic profiling in cultured fibroblast-like synoviocytes from rheumatoid arthritis. Joint Bone Spine. 2016;83:707–13.
22. Garcia-Carbonell R, Divakaruni AS, Lodi A, Vicente-Suarez I, Saha A, Cheroutre H, et al. Critical role of glucose metabolism in rheumatoid arthritis fibroblast-like synoviocytes. Arthritis Rheumatol. 2016;68:1614–26.
23. Guma M, Sanchez-Lopez E, Lodi A, Garcia-Carbonell R, Tiziani S, Karin M, et al. Choline kinase inhibition in rheumatoid arthritis. Ann Rheum Dis. 2015;74:1399–407.
24. Fujii W, Kawahito Y, Nagahara H, Kukida Y, Seno T, Yamamoto A, et al. Monocarboxylate transporter 4, associated with the acidification of synovial fluid, is a novel therapeutic target for inflammatory arthritis. Arthritis Rheumatol. 2015;67:2888–96.
25. Biniecka M, Canavan M, McGarry T, Gao W, McCormick J, Cregan S, et al. Dysregulated bioenergetics: a key regulator of joint inflammation. Ann Rheum Dis. 2016;75:2192–200.
26. Bian L, Josefsson E, Jonsson IM, Verdrengh M, Ohlsson C, Bokarewa M, et al. Dichloroacetate alleviates development of collagen II-induced arthritis in female DBA/1 mice. Arthritis Res Ther. 2009;11:R132.
27. Veras FP, Peres RS, Saraiva ALL, Pinto LG, Louzada-Junior P, Cunha TM, et al. Fructose 1,6-bisphosphate, a high-energy intermediate of glycolysis, attenuates experimental arthritis by activating anti-inflammatory adenosinergic pathway. Sci Rep. 2015;5:1517.
28. Seltzer MJ, Bennett BD, Joshi AD, Gao P, Thomas AG, Ferraris DV, et al. Inhibition of glutaminase preferentially slows growth of glioma cells with mutant IDH1. Cancer Res. 2010;70:8981–7.
29. Yang C, Sudderth J, Dang T, Bachoo RM, McDonald JG, DeBerardinis RJ. Glioblastoma cells require glutamate dehydrogenase to survive impairments of glucose metabolism or Akt signaling. Cancer Res. 2009;69:7986–93.

30. Wang JB, Erickson JW, Fuji R, Ramachandran S, Gao P, Dinavahi R, et al. Targeting mitochondrial glutaminase activity inhibits oncogenic transformation. Cancer Cell. 2010;18:207–19.

31. Tanaka K, Sasayama T, Irino Y, Takata K, Nagashima H, Satoh N, et al. Compensatory glutamine metabolism promotes glioblastoma resistance to mTOR inhibitor treatment. J Clin Invest. 2015;125:1591–602.

32. Arnett FC, Edworthy SM, Bloch DA, Mcshane DJ, Fries JF, Cooper NS, et al. The American Rheumatism Association 1987 revised criteria for the classification of rheumatoid arthritis. Arthritis Rheum. 1988;31:315–24.

33. Morinobu A, Wang B, Liu J, Yoshiya S, Kurosaka M, Kumagai S. Trichostatin A cooperates with Fas-mediated signal to induce apoptosis in rheumatoid arthritis synovial fibroblasts. J Rheumatol. 2006;33:1052–60.

34. Yoshida M, Hatano M, Nishimumi S, Irino Y, Izumi Y, Takenawa T, et al. Diagnosis of gastroenterological diseases by metabolome analysis using gas chromatography-mass spectrometry. J Gastroenterol. 2012;47:9–20.

35. Nakamizo S, Sasayama T, Shinohara M, Irino Y, Nishiumi S, Nishihara M, et al. GC/MS-based metabolomic analysis of cerebrospinal fluid (CSF) from glioma patients. J Neurooncol. 2013;113:65–74.

36. Makinoshima H, Takita M, Matsumoto S, Yagishita A, Owada S, Esumi H, et al. Epidermal growth factor receptor (EGFR) signaling regulates global metabolic pathways in EGFR-mutated lung adenocarcinoma. J Biol Chem. 2014;289:20813–23.

37. Yoshitomi H, Sakaguchi N, Kobayashi K, Brown GD, Tagami T, Sakihama T, et al. A role for fungal β-glucans and their receptor Dectin-1 in the induction of autoimmune arthritis in genetically susceptible mice. J Exp Med. 2005;201:949–60.

38. Sakaguchi N, Takahashi T, Hata H, Nomura T, Tagami T, Yamazaki S, et al. Altered thymic T-cell selection due to a mutation of the ZAP-70 gene causes autoimmune arthritis in mice. Nature. 2003;426:454–60.

39. Misaki K, Morinobu A, Saegusa J, Kasagi S, Fujita M, Miyamoto Y, et al. Histone deacetylase inhibition alters dendritic cells to assume a tolerogenic phenotype and ameliorates arthritis in SKG mice. Arthritis Res Ther. 2011;13:R77.

40. Colombo SL, Palacios-Callender M, Frakich N, Carcamo S, Kovacs I, Tudzarova S, et al. Molecular basis for the differential use of glucose and glutamine in cell proliferation as revealed by synchronized HeLa cells. Proc Natl Acad Sci U S A. 2011;108:21069–74.

41. Colombo SL, Palacios-Callender M, Frakich N, De Leon J, Schmitt CA, Boorn L, et al. Anaphase-promoting complex/cyclosome-Cdh 1 coordinates glycolysis and glutaminolysis with transition to S phase in human T lymphocytes. Proc Natl Acad Sci U S A. 2010;107:18868–73.

42. Bush A, Mateyak M, Dugan K, Obaya A, Adachi S, Sedivy J, et al. c-myc null cells misregulate cad and gadd45 but not other proposed c-Myc targets. Genes Dev. 1998;12:3797–802.

43. Trabandt A, Gay RE, Gay S. Oncogene activation in rheumatoid synovium. APMIS. 1992;100:861–75.

44. Qu Z, Garcia CH, O'Rourke LM, Planck SR, Kohli M, Rosenbaum JT. Local proliferation of fibroblast-like synoviocytes contributes to synovial hyperplasia. Results of proliferating cell nuclear antigen/cyclin, c-myc, and nucleolar organizer region staining. Arthritis Rheum. 1994;37:212–20.

45. Michael W, Alisa KE. Cell cycle implications in the pathogenesis of rheumatoid arthritis. Front Biosci. 2000;5:D594–601.

46. Yang W, Ramachandran A, You S, Jeong H, Morley S, Mulone MD, et al. Integration of proteomic and transcriptomic profiles identifies a novel PDGF-MYC network in human smooth muscle cells. Cell Commun Signal. 2014;12:44.

47. Xu M, Song ZG, Xu CX, Rong GH, Fan KX, Chen JY, et al. IL-17A stimulates the progression of giant cell tumors of bone. Clin Cancer Res. 2013;19:4697–705.

48. Straus DS. TNFα and IL-17 cooperatively stimulate glucose metabolism and growth factor production in human colorectal cancer cells. Mol Cancer. 2013;12:78.

49. Ye L, Huang Y, Zhao L, Li Y, Sun L, Zhou Y, et al. IL-1β and TNF-α induce neurotoxicity through glutamate production: a potential role for neuronal glutaminase. J Neurochem. 2013;125:897–908.

50. Li C, Deng M, Hu J, Li X, Chen L, Ju Y, et al. Chronic inflammation contributes to the development of hepatocellular carcinoma by decreasing miR-122 levels. Oncotarget. 2016;7:17021–34.

51. Wang R, Green DR. Metabolic checkpoints in activated T cells. Nat Immunol. 2012;13:907–15.

52. Palsson-McDermott EM, O'Neill LA. The Warburg effect then and now: from cancer to inflammatory diseases. Bioessays. 2013;35:965–73.

53. Ghesquière B, Wong BW, Kuchnio A, Carmeliet P. Metabolism of stromal and immune cells in health and disease. Nature. 2014;511:167–76.

54. Duarte J, Agua-Doce A, Oliveira VG, Fonseca JE, Graca L. Modulation of IL-17 and Foxp3 expression in the prevention of autoimmune arthritis in mice. PLoS One. 2010;5:e10558.

2

Endoplasmic reticulum stress cooperates with Toll-like receptor ligation in driving activation of rheumatoid arthritis fibroblast-like synoviocytes

Pawel A. Kabala[1,2,3,4,5], Chiara Angiolilli[1,2,3,4,5], Nataliya Yeremenko[2,3,4], Aleksander M. Grabiec[2,3,4,6], Barbara Giovannone[5,7], Desiree Pots[2,3,4], Timothy R. Radstake[1,5], Dominique Baeten[2,3,4*] and Kris A. Reedquist[1,5]

Abstract

Background: Endoplasmic reticulum (ER) stress has proinflammatory properties, and transgenic animal studies of rheumatoid arthritis (RA) indicate its relevance in the process of joint destruction. Because currently available studies are focused primarily on myeloid cells, we assessed how ER stress might affect the inflammatory responses of stromal cells in RA.

Methods: ER stress was induced in RA fibroblast-like synoviocytes (FLS), dermal fibroblasts, and macrophages with thapsigargin or tunicamycin alone or in combination with Toll-like receptor (TLR) ligands, and gene expression and messenger RNA (mRNA) stability was measured by quantitative polymerase chain reaction. Cellular viability was measured using cell death enzyme-linked immunosorbent assays and 3-(4,5-dimethylthiazol-2-yl)-2,5-diphenyltetrazolium bromide assays, and signaling pathway activation was analyzed by immunoblotting.

Results: No cytotoxicity was observed in FLS exposed to thapsigargin, despite significant induction of ER stress markers. Screening of 84 proinflammatory genes revealed minor changes in their expression (fold change 90th percentile range 2.8–8.3) by thapsigargin alone, but the vast majority were hyperinduced during combined stimulation with thapsigargin and TLR ligands (35% greater than fivefold vs lipopolysaccharide alone). The synergistic response could not be explained by quantitative effects on nuclear factor-κB and mitogen-activated protein kinase pathways alone, but it was dependent on increased mRNA stability. mRNA stabilization was similarly enhanced by ER stress in dermal fibroblasts but not in macrophages, correlating with minimal cooperative effects on gene induction in macrophages.

Conclusions: RA FLS are resistant to apoptosis induced by ER stress, but ER stress potentiates their activation by multiple TLR ligands. Interfering with downstream signaling pathway components of ER stress may be of therapeutic potential in the treatment of RA.

Keywords: ER stress, Rheumatoid arthritis, Fibroblast-like synoviocytes, Dermal fibroblasts, Macrophages, RNA stability, Inflammation

* Correspondence: d.l.baeten@amc.uva.nl
[2]Department of Clinical Immunology and Rheumatology, Academic Medical Centre/University of Amsterdam, Amsterdam, The Netherlands
[3]Amsterdam Rheumatology and Immunology Center, Amsterdam, The Netherlands
Full list of author information is available at the end of the article

Background

Genetic studies have shed light on our understanding of the causes of autoimmune diseases by identifying shared and unique risk loci among these diseases. However, in rheumatoid arthritis (RA), only a fraction of disease susceptibility can be explained by genetic variation [1], and the temporal link between the break of self-tolerance and development of clinical disease remains elusive because circulating autoantibodies are detectable long before the onset of arthritis [2]. In RA, stromal cells in the joint, fibroblast-like synoviocytes (FLS), exhibit an imprinted and epigenetically maintained aggressive phenotype, predisposing them to participate in an inflammatory positive feedback loop in response to the cues from the synovial environment [3]. Identifying local tissue conditions able to initiate and perpetuate the ensuing inflammatory cycle is therefore of critical importance to understanding and intervening in the disease process.

Endoplasmic reticulum (ER) stress is a common cellular response to many of the conditions RA FLS encounter in the inflamed synovium [4], and it occurs when the amount of newly synthesized proteins in the ER exceeds the organelle's capacity to ensure their proper folding. The resulting accumulation of misfolded proteins in the ER triggers a set of signals collectively referred to as the *unfolded protein response* (UPR), aimed at relieving the burden by slowing down the global translation rate while increasing production of a selected set of proteins, particularly ER chaperones [5]. The UPR depends upon the triggering of inositol-requiring enzyme 1α (IRE1α), protein kinase R-like endoplasmic reticulum kinase (PERK), and activating transcription factor 6, sensors embedded in the ER membrane, by unfolded protein aggregates in the lumen. In response, IRE1α homodimerizes and causes the unconventional splicing of X-box binding protein 1 (*XBP1*) messenger RNA (mRNA). This causes a frameshift mutation in *XBP1*, making it a powerful transcription factor instrumental in restoring homeostasis. Additional transcription factors are activated by the two other sensors [6].

Although primarily a safeguard for protein folding homeostasis, ER stress is tightly associated with immunological processes via crosstalk occurring between the UPR and inflammatory signaling pathways. For example, the decrease in translation rate caused by PERK activity limits expression of proteins with a short half-life, such as nuclear factor of kappa light polypeptide gene enhancer in B-cells inhibitor, alpha (IκBα), resulting in enhanced activation of the nuclear factor (NF)-κB pathway [7]. Autophosphorylated IRE1α interacts with the tumor necrosis factor receptor-associated factor 2 adaptor molecule, facilitating activation of NF-κB and mitogen-activated protein (MAP) kinase pathways [8]. Transcription factors involved in ER stress can directly drive expression of inflammatory gene products such as interleukin (IL)-6 and tumor necrosis factor (TNF) [9], and elements of the UPR are necessary for maturation of several immune cell populations [10, 11]. Consequently, ER stress has been linked to a number of human disease conditions, including autoimmunity, where it has been postulated to drive inflammatory activation, act as the source of or as an adjuvant for autoantigens, or contribute to pathology by modulating apoptotic pathways [12, 13].

Despite this, understanding of the relevance of ER stress to pathology in RA is largely incomplete. Analysis of publicly available datasets of microarrays performed on synovial tissue has identified genes related to ER stress and protein processing in the ER as those most significantly differentiating between RA and osteoarthritis (OA) synovia, whereas no such difference was observed between OA and normal synovia [14]. Prominent staining for ER stress markers was observed throughout RA synovial tissue, particularly in the lining layer, indicating that these differences were unlikely to reflect changes in numbers of minor cell populations. A similar enhancement of ER stress and ER stress signaling to the nucleus in synovial fluid macrophages has been observed, and the ER chaperone binding immunoglobulin protein (BiP) is an important regulator of synovial angiogenesis, synoviocyte proliferation and survival, and disease severity in animal models of RA [14]. In experimental arthritis, strong expression of ER stress markers is observed during disease development in both synovial macrophages and fibroblasts [15]. Whereas myeloid-specific targeting of UPR pathways resulted in decreased cytokine expression and ameliorated disease in K/BxN serum-induced arthritis [16], studies involving RA FLS focus predominantly on changes in cellular viability and their potential consequences for synovial hyperplasia [17]. Unlike other cell types, RA FLS are resistant to apoptosis induced by ER stress, likely due to enhanced rates of autophagy and proteasomal activity [18, 19]. However, little is known about how ER stress changes the potential of FLS to directly modulate synovial inflammation, and recent studies have indicated that splicing of *XBP1* may be associated with the activation of RA FLS by Toll-like receptor (TLR) signaling, IL-1β, and TNF [20]. The aim of this study was therefore to examine if ER stress could regulate inflammatory gene expression in RA FLS.

Methods

Patients and cells

FLS were derived from synovial biopsies obtained by needle arthroscopy from patients fulfilling the 2010 American College of Rheumatology/European League Against Rheumatism classification criteria for RA [21, 22] and isolated as previously described [23]. Healthy skin biopsies were obtained as resected material after cosmetic surgery, and dermal fibroblasts (DF) were isolated using the Whole Skin Dissociation Kit (Miltenyi Biotec, Leiden, The Netherlands) following the manufacturer's instructions. FLS and DF were cultured in DMEM (Gibco/ Thermo Fisher Scientific, Waltham, MA, USA) containing 10% FBS (Invitrogen/Thermo Fisher Scientific) and used for experiments between passages 5 and 10. Prior to stimulations, cells were incubated in medium containing 1% FBS overnight.

Monocytes were isolated from healthy donor buffy coats (Sanquin, Amsterdam, The Netherlands) using Lymphoprep (AXIS-SHIELD; Alere Technologies, Oslo, Norway) density gradient centrifugation followed by standard isotonic Percoll gradient centrifugation (GE Healthcare, Eindhoven, The Netherlands). Monocytes were plated in Iscove's modified Dulbecco's medium (IMDM; Invitrogen/Thermo Fisher Scientific), supplemented with 1% FBS, for 30 minutes at 37 °C, followed by the removal of nonadherent cells. Monocytes were differentiated into macrophages by 7 days of culture in IMDM containing 10% FBS, 100 μg/ml gentamicin, and 800 U/ml granulocyte-macrophage colony-stimulating factor (Tebu-Bio, Heerhugowaard, The Netherlands).

Cell stimulation
Escherichia coli 0111:B4 lipopolysaccharide (LPS) was ordered from Sigma-Aldrich (Zwijndrecht, The Netherlands) and used at 1 μg/ml. ER stress was induced by tunicamycin from *Streptomyces* sp. (10 μg/ml; Sigma-Aldrich) or thapsigargin at varying concentrations (Calbiochem/ Merck, Amsterdam-Zuidoost, The Netherlands). Other stimulants used included IL-1β (1 ng/ml; R&D Systems, Minneapolis, MN, USA), polyinosinic:polycytidylic acid (pI:C; TLR3 agonist, 25 μg/ml; InvivoGen, San Diego, CA, USA), Pam3CSK4 (TLR1/2 agonist, 5 μg/ml; InvivoGen), flagellin (TLR5 agonist, 200 ng/ml; InvivoGen), SB202190 (p38 inhibitor,10 μM; Tocris Bioscience, Bristol, UK), U0216 (extracellular signal-regulated kinase [ERK] inhibitor, 10 μM; Tocris Bioscience), and c-Jun N-terminal (JNK) inhibitor IX (20 μM; Calbiochem/Merck).

Gene expression measurement
Total RNA was isolated using an RNeasy Micro Kit (QIAGEN, Venlo, The Netherlands) according to the manufacturer's instructions and reverse-transcribed using a RevertAid First Strand cDNA Synthesis Kit (Thermo Fisher Scientific). Quantitative polymerase chain reaction (qPCR) reagents were purchased from Thermo Fisher Scientific, and reactions were performed using TaqMan probes and Master Mix (for detection of *HSPA5, DDIT3, ERN1*) or SYBR Select Master Mix (all other targets) (Applied Biosystems/Thermo Fisher Scientific, Foster City, CA, USA). Alternatively, gene expression was measured using qPCR-based low-density arrays (QIAGEN). The custom array in use was previously designed to cover 84 genes relevant to joint pathology and regulated by proinflammatory stimuli in RA FLS [24, 25].

Cell viability and apoptosis detection
RA FLS were exposed to thapsigargin at concentrations ranging from 10 nM to 1 μM for 4–24 h. Apoptosis induction was analyzed using the Cell Death Detection ELISA (enzyme-linked immunosorbent assay; Roche Diagnostics/ Sigma-Aldrich, Mannheim, Germany) according to the manufacturer's instructions. Viability was assessed by 3-(4,5-dimethylthiazol-2-yl)-2,5-diphenyltetrazolium bromide (MTT) assay. Following treatment, cells were incubated with 1 mg/ml thiazolyl blue tetrazolium bromide (Sigma-Aldrich) for 1 h at 37 °C. The water-insoluble reaction product was dissolved with isopropanol containing 5 mM HCl and 0.1% Nonidet P-40 and quantified by measuring absorbance at 595 nm.

ELISA
Cells were stimulated with 10 nM thapsigargin or 1 μg/ml LPS, alone or in combination, for 24 h. Cell-free supernatants were collected, and the concentrations of IL-6 and IL-8 were measured using PeliKine Compact human IL-6 and IL-8 ELISA kits (Sanquin) according to the manufacturer's instructions.

Immunoblotting
Cells were stimulated with 10 nM thapsigargin or 1 μg/ml LPS or a combination thereof for 30 minutes and 1, 2, 4, and 8 h, and then they were lysed in modified Laemmli buffer (120 mM Tris-HCl, pH 6.8, 4% SDS, 4% glycerol). Lysates were combined with loading buffer containing β-mercaptoethanol, heat-denatured at 95 °C, resolved by SDS-PAGE electrophoresis, and blotted onto polyvinylidene fluoride membranes. Membranes were blocked with 4% nonfat dry milk for 1 h, followed by overnight probing with primary antibodies recognizing histone 3, IκBα, and phosphorylated forms of JNK, p38 (all from Cell Signaling Technologies, Leiden, The Netherlands), and ERK (Santa Cruz Biotechnology, Dallas, TX, USA). HRP-conjugated secondary antibodies were purchased from Dako/Agilent Technologies (Santa Clara, CA, USA), and proteins were detected using Lumi-Light enhanced chemiluminescence substrate (Roche/Sigma-Aldrich) and the ChemiDoc imaging system (Bio-Rad Laboratories, Hercules, CA, USA). Densitometric analysis of bands was performed with ImageJ software (https://imagej.nih.gov/ij/). Band intensities were normalized to histone 3 signal in the sample and expressed relative to the unstimulated cells.

Statistical analysis

Data are presented as mean ± SEM. Statistical analysis was performed using Prism 6.02 software (GraphPad Software Inc., La Jolla, CA, USA). The number of replicates in the figure description refers to the number of different FLS donors included in the analysis. For comparison of multiple datasets with a single reference set, repeated measures analysis of variance followed by Dunnett's post hoc test was used. For comparison between two datasets only, a paired t test was used unless otherwise indicated. All tests were two-tailed, and p values <0.05 were considered significant.

Results

ER stress alone has limited impact on inflammatory gene expression in RA FLS

We initiated our studies by analyzing the effects of thapsigargin, a widely used ER stress inducer, on the expression of ER stress markers C/EBP homologous protein (CHOP; *DDIT3*) and BiP (*HSPA5*) in RA FLS. mRNA levels of these genes were significantly increased in a dose- and time-dependent manner following thapsigargin treatment (Fig. 1a). Induction was readily observed 2 h after treatment and continued to increase for as long as 24 h. Notably, although thapsigargin is typically used at micromolar concentrations [17, 19], 10 nM thapsigargin was sufficient for maximum induction of *DDIT3* and *HSPA5* in FLS. To quantitatively assess signaling emanating directly from the ER, we developed an assay in which expression of *XBP1* splice variants is followed by real-time PCR using primers recognizing only its IRE1α-processed (spliced) or unprocessed (unspliced) versions or detecting both variants indiscriminately (total). At baseline, most of *XBP1* was in its unspliced form, confirming a low level of IRE1α activity (Fig. 1b). The amount of spliced *XBP1* increased

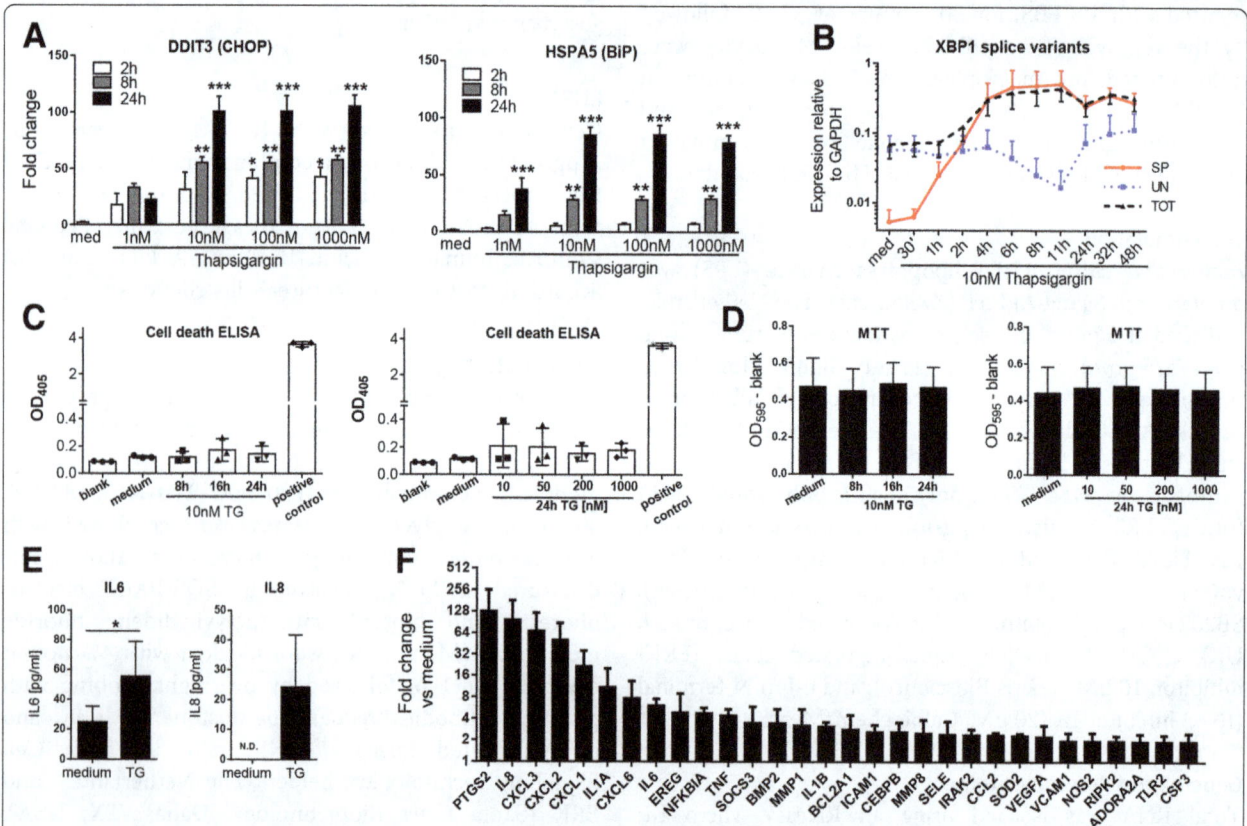

Fig. 1 Effects of ER stress on RA FLS inflammatory gene expression and cellular viability. **a, b** Expression of ER stress markers (**a**) and XBP1 splice variants (**b**) was measured in three FLS lines after exposure to increasing concentrations of TG (**a**) or constant 10 nM TG (**b**). The significance of changes relative to unstimulated controls was assessed by analysis of variance with post hoc Dunnett's test. * $p < 0.05$; ** $p < 0.01$; *** $p < 0.001$. **c, d** Apoptosis induction and cellular viability were measured using a cell death ELISA (**c**) and an MTT assay (**d**), respectively, after stimulation with 10 nM TG for 8, 16, or 24 h or with increasing concentrations of TG for 24 h. **e** IL-6 and IL-8 in cell culture supernatants ($n = 3$) were measured by ELISA after 24-h incubation with 10 nM TG. **f** FLS ($n = 3$) were incubated with 10 nM TG for 2 h, and expression of 84 inflammatory genes was analyzed by qPCR-based array. Shown are the top 20 genes ranked by mean fold change relative to unstimulated cells. *BiP* Binding immunoglobulin protein, *CHOP* C/EBP homologous protein, *ELISA* Enzyme-linked immunosorbent assay, *ER* Endoplasmic reticulum, *FLS* Fibroblast-like synoviocytes, *GAPDH* Glyceraldehyde 3-phosphate dehydrogenase, *IL* Interleukin, *MTT* 3-(4,5-dimethylthiazol-2-yl)-2,5-diphenyltetrazolium bromide, *N.D.* Not detectable, *OD* Optical density, *qPCR* Quantitative polymerase chain reaction, *RA* Rheumatoid arthritis, *TG* Thapsigargin, *TLR* Toll-like receptor, *TNF* Tumor necrosis factor, *XBP1* X-box binding protein 1

exponentially 30 minutes after stimulation with 10 nM thapsigargin and soon approximated the amount of total *XBP1*, indicating sustained and maximal UPR signaling. Consistent with previous studies [17–19], we observed no apoptotic effect of ER stress in RA FLS for up to 24 h after treatment with thapsigargin over a range of 10 nM to 1 µM (Fig. 1c). Similarly, thapsigargin had no effect on RA FLS cellular viability, as measured by MTT assay (Fig. 1d). Thus, RA FLS are biochemically and transcriptionally sensitive to ER stress in the absence of effects on cellular survival.

We next examined if ER stress leads to modulation of inflammatory gene expression in RA FLS. In initial experiments, we observed increased amounts of IL-6 and IL-8 protein present in the media of cells exposed to thapsigargin (Fig. 1e). Although statistically significant, the concentrations were low compared with cytokine production induced by agonists such as IL-1β, LPS, and TNF (*see below* and data not shown). We therefore analyzed the expression of 84 genes responsive to

proinflammatory stimuli in FLS. Surprisingly, only a few genes, such as *PTGS2*, *IL8*, and a subset of chemokine (C-X-C motif) ligand (CXCL) chemokines, appeared to be substantially regulated by thapsigargin treatment (Fig. 1f). We subsequently validated these results using tunicamycin, a molecule that causes ER stress by an unrelated mechanism, and obtained similarly modest changes in the gene expression pattern, despite clear induction of UPR signaling (Additional file 1).

ER stress cooperates with TLR signaling to regulate inflammatory gene expression
We next examined the capacity of ER stress to interact with other inflammatory stimuli by incubating RA FLS with IL-1β or LPS with or without thapsigargin. Thapsigargin alone again had significant, although minor, effects on *IL6* (Fig. 2a, *left panels*) and *IL8* (Fig. 2a, *right panels*) expression. However, we observed highly consistent trends toward higher expression of both analytes when LPS or IL-1β was used in combination with ER stress induction,

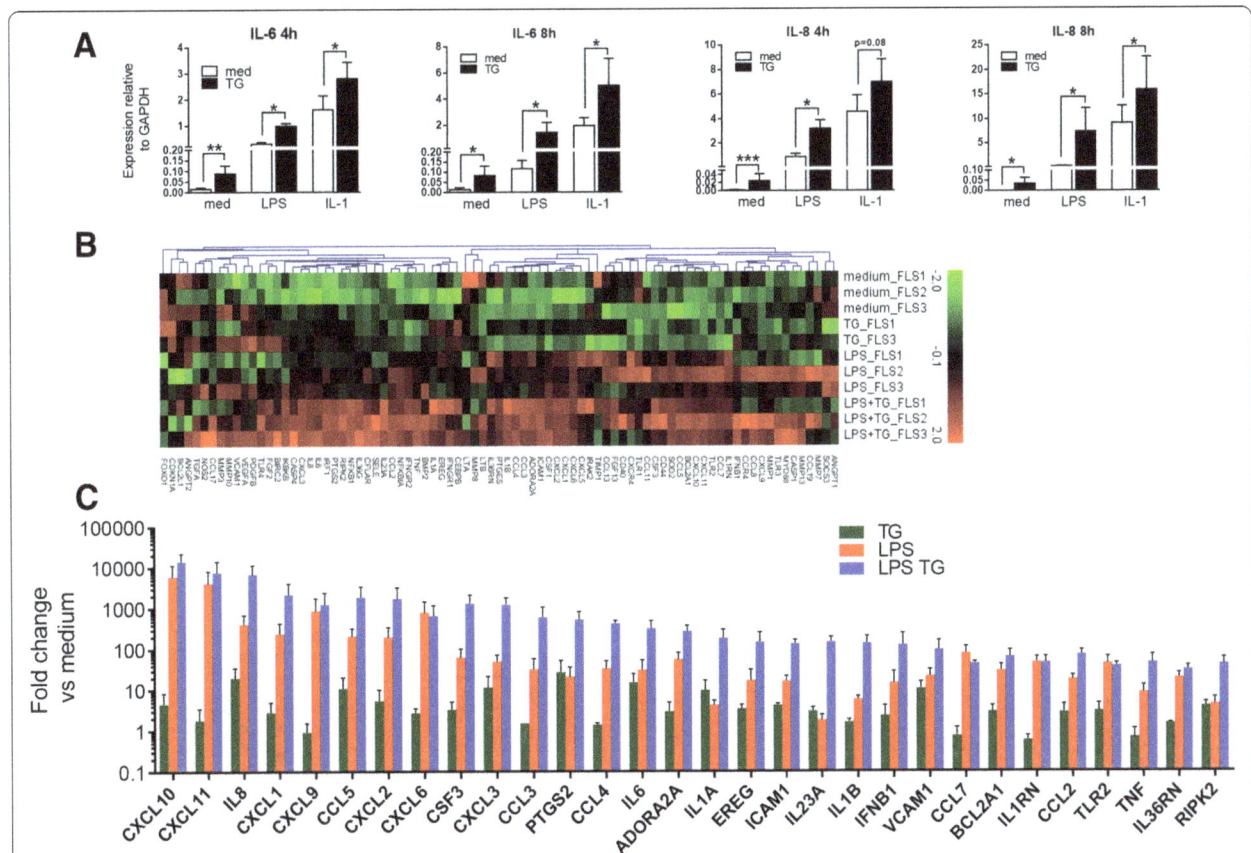

Fig. 2 Synergism between ER stress and other stimuli. **a** FLS (*n* = 4) were left untreated or stimulated with 1 µg/ml LPS or 1 ng/ml IL-1β in the presence or absence of 10 nM TG. Expression of *IL6* and *IL8* was measured by qPCR 4 h or 8 h after stimulation. **b, c** FLS (*n* = 3, *n* = 2 for TG alone) were stimulated with 10 nM TG or 1 µg/ml LPS in the presence or absence of 10 nM TG for 8 h. Expression of 84 inflammatory genes was monitored by qPCR-based array. Heat map (**b**) depicts per-gene z-scores of log-scaled expression values relative to GAPDH, and bar graph (**c**) presents fold changes relative to unstimulated cells for 30 genes with the highest overall level of regulation (mean across all conditions). *ER* Endoplasmic reticulum, *FLS* Fibroblast-like synoviocytes, *GAPDH* Glyceraldehyde 3-phosphate dehydrogenase, *IL* Interleukin, *LPS* Lipopolysaccharide, *qPCR* Quantitative polymerase chain reaction, *TG* Thapsigargin

with the differences particularly apparent in the context of LPS stimulation. Expanding our analyses to a larger set of genes, we found that ER stress enhanced the expression of most of the transcripts regulated by LPS (Fig. 2b). We observed that 53% of genes showed increased induction of greater than twofold relative to LPS alone, and over one-third (34.9%) of them showed greater than fivefold increases (Fig. 2c; note logarithmic scale). Finally, we examined whether synergistic regulation of gene expression by ER stress could also be observed for other TLR ligands (Fig. 3). Of genes for which strong synergism could be observed between ER stress and LPS, such as *IL6* (Fig. 3a), *IL8* (Fig. 3b), *CCL3*, *PTGS2*, *TNF*, and *IFNB* (data not shown), we observed a similar synergistic effect between ER stress and other TLR ligands, including pI:C, Pam3CSK4, and flagellin. Consistently, no combinatorial effect between TLR ligands and thapsigargin was observed for *CXCL10* (Fig. 3c) and other genes (data not shown) that were refractory to modulation by ER stress during LPS stimulation. Changes observed in LPS-induced gene transcription in the presence of ER stress were functionally relevant because we could detect significantly elevated levels of IL-6 and IL-8 in cell culture supernatants of RA FLS when cells were exposed to both LPS and thapsigargin (Fig. 3d).

Effects of ER stress on inflammatory gene expression in RA FLS depend primarily on changes in mRNA stability

We hypothesized that ER stress, while having little effect on its own, may act by increasing the magnitude or the duration of signaling initiated by other events. Using TLR4 stimulation as a model, we analyzed activation of NF-κB and MAP kinase pathways (Additional file 2: Figure S2a), but we failed to observe pronounced modulatory effects of thapsigargin, although quantitative analysis of multiple experiments demonstrated that p38 activation and degradation of IκBα were maintained longer during ER stress (Additional file 2: Figure S2b). Thus, although ER stress may lead to a slight prolongation of activation of inflammatory signaling pathways, the magnitude of these changes is insufficient to explain profound modulation of inflammatory gene expression.

Next, we examined whether differences in gene expression could be explained by differences in transcriptional activity at their loci. We used the amount of primary transcripts, nascent transcripts produced by RNA polymerase before intronic sequence excision, as a surrogate measure of the transcription rate and compared the kinetics of expression of the primary transcripts and mature mRNAs encoding *IL6* and *IL8*. After 8 h of stimulation, expression of mature forms of *IL6* and *IL8* was approximately 15 and 40 times higher, respectively, in cells treated with the

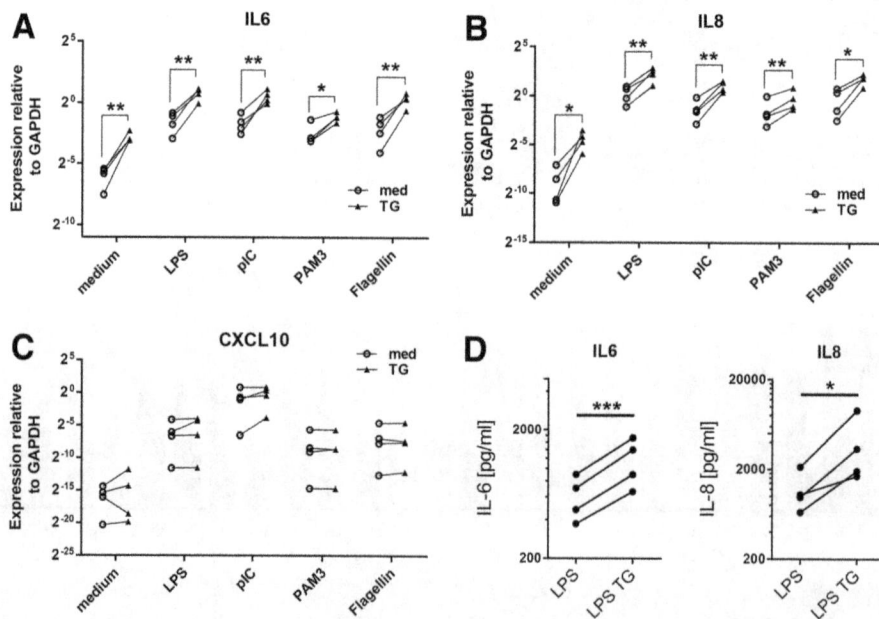

Fig. 3 Synergism between ER stress and multiple TLR ligands. mRNA expression of *IL6* (**a**), *IL8* (**b**), and *CXCL10* (**c**) in RA FLS was measured by qPCR after 4-h stimulation with the indicated TLR ligands in the presence or absence of 10 nM TG. **d** IL-6 and IL-8 protein production in response to combined treatment with LPS and TG was measured by ELISA. * *p* < 0.05; ** *p* < 0.01; *** *p* < 0.001. *CXCL* Chemokine (C-X-C motif) ligand, *ELISA* Enzyme-linked immunosorbent assay, *ER* Endoplasmic reticulum, *FLS* Fibroblast-like synoviocytes, *GAPDH* Glyceraldehyde 3-phosphate dehydrogenase, *IL* Interleukin, *LPS* Lipopolysaccharide, *mRNA* Messenger RNA, *pIC* Polyinosinic:polycytidylic acid, *qPCR* Quantitative polymerase chain reaction, *RA* Rheumatoid arthritis, *TG* Thapsigargin, *TLR* Toll-like receptor

combination of LPS and thapsigargin than with LPS alone (Fig. 4a). The corresponding values for the primary transcript were much lower indicating that an increase in the transcription rate can account for only a fraction of the elevated mRNA expression during combined LPS and thapsigargin treatment. Because these results pointed to the importance of posttranscriptional regulatory mechanisms, we investigated possible differences in mRNA decay rates. Cells were stimulated with LPS or LPS and thapsigargin for 4 h, at which point further transcription was blocked and the amount of mature mRNA remaining in the cells was followed over time. We observed that the rates of mRNA decay of genes synergistically regulated by LPS and ER stress, including *IL6*, *IL8*, *CCL3*, and *PTGS2*, were significantly slowed by ER stress as compared with rates observed with LPS alone (Fig. 4b and c). In contrast, ER stress had little to no effect on the stability of mRNA encoding genes refractory to modulation by thapsigargin, such as *CXCL10* or *CXCL11* (Fig. 4b and c). By using tunicamycin as an alternative ER stress inducer, we validated that both the observed synergy and stabilization of cytokine mRNAs are caused by the ER

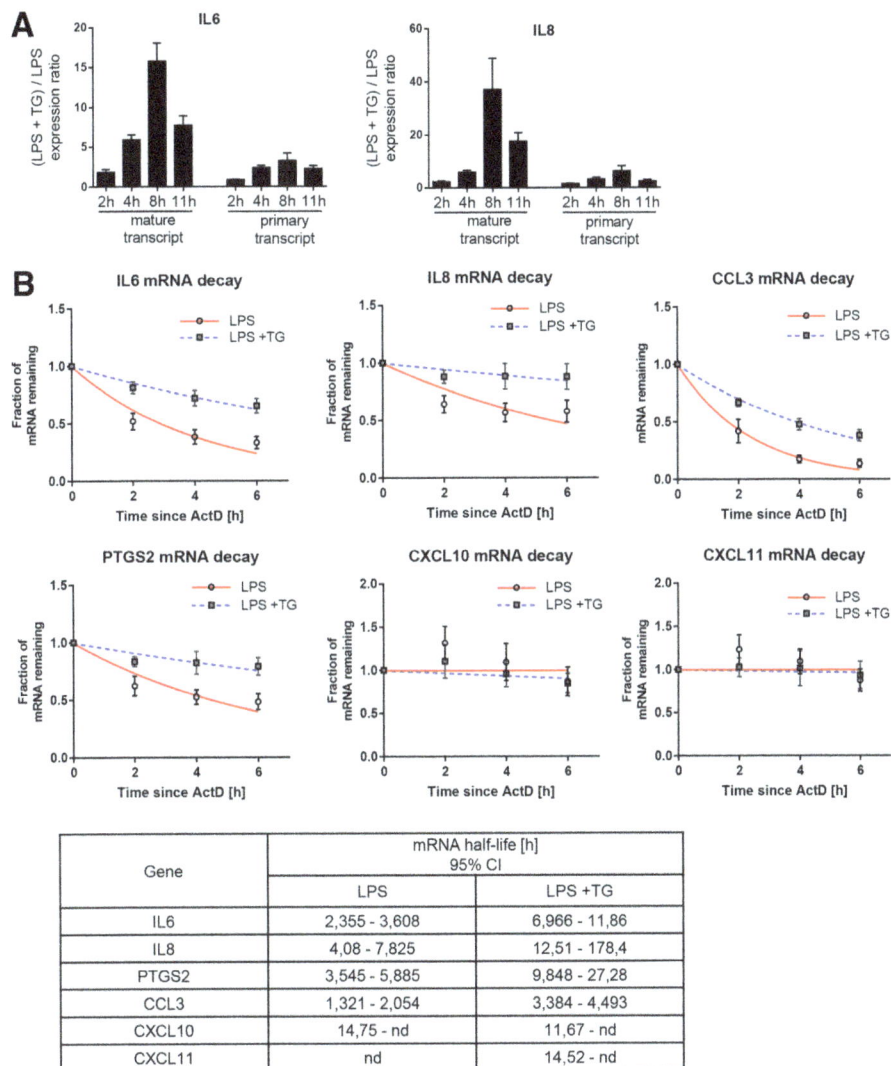

Gene	mRNA half-life [h] 95% CI	
	LPS	LPS +TG
IL6	2,355 - 3,608	6,966 - 11,86
IL8	4,08 - 7,825	12,51 - 178,4
PTGS2	3,545 - 5,885	9,848 - 27,28
CCL3	1,321 - 2,054	3,384 - 4,493
CXCL10	14,75 - nd	11,67 - nd
CXCL11	nd	14,52 - nd

Fig. 4 Effects of ER stress on gene transcription and mRNA stability in RA FLS. **a** FLS (*n* = 3) were stimulated with 1 μg/ml LPS in the presence or absence of 10 nM TG for the indicated amount of time. mRNA expression of mature and primary forms of transcripts of *IL6* and *IL8* was measured by qPCR. Shown is the ratio between expression observed in both experimental conditions at each time point. **b** FLS (*n* = 8) were stimulated with 1 μg/ml LPS in the presence or absence of 10 nM TG for 4 h, followed by incubation with 10 μg/ml ActD to induce transcriptional block. Cells were lysed at the indicated time points after addition of ActD, and the amount of transcript for each gene remaining in cells was analyzed by qPCR. Data are presented as a fraction of transcript detectable at each time point relative to the moment immediately after addition of ActD. Table shows 95% CIs of transcript half-life calculated using Prism software (GraphPad Software). *ActD* Actinomycin D; *CXCL* Chemokine (C-X-C motif) ligand, *ER* Endoplasmic reticulum, *FLS* Fibroblast-like synoviocytes, *IL* Interleukin, *LPS* Lipopolysaccharide, *mRNA* Messenger RNA, *qPCR* Quantitative polymerase chain reaction, *RA* Rheumatoid arthritis, *TG* Thapsigargin

stress itself and not by compound-specific effects of thapsigargin (Additional file 3: Figure S3).

Because regulation of mRNA decay in response to inflammatory stimuli is known to be strongly influenced by MAP kinase signaling tone [26], we decided to reexamine MAP kinases' potential involvement. SB202190, a specific p38 inhibitor, significantly accelerated mRNA decay in cells exposed to both LPS alone and LPS in combination with thapsigargin (Additional file 4: Figure S4a). It was, however, insufficient to equalize the observed decay rates, suggesting that the contribution of ER stress to mRNA stabilization does not rely on changes in p38 activity. Inhibition of the JNK and ERK pathways had similarly little effect on narrowing the differences in the fraction of

mRNA detectable in cells after 2 h of actinomycin D chase (Additional file 4: Figure S4b).

Enhanced mRNA stability of proinflammatory genes during ER stress is observed in stromal but not myeloid cells

To establish whether the ability of ER stress to regulate inflammatory gene expression was limited to FLS, we analyzed the effects of LPS treatment combined with ER stress in DF, representing another fibroblastic cell, and macrophages, representing both an unrelated lineage and a major cellular constituent of the inflamed synovial membrane. In DF, coincubation of cells with thapsigargin and LPS resulted in enhanced expression of *IL6* and *IL8* similar to that observed in FLS (Fig. 5a). Also,

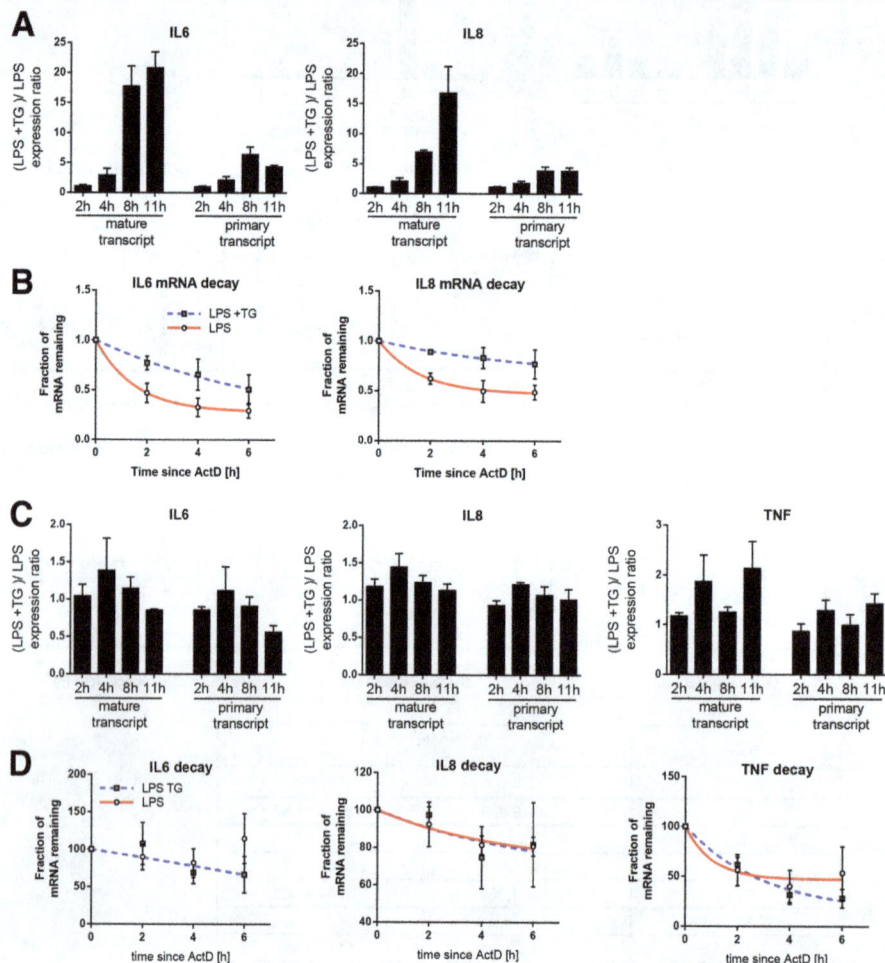

Fig. 5 Synergism between ER stress and LPS in dermal fibroblasts and macrophages. **a**, **c** Human dermal fibroblasts (**a**, *n* = 3) or GM-CSF-differentiated macrophages (**c**, *n* = 3) were stimulated with 1 μg/ml LPS in the presence or absence of 10 nM TG for the indicated amount of time. mRNA expression of mature and primary forms of transcripts of *IL6*, *IL8*, and *TNF* was measured by qPCR. Shown is the ratio between expression observed in both experimental conditions at each time point. **b**, **d** Human dermal fibroblasts (**b**, *n* = 3) or GM-CSF-differentiated macrophages (**d**, *n* = 3) were stimulated with 1 μg/ml LPS in the presence or absence of 10 nM TG for 4 h, followed by incubation with 10 μg/ml ActD to induce transcriptional block. Cells were lysed at the indicated time points after addition of ActD, and the amount of transcript for each gene remaining in cells was analyzed by qPCR. Data are presented as a fraction of transcript detectable at each time point relative to the moment immediately after addition of ActD. *ActD* Actinomycin D, *ER* Endoplasmic reticulum, *GM-CSF* Granulocyte-macrophage colony-stimulating factor, *IL* Interleukin, *LPS* Lipopolysaccharide, *mRNA* Messenger RNA, *qPCR* Quantitative polymerase chain reaction, *TG* Thapsigargin, *TNF* Tumor necrosis factor

although the kinetics of primary transcript expression failed to explain the level of synergy in the mature transcript (Fig. 5a), we again observed increased mRNA stability of these cytokines (Fig. 5b). The presence of thapsigargin did not result in similarly high changes in the expression of *IL6*, *IL8*, and *TNF* in macrophages (Fig. 5c). The transcription rate was only marginally affected, and no discordance between primary and mature transcript kinetics was observed. In line with these results, we failed to observe stabilization of mRNA in macrophages treated with LPS and thapsigargin (Fig. 5d). Also, at higher concentrations of thapsigargin, we did not notice synergistic effects with LPS, but we observed strong cytotoxic effects in macrophages (data not shown). Our results suggest that in RA synovial tissue, ER stress contributes to local inflammation primarily through its effects on FLS, rather than myeloid cells, by promoting mRNA stabilization of genes relevant to pathology.

Discussion

ER stress plays an important role in both physiological and pathological immune responses, and RA and OA synovia are distinguished by a strong UPR signature [14]. Similarly, macrophages isolated from RA patient synovial fluid were demonstrated by several groups to bear signs of ER stress, as compared with both peripheral blood monocyte-derived macrophages or macrophages isolated from OA patient synovial fluid [14, 16]. In the present study, we demonstrate that also stromal cells, FLS, are readily responsive to ER stress induction, but by itself this has little significant effect on cellular activation, nor does it affect viability. Instead, ER stress primes stromal cells for enhanced cytokine and chemokine production in the presence of other agonistic signals. The magnitude and range of this synergistic response are in stark contrast with the negligible changes in cytokine expression induced by thapsigargin alone, and they are a result of effects on transcriptional rates, to some extent, and primarily on mRNA decay rates of inflammatory genes.

In regard to cell survival, RA FLS were previously described as more resistant to such challenge than OA FLS, with altered expression of CHOP and synoviolin postulated as possible mechanisms [17, 18]. Similarly, the ER chaperone BiP has been identified as an important survival factor for stressed synoviocytes, and its expression regulates joint destruction in animal models [14]. On the other hand, inflammatory responses to ER stress in FLS have been scarcely studied so far. Contrary to freshly isolated synovial fluid macrophages, cultured RA FLS do not show signs of increased ER stress [20], although they upregulate UPR-related genes more readily than OA FLS in response to a variety of stimuli [14]. Analogously to similar observations in macrophages [9],

a possible effect of TLR-dependent XBP1 activation on gene expression has been proposed in RA FLS [20]. However, following stimulation with LPS alone, we have observed only minor differences in the amount and fraction of *XBP1* existing in the spliced form, indicating no significant changes in UPR signaling (data not shown).

Our data suggest that enhanced mRNA stability is a major contributor to the increased level of gene expression during ER stress. A growing number of reports underscore the importance of mRNA stability regulation during chronic synovitis in RA. In particular, Loupasakis et al. [27] recently demonstrated mRNA stabilization as a crucial factor shaping the FLS transcriptome during long-term exposure to TNF, with a strong influence on *IL6*, *IL8*, *CCL2*, *PTGS2*, and other genes with pathogenic potential.

Intriguingly, ER stress has long been known to impact the mRNA stability of certain genes via regulated IRE1α-dependent degradation [28]. In such cases, activated IRE1α was shown to splice not only *XBP1* but also several other mRNAs, resulting in their accelerated decay. However, the idea that ER stress might conversely contribute to inflammation by stabilizing cytokine mRNA has not previously been explored. Regulation of cytokine expression through changes in mRNA stability depends primarily on the presence of adenylate- and uridylate-rich elements in their sequences. These are recognized by adenylate- and uridylate-rich element-binding proteins (ABPs) whose expression and activity are tightly regulated and can lead to both positive and negative regulation of mRNA half-life [29]. We have screened possible candidate ABPs, including BRF1 (*ZFP36L1*), BRF2 (*ZFP36L2*), AUF1 (*HNRNPD*), TTP (*ZFP36*), HuR (*ELAVL1*) and *KHSRP*, using small interfering RNA-mediated knockdown (data not shown), but we were unsuccessful in mimicking or significantly modulating the effects of combined LPS and thapsigargin stimulation by their independent targeting. Additionally, inhibition of conventional pathways involved in ABP-mediated decay [26], such as p38, ERK, and JNK, did not block a positive effect of ER stress on mRNA stability. These observations indicate that additional regulatory layers, such as micro-RNAs or components of nonsense-mediated decay, may be implicated.

The observation that ER stress regulates mRNA stability in DF is similarly novel, suggesting a shared mode of stromal cell response to suspected injury by preparing to mount a rapid inflammatory response if further danger signals appear in the environment. This may be relevant to rheumatic diseases other than RA characterized by skin involvement, such as psoriatic arthritis and systemic sclerosis. In this regard, the role of TLR ligands and ER stress in systemic sclerosis has been described extensively (reviewed in [30, 31]), and it will be of interest to determine whether ER stress-dependent regulation of gene expression contributes to the acquisition of the profibrotic phenotype in these patients.

Our inability to observe a similar effect of ER stress on mRNA stability in macrophages was surprising, given the available literature. For example, the IRE1α-XBP1 signaling pathway was shown to be a critical element of macrophage responses to TLR ligation [9], and myeloid-specific knockout of IRE1α ameliorated disease severity in the K/BxN serum-induced arthritis model [16]. Although the primary focus of these previous studies was the role of IRE1α during TLR stimulation alone, an enhancement of LPS-induced cytokine expression during ER stress in murine bone marrow-derived macrophages was noted, and a similar finding was observed in human macrophages [9]. The discrepancy in macrophage responses to ER stress between these studies and ours, where we also noted a sensitivity of macrophages to LPS and ER stress-induced apoptosis, may be a result of differences in tissue- and polarization-specific macrophage responses. In line with this, it was previously observed that resident and thioglycolate-elicited peritoneal macrophages show opposite patterns of regulation of *CXCL1* during stimulation with LPS and thapsigargin [32]. Our results suggest that in RA synovial tissue, the IRE1α-XBP1 axis might contribute to macrophage responses to TLR signaling in the absence of induction of ER stress, whereas in stromal cells, TLR stimulation in the presence of ER stress amplifies cytokine and chemokine production.

Conclusions

Whereas a strong ER stress signature is a distinguishing feature of RA synovium, the understanding of its capacity to influence pathological processes was incomplete. Specifically in the case of stromal cells, the effects of ER stress reported in the literature that could be relevant in a disease setting are linked to the RA FLS intrinsic resistance to apoptosis and were not known to contain an inflammatory component. In our present study, however, we identify a novel regulatory mechanism relying on interactions between stromal cells, ER stress, and molecular danger signals with potential to profoundly affect the course of the locally developed inflammation. We propose a model in which cytokine transcription is initiated by an external trigger rather than by ER stress itself, with the latter being instead responsible for promoting mRNA stability. Combination of both inputs leads to significant augmentation of the overall response in stressed cells. Further characterization of this mechanism may lead to identification of molecular targets relevant for a range of immune-mediated inflammatory diseases characterized by synovial and connective tissue involvement.

Abbreviations

ABP: Adenylate- and uridylate-rich element-binding protein; ActD: Actinomycin D; BiP: Binding immunoglobulin protein; CHOP: C/EBP homologous protein; CXCL: Chemokine (C-X-C motif) ligand; DF: Dermal fibroblasts; ELISA: Enzyme-linked immunosorbent assay; ER: Endoplasmic reticulum; ERK: Extracellular signal-regulated kinase; FLS: Fibroblast-like synoviocytes; GAPDH: Glyceraldehyde 3-phosphate dehydrogenase; GM-CSF: Granulocyte-macrophage colony-stimulating factor; IκBα: Nuclear factor of kappa light polypeptide gene enhancer in B-cells inhibitor, alpha; IL: Interleukin; IMDM: Iscove's modified Dulbecco's medium; IRE1α: Inositol-requiring enzyme 1α; JNK: c-Jun N-terminal kinase; LPS: Lipopolysaccharide; MAP: Mitogen-activated protein; mRNA: Messenger RNA; MTT: 3-(4,5-dimethylthiazol-2-yl)-2,5-diphenyltetrazolium bromide; NF-κB: Nuclear factor-κB; OA: Osteoarthritis; OD: Optical density; PERK: Protein kinase R-like endoplasmic reticulum kinase; pI:C: Polyinosinic:polycytidylic acid; qPCR: Quantitative polymerase chain reaction; RA: Rheumatoid arthritis; TG: Thapsigargin; TLR: Toll-like receptor; TNF: Tumor necrosis factor; UPR: Unfolded protein response; XBP1: X-box binding protein 1

Acknowledgements

Not applicable.

Funding

This research was supported in part by a research grant from the Dutch Arthritis Association (11-1-403) (to KAR). TRR is supported by a grant (Circumvent) from the European Research Council (ERC). DB is supported by a Vici grant from the Netherlands Scientific Organization (NWO) and a consolidator grant from the ERC (Inflammostrome).

Authors' contributions

PAK designed the experiments, acquired and interpreted the data, and drafted the manuscript. CA, NY, AMG, and DP substantially contributed to the study design as well as data acquisition and interpretation throughout the study. BG made a substantial contribution to the experiments involving dermal fibroblasts. TRR, DB, and KAR substantially contributed to the study design, interpretation of data, and writing of the manuscript. All authors were involved in critical revision of the manuscript, and all authors read and approved the final version to be published.

Competing interests

The authors declare that they have no competing interests.

Author details

[1]Department of Rheumatology and Clinical Immunology, University Medical Center Utrecht, Utrecht, The Netherlands. [2]Department of Clinical Immunology and Rheumatology, Academic Medical Centre/University of Amsterdam, Amsterdam, The Netherlands. [3]Amsterdam Rheumatology and Immunology Center, Amsterdam, The Netherlands. [4]Department of Experimental Immunology, Academic Medical Centre/University of Amsterdam, Amsterdam, The Netherlands. [5]Laboratory of Translational Immunology, University Medical Center Utrecht, Utrecht, The Netherlands. [6]Department of Microbiology, Faculty of Biochemistry, Biophysics and Biotechnology, Jagiellonian University, Krakow, Poland. [7]Division of Internal Medicine and Dermatology, Department of Dermatology/Allergology, University Medical Center Utrecht, Utrecht, The Netherlands.

References

1. Eyre S, Bowes J, Diogo D, Lee A, Barton A, Martin P, et al. High-density genetic mapping identifies new susceptibility loci for rheumatoid arthritis. Nat Genet. 2012;44(12):1336–40.
2. Nielen MMJ, van Schaardenburg D, Reesink HW, van de Stadt RJ, van der Horst-Bruinsma IE, de Koning MHMT, et al. Specific autoantibodies precede the symptoms of rheumatoid arthritis: a study of serial measurements in blood donors. Arthritis Rheum. 2004;50(2):380–6.

3. Bottini N, Firestein GS. Duality of fibroblast-like synoviocytes in RA: passive responders and imprinted aggressors. Nat Rev Rheumatol. 2012;9(1):24–33.

4. Grootjans J, Kaser A, Kaufman RJ, Blumberg RS. The unfolded protein response in immunity and inflammation. Nat Rev Immunol. 2016;16(8):469–84.

5. Zhang K, Kaufman RJ. From endoplasmic-reticulum stress to the inflammatory response. Nature. 2008;454(7203):455–62.

6. Moore KA, Hollien J. The unfolded protein response in secretory cell function. Annu Rev Genet. 2012;46:165–83.

7. Hu P, Han Z, Couvillon AD, Kaufman RJ, Exton JH. Autocrine tumor necrosis factor α links endoplasmic reticulum stress to the membrane death receptor pathway through IRE1α-mediated NF-κB activation and down-regulation of TRAF2 expression. Mol Cell Biol. 2006;26(8):3071–84.

8. Urano F, Wang X, Bertolotti A, Zhang Y, Chung P, Harding HP, et al. Coupling of stress in the ER to activation of JNK protein kinases by transmembrane protein kinase IRE1. Science. 2000;287(5453):664–6.

9. Martinon F, Chen X, Lee AH, Glimcher LH. TLR activation of the transcription factor XBP1 regulates innate immune responses in macrophages. Nat Immunol. 2010;11(5):411–8.

10. Todd DJ, McHeyzer-Williams LJ, Kowal C, Lee AH, Volpe BT, Diamond B, et al. XBP1 governs late events in plasma cell differentiation and is not required for antigen-specific memory B cell development. J Exp Med. 2009; 206(10):2151–9.

11. Bettigole SE, Lis R, Adoro S, Lee AH, Spencer LA, Weller PF, et al. The transcription factor XBP1 is selectively required for eosinophil differentiation. Nat Immunol. 2015;16(8):829–37.

12. Todd DJ, Lee AH, Glimcher LH. The endoplasmic reticulum stress response in immunity and autoimmunity. Nat Rev Immunol. 2008;8(9):663–74.

13. Navid F, Colbert RA. Causes and consequences of endoplasmic reticulum stress in rheumatic disease. Nat Rev Rheumatol. 2017;13(1):25–40.

14. Yoo SA, You S, Yoon HJ, Kim DH, Kim HS, Lee K, et al. A novel pathogenic role of the ER chaperone GRP78/BiP in rheumatoid arthritis. J Exp Med. 2012;209(4):871–86.

15. Feng LJ, Jiang TC, Zhou CY, Yu CL, Shen YJ, Li J, et al. Activated macrophage-like synoviocytes are resistant to endoplasmic reticulum stress-induced apoptosis in antigen-induced arthritis. Inflamm Res. 2014;63(5):335–46.

16. Qiu Q, Zheng Z, Chang L, Zhao YS, Tan C, Dandekar A, et al. Toll-like receptor-mediated IRE1α activation as a therapeutic target for inflammatory arthritis. EMBO J. 2013;32(18):2477–90.

17. Yamasaki S, Yagishita N, Tsuchimochi K, Kato Y, Sasaki T, Amano T, et al. Resistance to endoplasmic reticulum stress is an acquired cellular characteristic of rheumatoid synovial cells. Int J Mol Med. 2006;18(1):113–7.

18. Shin YJ, Han SH, Kim DS, Lee GH, Yoo WH, Kang YM, et al. Autophagy induction and CHOP under-expression promotes survival of fibroblasts from rheumatoid arthritis patients under endoplasmic reticulum stress. Arthritis Res Ther. 2010;12(1):R19.

19. Kato M, Ospelt C, Gay RE, Gay S, Klein K. Dual role of autophagy in stress-induced cell death in rheumatoid arthritis synovial fibroblasts. Arthritis Rheum. 2013;66(1):40–8.

20. Savic S, Ouboussad L, Dickie LJ, Geiler J, Wong C, Doody GM, et al. TLR dependent XBP-1 activation induces an autocrine loop in rheumatoid arthritis synoviocytes. J Autoimmun. 2014;50:59–66.

21. Aletaha D, Neogi T, Silman AJ, Funovits J, Felson DT. Bingham 3rd CO, et al. 2010 Rheumatoid arthritis classification criteria: an American College of Rheumatology/European League Against Rheumatism collaborative initiative. Arthritis Rheum. 2010;62(9):2569–81.

22. Aletaha D, Neogi T, Silman AJ, Funovits J, Felson DT, Bingham III CO, et al. Rheumatoid arthritis classification criteria: an American College of Rheumatology/European League Against Rheumatism collaborative initiative. Ann Rheum Dis. 2010;69(9):1580–8.

23. van de Sande MGH, Gerlag DM, Lodde BM, van Baarsen LGM, Alivernini S, Codullo V, et al. Evaluating antirheumatic treatments using synovial biopsy: a recommendation for standardisation to be used in clinical trials. Ann Rheum Dis. 2011;70(3):423–7.

24. Klein K, Kabala PA, Grabiec AM, Gay RE, Kolling C, Lin LL, et al. The bromodomain protein inhibitor I-BET151 suppresses expression of inflammatory genes and matrix degrading enzymes in rheumatoid arthritis synovial fibroblasts. Ann Rheum Dis. 2016;75(2):422–9.

25. Angiolilli C, Kabala PA, Grabiec AM, Van Baarsen IM, Ferguson BS, García S, et al. Histone deacetylase 3 regulates the inflammatory gene expression programme of rheumatoid arthritis fibroblast-like synoviocytes. Ann Rheum Dis. 2017;76(1):277–85.

26. Tiedje C, Holtmann H, Gaestel M. The role of mammalian MAPK signaling in regulation of cytokine mRNA stability and translation. J Interferon Cytokine Res. 2014;34(4):220–32.

27. Loupasakis K, Kuo D, Sohn C, Syracuse B, Giannopoulou EG, Park SH, et al. 04.10 Chronic inflammation regulates the mRNA stabilome in rheumatoid arthritis fibroblast-like synoviocytes [abstract]. Ann Rheum Dis. 2017;76 Suppl 1:A45–6.

28. Maurel M, Chevet E, Tavernier J, Gerlo S. Getting RIDD of RNA: IRE1 in cell fate regulation. Trends Biochem Sci. 2014;39(5):245–54.

29. Schoenberg DR, Maquat LE. Regulation of cytoplasmic mRNA decay. Nat Rev Genet. 2012;13(4):246–59.

30. Bhattacharyya S, Varga J. Emerging roles of innate immune signaling and Toll-like receptors in fibrosis and systemic sclerosis. Curr Rheumatol Rep. 2015;17(1):474.

31. Lenna S, Trojanowska M. The role of endoplasmic reticulum stress and the unfolded protein response in fibrosis. Curr Opin Rheumatol. 2012;24(6):663–8.

32. Zhao C, Pavicic Jr PG, Datta S, Sun D, Novotny M, Hamilton TA. Cellular stress amplifies TLR3/4-induced CXCL1/2 gene transcription in mononuclear phagocytes via RIPK1. J Immunol. 2014;193(2):879–88.

3

Biological function integrated prediction of severe radiographic progression in rheumatoid arthritis

Young Bin Joo[1†], Yul Kim[2†], Youngho Park[3], Kwangwoo Kim[4], Jeong Ah Ryu[5], Seunghun Lee[5], So-Young Bang[3], Hye-Soon Lee[3*], Gwan-Su Yi[2*] and Sang-Cheol Bae[3*] (ID)

Abstract

Background: Radiographic progression is reported to be highly heritable in rheumatoid arthritis (RA). However, previous study using genetic loci showed an insufficient accuracy of prediction for radiographic progression. The aim of this study is to identify a biologically relevant prediction model of radiographic progression in patients with RA using a genome-wide association study (GWAS) combined with bioinformatics analysis.

Methods: We obtained genome-wide single nucleotide polymorphism (SNP) data for 374 Korean patients with RA using Illumina HumanOmni2.5Exome-8 arrays. Radiographic progression was measured using the yearly Sharp/van der Heijde modified score rate, and categorized in no or severe progression. Significant SNPs for severe radiographic progression from GWAS were mapped on the functional genes and reprioritized by post-GWAS analysis. For robust prediction of radiographic progression, tenfold cross-validation using a support vector machine (SVM) classifier was conducted. Accuracy was used for selection of optimal SNPs set in the Hanyang Bae RA cohort. The performance of our final model was compared with that of other models based on GWAS results and SPOT (one of the post-GWAS analyses) using receiver operating characteristic (ROC) curves. The reliability of our model was confirmed using GWAS data of Caucasian patients with RA.

Results: A total of 36,091 significant SNPs with a p value <0.05 from GWAS were reprioritized using post-GWAS analysis and approximately 2700 were identified as SNPs related to RA biological features. The best average accuracy of ten groups was 0.6015 with 85 SNPs, and this increased to 0.7481 when combined with clinical information. In comparisons of the performance of the model, the 0.7872 area under the curve (AUC) in our model was superior to that obtained with GWAS (AUC 0.6586, p value 8.97×10^{-5}) or SPOT (AUC 0.7449, p value 0.0423). Our model strategy also showed superior prediction accuracy in Caucasian patients with RA compared with GWAS (p value 0.0049) and SPOT (p value 0.0151).

Conclusions: Using various biological functions of SNPs and repeated machine learning, our model could predict severe radiographic progression relevantly and robustly in patients with RA compared with models using only GWAS results or other post-GWAS tools.

Keywords: Rheumatoid arthritis, Radiographic progression, Bioinformatic analysis, GWAS, Post-GWAS analysis

* Correspondence: lhsberon@hanyang.ac.kr; lhsberon@hanyang.ac.kr; gwansuyi@kaist.ac.kr; scbae@hanyang.ac.kr
†Equal contributors
[3]Department of Rheumatology, Hanyang University Hospital for Rheumatic Diseases, Seoul, Republic of Korea
[2]Department of Bio and Brain Engineering, Korea Advanced Institute of Science and Technology, Daejeon, Republic of Korea
Full list of author information is available at the end of the article

Background

The marked success of genome-wide association studies (GWAS) has led to the discovery of numerous novel genetic loci. To date, nearly 100 susceptibility loci of rheumatoid arthritis (RA) have been identified [1]. Recently, the role of post-GWAS analysis, which prioritizes GWAS signals by incorporating diverse biological and functional evidence, has been highlighted in the identification of causal loci and for prediction of phenotypic traits [2]. Most genome-wide association loci are in noncoding regions of the genome and might not directly implicate functional variants, whereas the prioritized loci in post-GWAS analysis are biologically relevant variants and more likely to be truly associated with phenotypic traits [2].

Radiographic severity is a pivotal outcome of RA. Prediction of patients who will ultimately develop severe radiographic progression in the initial stage of the disease course is important for better outcomes and necessary for precision medicine. As radiographic severity is reported to be highly heritable (45–58%) [3], genetic loci or genes could be helpful in the prediction of radiographic severity. However, there is currently a lack of genetic information for prediction of radiographic damage. According to a report by van Steenbergen et al., prediction accuracy of severe radiographic progression reached only 62% using a model consisting of 17 known genetic loci from several replication studies and meta-analysis and clinical factors [4].

Therefore, we sought to develop a more accurate and reliable prediction model for radiographic progression using a comprehensive approach consisting of GWAS, post-GWAS analysis, and bioinformatics. We first conducted GWAS of radiographic progression in Korean patients with early RA. Next, single nucleotide polymorphisms (SNPs) conferred by GWAS were mapped and prioritized according to their biological features through a post-GWAS approach and an optimal set of SNPs for prediction of radiographic progression was selected via tenfold cross-validation using a support vector machine (SVM). Next, a prediction model for radiographic progression was generated by the ensemble approach using genetic and clinical factors. Finally, we confirmed the usefulness of post-GWAS prioritization and our model strategy for prediction of radiographic progression in an independent cohort of Caucasian patients with RA.

Methods

Patients

All patients fulfilled the 1987 revised American College of Rheumatology criteria [5], and were recruited after providing informed consent and with ethical approval from the Institutional Review Board of Hanyang University Hospital (HYG-14-032-1).

Two cohorts were used to establish the prediction model of severe radiographic progression and their clinical characteristics are shown in Additional file 1: Table S1. First, 374 patients with early RA from the Hanyang Bae RA cohort of Hanyang University Hospital for Rheumatic Diseases [6] with two hand X-rays were included for the initial approach of post-GWAS analysis and construction of a prediction model. Next, reliability of post-GWAS prioritization for prediction of severe radiographic progression was evaluated in 399 patients with RA from the North American Rheumatoid Arthritis Consortium (NARAC) [7] with one hand X-ray per person.

Radiographic outcome

Radiographic joint damage was measured using the Sharp/Van der Heijde modified score (SHS) from hand radiographs [8]. For analysis of the Hanyang Bae RA cohort with two hand X-rays, the yearly radiographic joint damage rate (ΔSHS/year) was calculated as the difference in SHS between baseline and follow-up radiographs, divided by the duration between the two X-rays. Two independent expert radiologists scored the radiographs and the interclass observer correlation coefficient was 0.89 for the total score. For analysis of the NARAC cohort with one X-ray, the estimated yearly progression rate was calculated (total SHS/disease years at time of X-ray) as explained in a previous study [9]. Trained readers at the Leiden University Medical Center scored radiographs and the intra-observer reliability was 0.99 [10]. Patients with RA were classified into three groups of low, middle, and high tertiles based on their radiographic severity. Only the two groups of low tertile (no progression) and high tertile (severe progression) were used for analysis.

Genotyping

In the Hanyang Bae RA cohort, genotyping was conducted with Illumina HumanOmni2.5Exome-8 BeadChips at SNP Genetics Inc. (Seoul, South Korea). All subjects were successfully genotyped for >2.5 million markers with reliable genotyping call rates per sample ≥95%. After the quality control, approximately 1.4 million markers with minor allele frequency (MAF) ≥0.5%, genotyping call rates per each marker ≥95%, and Hardy Weinberg equilibrium (HWE) >5×10^{-7} were used in subsequent analyses. Genetic relationship analysis performed to identify cryptic relatedness among the subjects did not find any duplicates, twins, or first-degree relatives. Principal component (PC) analysis was performed to obtain PCs and assess population stratification among the subjects. We noted that there were no genetic outliers of >6 standard deviations for each of the top ten PCs.

In the NARAC cohort, genotyping was conducted with Illumina BeadChips (HumanHap 550 k) [7]. As reported in a previous study [10], 391,733 SNPs with reliable geno-typing success rate (>98%), MAF >0.1%, and $>1 \times 10^{-5}$ were used in analyses.

Genome-wide association study and genome mapping based on functional regions and eQTL data

A comprehensive approach including GWAS, post-GWAS analysis, repeated machine learning using SVM, and ensemble model was conducted to identify a prediction model for severe radiographic progression. The study workflow is presented in Fig. 1.

First, GWAS was performed in a nested case-control design, yielding genetic predictors for severe radiographic progression. Next, we mapped the statistically significant SNPs (p value <0.05 in GWAS analysis) with their biologically related genes based on the functional regions these SNPs map to. For this, we collected functional regions of SNPs from several public databases and obtained a total of 43,011 enhancer regions and associated genes retrieved from the FANTOM5 consortium [11]. A total of 50,900 gene regions, including both coding and intron regions and promoter regions, defined as 2 k bases upstream from the transcription start site, were downloaded from the UCSC table browser [12]. In addition, we collected 4666 miRNA regions from miR-base [13] and their target genes from miRTarBase [14]. Moreover, we assessed cis and trans-expression quantitative trait loci (eQTL) effects by reference to four publicly available datasets [15–18]. We integrated eQTL information tested in peripheral blood mononuclear cells (PBMCs), monocytes, CD4+ T cells, and lymphoblastoids with significance threshold defined in reference papers. When mapping the SNPs, we also considered their proxy SNPs with r2 > 0.8. Reference pair-wise linkage disequilibrium (LD) information was retrieved from HapMap genotype information of Japanese and Han Chinese populations.

SNP reprioritization based on RA network

We reprioritized the statistically significant SNPs in GWAS based on RA correlation scores of their related genes. To measure the RA correlation of the genes, we first constructed a RA gene network by propagation of prior RA information to their interaction partners (Fig. 2a). To construct the network, we used an integrated gene interaction database called HIPPIE [19], which provided 221,331 interactions between 15,615 genes. We collected prior gene-disease association (GDA) from DisGeNet [20] and disease similarity (DS) from MimMiner [21] to consider not only RA genes, but also genes for RA-related diseases. Next, for a gene v in the Y was assigned as below:

$$Y(v) = Max(GDA\_(v, d) \times DS\_(d, RA)),$$

where d represents all disease that is associated with gene v. With assignment of prior RA information, we propagated the information using the PRINCE method [22] and calculated RA correlation scores of all genes in the network. With the RA correlation scores of genes,

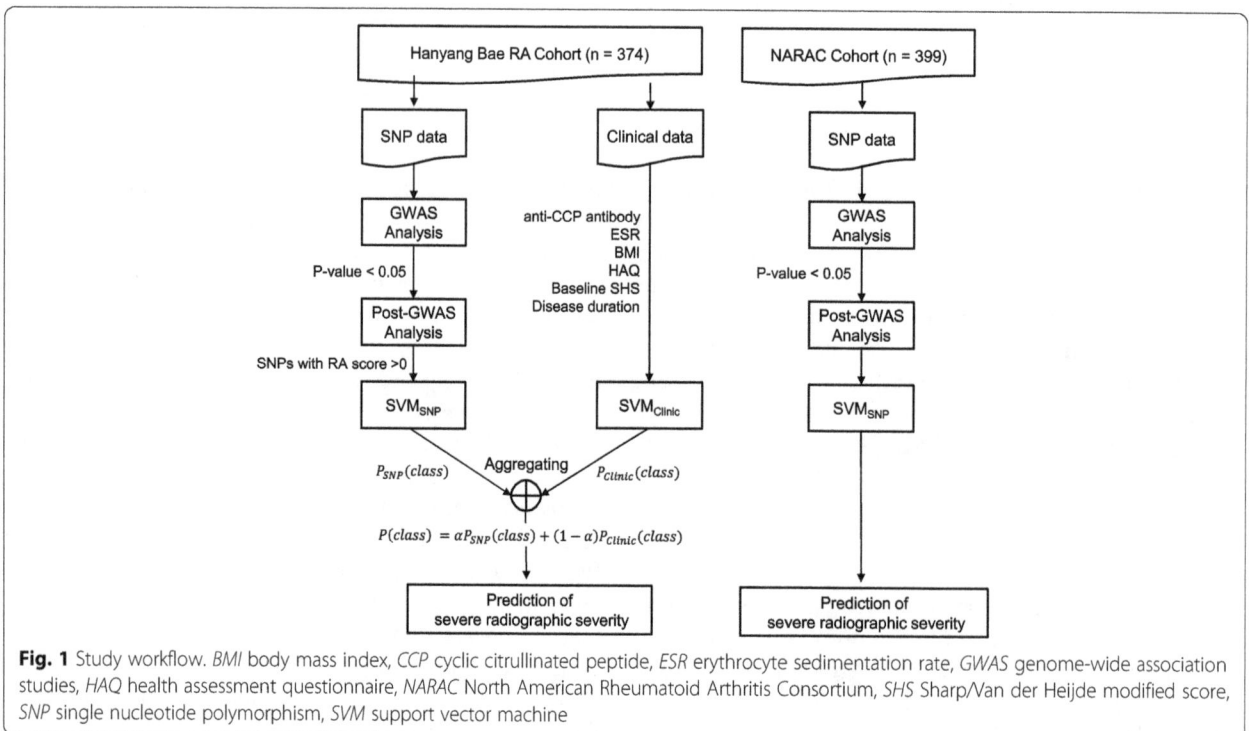

Fig. 1 Study workflow. *BMI* body mass index, *CCP* cyclic citrullinated peptide, *ESR* erythrocyte sedimentation rate, *GWAS* genome-wide association studies, *HAQ* health assessment questionnaire, *NARAC* North American Rheumatoid Arthritis Consortium, *SHS* Sharp/Van der Heijde modified score, *SNP* single nucleotide polymorphism, *SVM* support vector machine

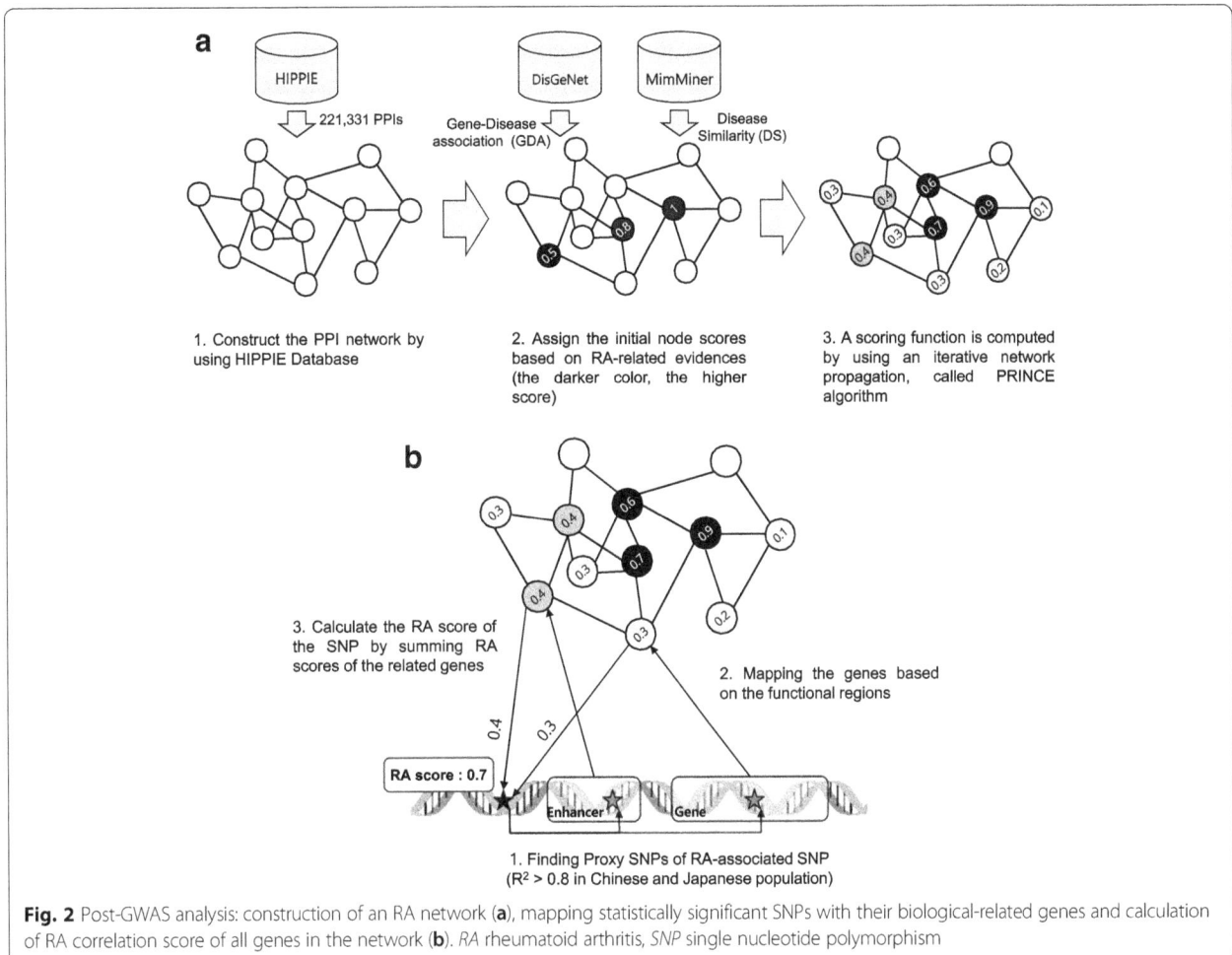

Fig. 2 Post-GWAS analysis: construction of an RA network (**a**), mapping statistically significant SNPs with their biological-related genes and calculation of RA correlation score of all genes in the network (**b**). *RA* rheumatoid arthritis, *SNP* single nucleotide polymorphism

we finally reprioritized SNPs by the sum of RA correlation scores of their related genes (Fig. 2b). We also collected SNP sets that were prioritized by *p* value in GWAS analysis and by SPOT analysis [23] for the comparison of prediction powers.

Prediction model for radiographic severity using ensemble approach

The final prediction model for severe radiographic progression consisted of an ensemble approach that combined two classification models: one was based on the SNPs that we selected and the other was based on clinical information. Each model was constructed by using SVM, which is a supervised machine learning algorithm to classify multiclasses based on a hyperplane that differentiate the classes on the n-dimensional space. We used six clinical predictive factors that we investigated in another study [24]: baseline SHS, disease duration, health assessment questionnaire (HAQ) index, anti-cyclic citrullinated peptide (CCP) antibody, body mass index (BMI), and erythrocyte sedimentation rate (ESR). The final decision for severe radiographic progression

was calculated as the weight sum of probabilities in each model.

Post-GWAS prioritization in an independent cohort of Caucasian patients with RA

To confirm the reliability of post-GWAS prioritization and SVM-based prediction of severe radiographic progression, we conducted GWAS, post-GWAS analysis, and machine learning using SVM in consecutive order. As there was limited clinical information in the NARAC cohort, only SNPs were used for prediction of severe radiographic progression.

Statistical analysis

The multivariate logistic regression model was used to investigate the association between SNPs and radiographic severity (no progression vs. severe progression) in GWAS, adjusted for anti-CCP antibody positivity, ESR, BMI, HAQ score, baseline SHS, disease duration, and the top ten principal components using PLINK v1.07.

Accuracy is a measure of the proportion of samples that are correctly predicted among all the test samples, and it is easy to intuitively understand the model performance at a glance. Thus, accuracy was used for selection of optimal SNPs set in the Hanyang Bae RA cohort and NARAC cohort, according to the standard method as follows:

$$Accuracy = \frac{\sum True\ positive + \sum True\ negative}{\sum True\ population}$$

Classification accuracy is typically not enough information to evaluate the performance of the model. To evaluate the robustness of a model, more performance measures are needed. The area under the curve (AUC) of the receiver operating characteristic (ROC) curve measures the performance of the markers with the total sum of performance at all thresholds. Based on the diversity of populations and the characteristics of SNP markers that should be evaluated with a limited number of samples, it would be more reliable to compare all the performance that the set could have, rather than looking for the best accuracy it could have, with expectations for performance for various unknown samples. In this reason, we further analyzed the performance of the model in the Hanyang Bae RA cohort using AUC according to the standard method as follows:

$$AUC = \frac{\sum Rank(pos) - \#pos \times (\#pos + 1)/2}{\#pos + \#neg}$$

Where $\sum Rank(pos)$ means the sum of the ranks of all positively classified examples, #pos means the number of positive examples in the dataset, and #neg means the number of negative examples in the dataset.

Results

Findings of GWAS for radiographic progression in Korean RA patients

After quality control, a total of 1,343,748 SNPs were available for comparison in 118 patients with no progression [age 49.5 ± 11.8 (mean ± standard deviation), female = 83.9%] and 120 patients with severe progression [age 47.7 ± 12.6, female = 85.0%] (Additional file 1: Table S1). In the single association analysis, none of the SNPs reached the significance threshold after Bonferroni correction. The SNPs with $p < 1.0 \times 10^{-3}$ and their related genes are listed in Additional file 1: Table S2.

Optimal SNP set selection using post-GWAS scoring

To determine the optimal number of SNPs for the prediction model, we tested the accuracy of the prediction model by adding 5 SNPs from the top ten scored SNPs. For this, we performed tenfold cross-validation by grouping the patients into ten groups. Of the ten groups, nine groups were used as the training set in GWAS and post-GWAS analysis for selection of the SNPs and construction of a SVM model using radial basis function Kernel. The remaining group was used as a test set and we calculated the average accuracies of ten test sets. Our results showed that the best accuracy was 0.6015 when the top 85 SNPs were used (Fig. 3a). Therefore, we defined the optimal number of SNPs as 85. Our method showed superior accuracy compared with SNPs selected based on p-value of GWAS and by SPOT analysis (p value 1.06×10^{-06} and 6.25×10^{-03}, respectively). The list of 85 SNPs and their related genes are described in Additional file 1: Table S3.

Interestingly, SNPs that had low p values in GWAS analysis showed the lowest accuracy. To investigate further, we compared the overlapping ratio of the top 85 SNPs selected by different methods between ten training sets (Fig. 3b). The results showed that the overlap ratio between SNPs selected by low p value was only 0.2403, whereas the overlap ratio of our method was more than two times higher (0.5627). It seems that the SNPs selected in each training set by tenfold cross-validation based on GWAS p value are likely to be biased in each training sample itself and could cause lower overlap ratio between groups. On other hand, post-GWAS analysis which integrated the biological meaning to the analysis is less likely to select the SNPs that were biased in the sample group, unlike the GWAS which depends only on the simple p value.

Comparison of the prediction accuracy among different models

The final ensemble model was composed of two different SVM models: one is based on 85 SNPs selected by post-GWAS analysis and the other is based on information on six clinical factors. We calculated a weighted sum of probabilities of these two models to predict severe radiographic progression. The best average accuracy of our model was 0.7481 with 0.27 of weight to SVM model using SNPs (Additional file 2: Figure S1). In the process of optimizing the weight, all tenfold cross-validation tests were performed on the test set, to avoid overfitting as much as possible. We compared the ROC curve of our ensemble model with other ensemble models that used 85 SNPs selected by GWAS p value or by SPOT analysis as well as clinical information (Fig. 4). The AUC of our model was 0.7872 (sensitivity 0.7644, specificity 0.7318, and positive predictive value 0.7445, Additional file 1: Table S4), which was significantly better than that of the ensemble model with GWAS (8.97X10E-5) and SPOT (0.0423).

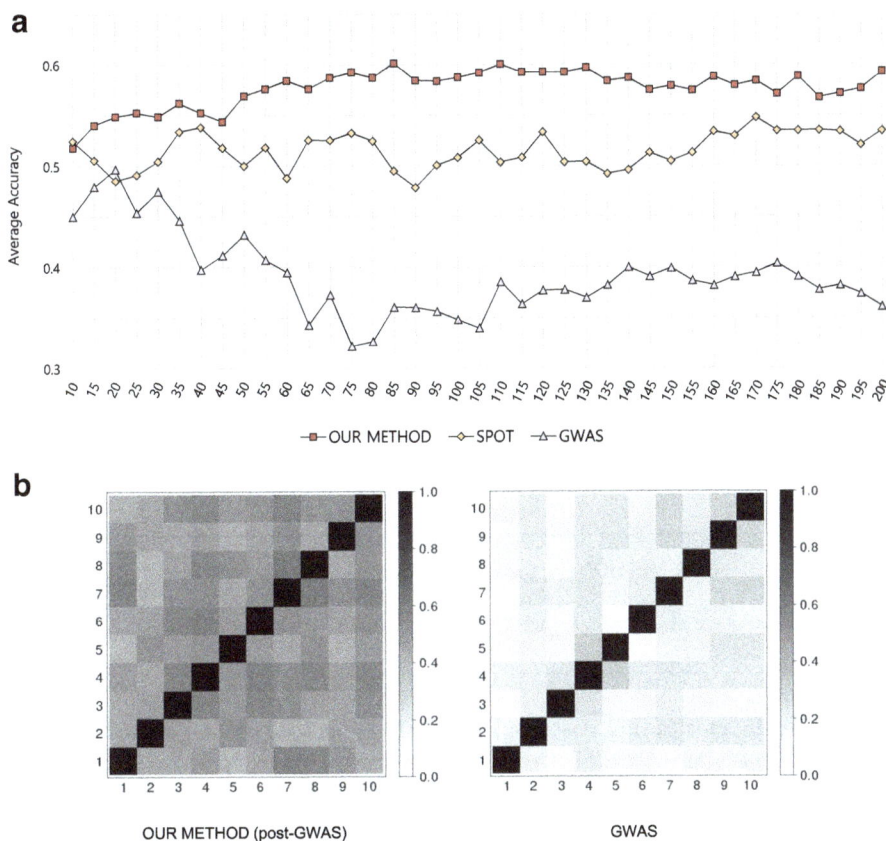

Fig. 3 Prediction accuracy of radiographic progression using SNPs obtained via post-GWAS, GWAS, and SPOT analysis: optimal number of SNPs for the prediction model (**a**), and overlapping ratio between 85 SNPs selected by post-GWAS and GWAS analysis (**b**). *GWAS* genome-wide association studies

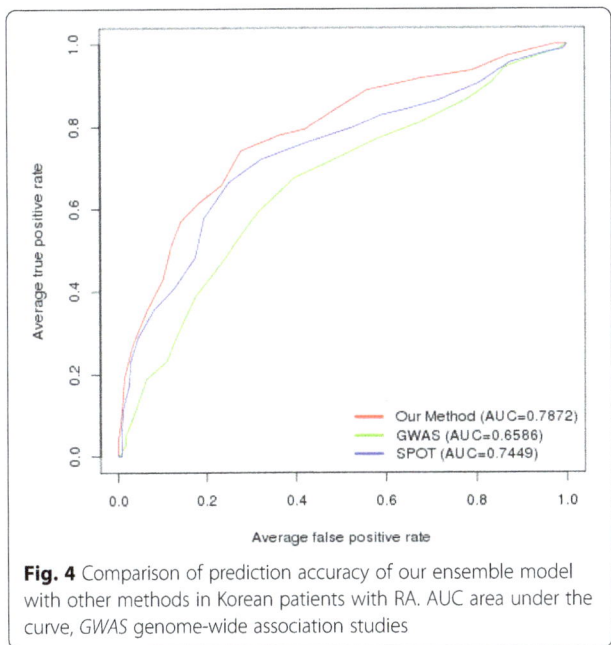

Fig. 4 Comparison of prediction accuracy of our ensemble model with other methods in Korean patients with RA. AUC area under the curve, *GWAS* genome-wide association studies

Reliability of post-GWAS prioritization in the independent cohort

By applying the same methods of post-GWAS prioritization and tenfold cross-validation using SVM to the NARAC cohort (68 patients with no progression and 86 patients with severe progression), we were able to confirm that the SNPs selected by post-GWAS analysis were more accurate than those selected by statistical significance in GWAS for prediction of severe radiographic progression. In the NARAC cohort the average accuracy was 0.6143 with SNPs selected by post-GWAS analysis, which was superior to that using SNPs selected by statistical significance in GWAS (average accuracy 0.3875) or by SPOT analysis (average accuracy 0.4563) (Fig. 5).

After quality control, a total of 1,343,748 SNPs were available for comparison in 118 patients with no progression [age 49.5 ± 11.8 (mean ± standard deviation), female = 83.9%] and 120 patients with severe progression [age 47.7 ± 12.6, female = 85.0%] (Additional file 1: Table S1).

Discussion

As hypothesized in this study, our new model allowed us to conduct more relevant and robust prediction of

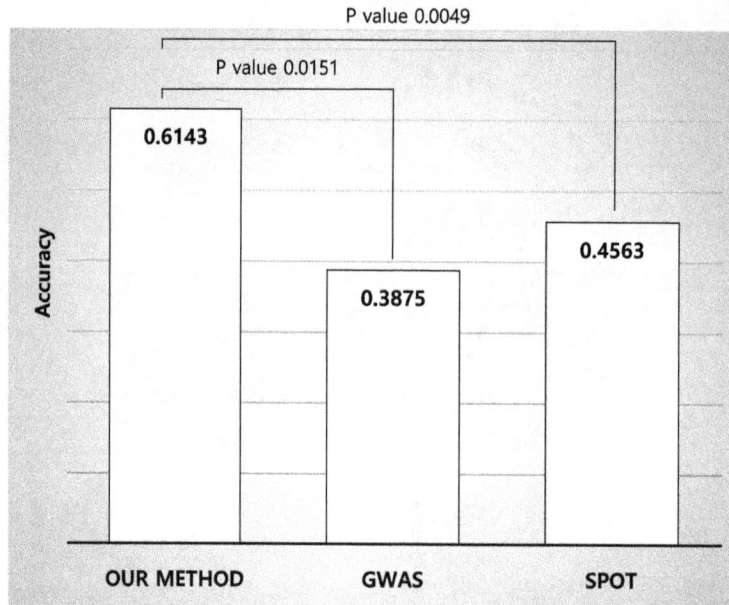

Fig. 5 Comparison of prediction accuracy of our model with other methods in an independent Caucasian cohort. *GWAS* genome-wide association studies

radiographic severity in RA. In short, using post-GWAS analysis we identified biologically relevant SNPs related to RA progression in patients with early RA. Our final model composed of SNPs combined with clinical factors could satisfactorily discriminate severe progression from the absence of progression, showing an average AUC of 0.78 in tenfold cross-validation. This result was superior to those obtained using data from GWAS (AUC = 0.59) or SPOT (AUC = 0.67), one of the methods of post-GWAS analysis. The superior effectiveness of our prediction model was also successfully reproduced in an independent cohort.

We initially thought that biological function-enriched prediction of radiographic severity would overcome the overfitting effect although the prediction accuracy would be similar to that using only GWAS results. Interestingly, however, the prediction accuracy was also improved compared with that using data of GWAS. Selection of biologically relevant variants based on post-GWAS analysis, in addition to p value in GWAS, and use of a machine learning algorithm such as SVM enabled more accurate and robust prediction of radiographic severity despite the limited sample size.

Regarding post-GWAS analysis, there have been examples of effective integration of biological database information of SNPs with GWAS results to identify causal SNPs in colorectal cancer [25] and chronic lymphocytic lymphoma [26]. We used information on various functional regions associated with SNPs and related genes such as enhancer region, mRNA, promoter region, miRNA region, and posttranscriptional modification

(PTM), in addition to expression of quantitative traits, and gave a higher priority to SNPs with greater involvement with these genes. Thus, SNPs with higher biological relevance obtained a higher reprioritization score and might be used in prediction of radiographic severity.

The SVM algorithm also contributed to increased prediction accuracy. It is one of the popular supervised learning techniques in classification. In the SVM algorithm, each patient is represented in n-dimensional space where n is the number of SNPs. After that, it finds a hyperplane that can separate patients' classes with maximum margin. We also used Kernel trick that mapped original dimensional space into a much higher-dimensional space. It can help to do a nonlinear classification more efficiently. This learning machine technique could discover new patterns for input features via investigation of complex relationships among SNPs, and thus increase the explanation power for prediction of radiographic severity in RA [27]. Many examples of outcome prediction with high predictive accuracy using SVM algorithms have been reported, such as in breast cancer [28], nasopharyngeal carcinoma [29], and severe radiation-induced pneumonitis in lung cancer [30–32]. Similarly, we could predict severe radiographic progression with high predictive accuracy via a SVM-based ensemble model that integrated multidimensional SNP data and clinical factors.

It is interesting that our model was superior to SPOT, which is also a method of SNP prioritization [23]. However, there were some differences between our SNP prioritization method and SPOT. Information on functional properties used in annotation was not the same;

our method used more varied biological information related to SNPs and genes including transcription factor binding sites, micro RNA regions, PTM, and eQTL. An eQTL study was able to explain the functional basis of up to 50% of SNPs related to immune-mediated disease [33] and therefore might be very useful in predicting the outcome of RA. Another important difference is the characteristics of the network used for scoring. In contrast to SPOT, we used a disease-specific gene database during construction of the network based on the concept that a RA susceptibility gene is also associated with phenotype. This is the first RA-specific network constructed based on network propagation and might give more accurate and stable relationship information to reprioritize the SNPs conferred by GWAS.

This study has some limitations. First, the sample size used in the analysis was small, which could lead to lower predictive accuracy of GWAS. However, as we applied the results of GWAS to post-GWAS analysis and tenfold cross-validation we could achieve higher predictive accuracy of radiographic progression and robustness of top SNPs in each of the ten groups. This meant that post-GWAS could take advantage of the small sample size of subjects in contrast to GWAS, which needs numerous samples to identify disease-specific loci. Second, we did not use the 85 SNPs selected in the Korean cohort in the analysis of the Caucasian cohort. Rather, we reproduced all courses of analysis from GWAS to using the SVM classifier in the Caucasian cohort to show the advantage of a post-GWAS approach over GWAS as a method of prediction. When we validated the final SNPs from the Hanyang Bae RA cohort in the NARAC cohort, the performance of the model using the final SNPs was unsatisfactory. Among the 85 SNPs, 72 SNPs were identified in the NARAC cohort and the accuracy (standard deviation) of the model was 0.5062 (0.1239) and the AUC was 0.4739 (Additional file 2: Figure S2). It seems that the same SNPs are not useful across ethnic groups for many reasons, such as ethnicity-specific SNPs or different allele frequency, or linkage disequilibrium.

Conclusions

We demonstrated that biologically relevant SNPs could provide more accurate and robust prediction of severe radiographic progression in Korean and Caucasian cohorts. Biologically relevant prediction of radiographic progression was possible through a bioinformatics approach including post-GWAS, which was conducted with functional annotation of the genome gathered from GWA studies, a RA network with propagation, and machine learning algorithm. This approach worked better than the GWAS approach alone. SNPs and genes selected in this approach could be targets for further functional studies and might be a basis of individual precision medicine.

Abbreviations
AUC: Area under the curve; BMI: Body mass index; CCP: Cyclic citrullinated peptide; eQTL: Expression quantitative trait loci; ESR: Erythrocyte sedimentation rate; GWAS: Genome-wide association studies; HAQ: health assessment questionnaire; HWE: Hardy Weinberg equilibrium; MAF: Minor allele frequency; NARAC: North American Rheumatoid Arthritis Consortium; PC: Principal component; PTM: posttranscriptional modification; RA: Rheumatoid arthritis; ROC: Receiver operating characteristic; SHS: Sharp/Van der Heijde modified score; SNP: Single nucleotide polymorphisms; SVM: Support vector machine

Acknowledgements
The authors would like to thank Dr. Gregersen PK for kindly providing the X-rays and clinical data from the North American Rheumatoid Arthritis Consortium (NARAC).

Funding
This work was supported by grants from the Korea Healthcare Technology R&D Project of the Ministry for Health & Welfare (HI13C2124) and the Bio-Synergy Research Project (NRF-2012M3A9C4048759) of the Ministry of Science, ICT and Future Planning through the National Research Foundation.

Authors' contributions
YBJ, YK, G-SY, H-SL, and S-CB designed the study. JAR and SL scored all radiographs, YK and YP analyzed the data. YBJ, YK, KK, and S-YB interpreted the data. YBJ, YK, and S-CB wrote the manuscript. All authors reviewed and approved the manuscript.

Competing interests
The authors declare that they have no competing interests.

Author details
[1]Department of Rheumatology, St. Vincent's Hospital, The Catholic University of Korea, Suwon, Republic of Korea. [2]Department of Bio and Brain Engineering, Korea Advanced Institute of Science and Technology, Daejeon, Republic of Korea. [3]Department of Rheumatology, Hanyang University Hospital for Rheumatic Diseases, Seoul, Republic of Korea. [4]Department of Biology, Kyung Hee University, Seoul, Republic of Korea. [5]Department of Radiology, Hanyang University Hospital, Seoul, Republic of Korea.

References
1. Kim K, Bang SY, Lee HS, Bae SC. Update on the genetic architecture of rheumatoid arthritis. Nat Rev Rheumatol. 2017;13:13–24.
2. Hou L, Zhao H. A review of post-GWAS prioritization approaches. Front Genet. 2013;4:280.
3. Knevel R, Grondal G, Huizinga TW, Visser AW, Jonsson H, Vikingsson A, Geirsson AJ, Steinsson K, van der Helm-van Mil AH. Genetic predisposition of the severity of joint destruction in rheumatoid arthritis: a population-based study. Ann Rheum Dis. 2012;71:707–9.
4. van Steenbergen HW, Tsonaka R, Huizinga TW, le Cessie S, van der Helm-van Mil AH. Predicting the severity of joint damage in rheumatoid arthritis; the contribution of genetic factors. Ann Rheum Dis. 2015;74:876–82.
5. Arnett FC, Edworthy SM, Bloch DA, McShane DJ, Fries JF, Cooper NS, Healey LA, Kaplan SR, Liang MH, Luthra HS, et al. The American Rheumatism Association 1987 revised criteria for the classification of rheumatoid arthritis. Arthritis Rheum. 1988;31:315–24.
6. Kim YJ, Choi CB, Sung YK, Lee HS, Bae SC. Characteristics of Korean patients with RA: a single center cohort study. J Korean Rheum Assoc. 2009;16:204–12.

7. Plenge RM, Seielstad M, Padyukov L, Lee AT, Remmers EF, Ding B, Liew A, Khalili H, Chandrasekaran A, Davies LR, et al. TRAF1-C5 as a risk locus for rheumatoid arthritis--a genomewide study. N Engl J Med. 2007;357:1199–209.

8. van der Heijde D. How to read radiographs according to the Sharp/van der Heijde method. J Rheumatol. 2000;27:261–3.

9. Strand V, Landewe R, van der Heijde D. Using estimated yearly progression rates to compare radiographic data across recent randomised controlled trials in rheumatoid arthritis. Ann Rheum Dis. 2002;61 Suppl 2:ii64–66.

10. Knevel R, Klein K, Somers K, Ospelt C, Houwing-Duistermaat JJ, van Nies JA, de Rooy DP, de Bock L, Kurreeman FA, Schonkeren J, et al. Identification of a genetic variant for joint damage progression in autoantibody-positive rheumatoid arthritis. Ann Rheum Dis. 2014;73:2038–46.

11. Forrest AR, Kawaji H, Rehli M, Baillie JK, de Hoon MJ, Haberle V, Lassmann T, Kulakovskiy IV, Lizio M, Itoh M, et al. A promoter-level mammalian expression atlas. Nature. 2014;507:462–70.

12. Karolchik D, Baertsch R, Diekhans M, Furey TS, Hinrichs A, Lu YT, Roskin KM, Schwartz M, Sugnet CW, Thomas DJ, et al. The UCSC Genome Browser Database. Nucleic Acids Res. 2003;31:51–4.

13. Griffiths-Jones S, Grocock RJ, van Dongen S, Bateman A, Enright AJ. miRBase: microRNA sequences, targets and gene nomenclature. Nucleic Acids Res. 2006;34:D140–4.

14. Hsu SD, Lin FM, Wu WY, Liang C, Huang WC, Chan WL, Tsai WT, Chen GZ, Lee CJ, Chiu CM, et al. miRTarBase: a database curates experimentally validated microRNA-target interactions. Nucleic Acids Res. 2011;39:D163–169.

15. Xia K, Shabalin AA, Huang S, Madar V, Zhou YH, Wang W, Zou F, Sun W, Sullivan PF, Wright FA. seeQTL: a searchable database for human eQTLs. Bioinformatics. 2012;28:451–2.

16. GTEx Consortium. The Genotype-Tissue Expression (GTEx) project. Nat Genet. 2013;45:580–5.

17. Westra HJ, Arends D, Esko T, Peters MJ, Schurmann C, Schramm K, Kettunen J, Yaghootkar H, Fairfax BP, Andiappan AK, et al. Cell specific eQTL analysis without sorting cells. PLoS Genet. 2015;11:e1005223.

18. De Jager PL, Hacohen N, Mathis D, Regev A, Stranger BE, Benoist C. ImmVar project: Insights and design considerations for future studies of "healthy" immune variation. Semin Immunol. 2015;27:51–7.

19. Schaefer MH, Fontaine JF, Vinayagam A, Porras P, Wanker EE, Andrade-Navarro MA. HIPPIE: Integrating protein interaction networks with experiment based quality scores. PLoS One. 2012;7:e31826.

20. Pinero J, Queralt-Rosinach N, Bravo A, Deu-Pons J, Bauer-Mehren A, Baron M, Sanz F, Furlong LI. DisGeNET: a discovery platform for the dynamical exploration of human diseases and their genes. Database (Oxford). 2015;2015:bav028.

21. van Driel MA, Bruggeman J, Vriend G, Brunner HG, Leunissen JA. A text-mining analysis of the human phenome. Eur J Hum Genet. 2006;14:535–42.

22. Vanunu O, Magger O, Ruppin E, Shlomi T, Sharan R. Associating genes and protein complexes with disease via network propagation. PLoS Comput Biol. 2010;6:e1000641.

23. Saccone SF, Bolze R, Thomas P, Quan J, Mehta G, Deelman E, Tischfield JA, Rice JP. SPOT: a web-based tool for using biological databases to prioritize SNPs after a genome-wide association study. Nucleic Acids Res. 2010;38:W201–209.

24. Joo YB, Bang SY, Ryu JA, Lee S, Lee HS, Bae SC. Predictors of severe radiographic progression in patients with early rheumatoid arthritis: Prospective observational cohort study. Int J Rheum Dis. 2017. doi:10.1111/1756-185X.13054. [Epub ahead of Print]

25. Wang HM, Chang TH, Lin FM, Chao TH, Huang WC, Liang C, Chu CF, Chiu CM, Wu WY, Chen MC, et al. A new method for post Genome-Wide Association Study (GWAS) analysis of colorectal cancer in Taiwan. Gene. 2013;518:107–13.

26. Sille FC, Thomas R, Smith MT, Conde L, Skibola CF. Post-GWAS functional characterization of susceptibility variants for chronic lymphocytic leukemia. PLoS One. 2012;7(e29632).

27. Klement RJ, Allgauer M, Appold S, Dieckmann K, Ernst I, Ganswindt U, Holy R, Nestle U, Nevinny-Stickel M, Semrau S, et al. Support vector machine-based prediction of local tumor control after stereotactic body radiation therapy for early-stage non-small cell lung cancer. Int J Radiat Oncol Biol Phys. 2014;88:732–8.

28. Nimeus-Malmstrom E, Krogh M, Malmstrom P, Strand C, Fredriksson I, Karlsson P, Nordenskjold B, Stal O, Ostberg G, Peterson C, et al. Gene expression profiling in primary breast cancer distinguishes patients developing local recurrence after breast-conservation surgery, with or without postoperative radiotherapy. Breast Cancer Res. 2008;10:R34.

29. Wan XB, Zhao Y, Fan XJ, Cai HM, Zhang Y, Chen MY, Xu J, Wu XY, Li HB, Zeng YX, et al. Molecular prognostic prediction for locally advanced nasopharyngeal carcinoma by support vector machine integrated approach. PLoS One. 2012;7(e31989).

30. Naqa IE, Deasy JO, Mu Y, Huang E, Hope AJ, Lindsay PE, Apte A, Alaly J, Bradley JD. Datamining approaches for modeling tumor control probability. Acta Oncol. 2010;49:1363–73.

31. Chen S, Zhou S, Yin FF, Marks LB, Das SK. Investigation of the support vector machine algorithm to predict lung radiation-induced pneumonitis. Med Phys. 2007;34:3808–14.

32. Das SK, Chen S, Deasy JO, Zhou S, Yin FF, Marks LB. Combining multiple models to generate consensus: application to radiation-induced pneumonitis prediction. Med Phys. 2008;35:5098–109.

33. Kumar V, Wijmenga C, Xavier RJ. Genetics of immune-mediated disorders: from genome-wide association to molecular mechanism. Curr Opin Immunol. 2014;31:51–7.

4

Patient-provider discordance between global assessments of disease activity in rheumatoid arthritis: a comprehensive clinical evaluation

Divya N. Challa[1], Zoran Kvrgic[1], Andrea L. Cheville[2], Cynthia S. Crowson[3], Tim Bongartz[4], Thomas G. Mason II[1], Eric L. Matteson[1], Clement J. Michet Jr[1], Scott T. Persellin[1], Daniel E. Schaffer[1], Theresa L. Wampler Muskardin[1], Kerry Wright[1] and John M. Davis III[1]*

Abstract

Background: Discordance between patients with rheumatoid arthritis (RA) and their rheumatology health care providers is a common and important problem. The objective of this study was to perform a comprehensive clinical evaluation of patient-provider discordance in RA.

Methods: A cross-sectional observational study was conducted of consecutive RA patients in a regional practice with an absolute difference of ≥ 25 points between patient and provider global assessments (possible points, 0–100). Data were collected for disease activity measures, clinical characteristics, comorbidities, and medications. In a prospective substudy, participants completed patient-reported outcome measures and underwent ultrasonographic assessment of synovial inflammation. Differences between the discordant and concordant groups were tested using χ^2 and rank sum tests. Multivariable logistic regression was used to develop a clinical model of discordance.

Results: Patient-provider discordance affected 114 (32.5%) of 350 consecutive patients. Of the total population, 103 patients (29.5%) rated disease activity higher than their providers (i.e., 'positive' discordance); only 11 (3.1%) rated disease activity lower than their providers and were excluded from further analysis. Positive discordance correlated with negative rheumatoid factor and anticyclic citrullinated peptide antibodies, lack of joint erosions, presence of comorbid fibromyalgia or depression, and use of opioids, antidepressants, or anxiolytics, or fibromyalgia medications. In the prospective study, the group with positive discordance was distinguished by higher pain intensity, neuropathic type pain, chronic widespread pain and associated polysymptomatic distress, and limited functional health status. Depression was found to be an important mediator of positive discordance in low disease activity whereas the widespread pain index was an important mediator of positive discordance in moderate-to-high disease activity states. Ultrasonography scores did not reveal significant differences in synovial inflammation between discordant and concordant groups.

Conclusions: The findings provide a deeper understanding of patient-provider discordance than previously known. New insights from this study include the evidence that positive discordance is not associated with unrecognized joint inflammation by ultrasonography and that depression and fibromyalgia appear to play distinct roles in determining positive discordance. Further work is necessary to develop a comprehensive framework for patient-centered evaluation and management of RA and associated comorbidities in patients in the scenario of patient-provider discordance.

Keywords: Depression, Disease activity, Fibromyalgia, Patient-reported outcomes, Rheumatoid arthritis

* Correspondence: davis.john4@mayo.edu
[1]Division of Rheumatology, Mayo Clinic, 200 First St. SW, Rochester, MN 55905, USA
Full list of author information is available at the end of the article

Table 1 Association of patient characteristics with patient-provider discordance in global assessments of disease activity in the total study population

Characteristic	All patients (N = 339)	Concordant group (n = 236)	Discordant group[a] (n = 103)	P value
Age, years	63.5 (55.1–72.8)	62.4 (55.1–73.8)	63.5 (54.9–72.0)	.79
Sex				.15
Female	235 (69)	158 (67)	77 (75)	
Male	104 (31)	78 (33)	26 (25)	
Disease duration, years	7.0 (2.7, 11.4)	7.4 (3.5, 11.7)	6.3 (2.2, 8.8)	.53
Provider type				.63
NP/PA	230 (68)	160 (68)	70 (68)	
Physician	90 (27)	61 (26)	29 (28)	
Fellow	19 (6)	15 (6)	4 (4)	
Comorbidity				
Fibromyalgia	28 (8)	10 (4)	18 (17)	< .001
Depression	101 (30)	61 (26)	40 (39)	.02
Osteoarthritis	184 (54)	121 (51)	63 (61)	.09
Sleep apnea	63 (19)	47 (20)	16 (16)	.34
Obesity (BMI ≥ 30 kg/m²)	130 (42)	87 (39)	43 (47)	.19
BMI, kg/m²	28.5 (25.1–33.7)	28.4 (24.2–32.9)	29.4 (26.5–35.4)	.03
Disease assessment				
Patient global, 0-100	33 (11–57)	20 (6–44)	57 (46–72)	< .001
Provider global, 0-100	15 (5–30)	15 (5–40)	15 (10–20)	.20
Pain VAS, 0-100	38 (15–63)	24 (9–50)	60 (44–73)	< .001
Tender joint count ≥ 2	121 (36)	75 (32)	46 (45)	.02
Swollen joint count ≥ 2	122 (36)	82 (35)	40 (39)	.47
DAS28-CRP	3.0 (2.2–4.4)	2.6 (1.9–4.1)	3.7 (2.7–4.7)	.004
CDAI	7.5 (3.0–14.5)	5.6 (2.0–13.8)	9.8 (6.5–15.6)	< .001
Remission, < 2.8	80 (24)	78 (33)	2 (2)	< .001
LDA, ≥ 2.8 to < 10.0	130 (38)	79 (33)	51 (50)	
MDA, ≥ 10.0 to < 22.0	89 (26)	51 (22)	38 (37)	
HDA, ≥ 22.0	40 (12)	28 (12)	12 (12)	
Laboratory assessment				
CRP, mg/L	3.2 (2.9–9.2)	3.3 (2.9–9.4)	3.2 (2.9–9.2)	.96
RF positivity	233 (71)	173 (75)	60 (61)	.01
Anti-CCP antibody positivity	201 (67)	146 (71)	55 (59)	.045
Radiographic joint erosion	172 (52)	133 (57)	39 (39)	.002
Medication use				
Prednisone	150 (44)	101 (43)	49 (48)	.42
Methotrexate	215 (63)	148 (63)	67 (65)	.68
Biologics	125 (37)	83 (35)	42 (41)	.33
Change of RA medications at index visit	91 (27)	69 (29)	22 (21)	.13
Opioid	78 (23)	45 (19)	33 (32)	.009

Table 1 Association of patient characteristics with patient-provider discordance in global assessments of disease activity in the total study population *(Continued)*

Fibromyalgia med	33 (10)	16 (7)	17 (17)	.005
Sleep aid	36 (11)	18 (8)	18 (17)	.007
Antidepressant or anxiolytic	80 (24)	45 (19)	35 (34)	.003

[a]Values are presented as median (interquartile range) or number (percentage)
[b]Discordant group contains only those patients with a global assessment greater than the physician global assessment
anti-CCP anticyclic citrullinated peptide, *BMI* body mass index, *CDAI* Clinical Disease Activity Index, *CRP* C-reactive protein, *DAS28-CRP* Disease Activity Score in 28 joints using C-reactive protein, *DMARD* disease-modifying antirheumatic drug, *HDA* high disease activity, *LDA* low disease activity, *MDA* moderate disease activity, *NP* nurse practitioner, *PA* physician assistant, *RA* rheumatoid arthritis, *RF* rheumatoid factor

According to the CDAI, a smaller proportion of patients in the discordant group was in remission than in the concordant group (2% vs. 33%), and greater proportions of patients in the discordant group were in LDA (50% vs. 33%) and MDA (37% vs. 22%) categories than in the concordant groups ($P < .001$), while proportions of patients with HDA were similar between groups.

Comparison of patient characteristics between concordant and discordant groups showed no significant differences in age, sex, or provider type (Table 1). The discordant group reported higher pain by VAS than the concordant group (median 60.0 vs. 23.5; $P < .001$). Negative results for RF ($P = .01$) and anti-CCP antibodies ($P = .045$), lack of radiographic joint erosions ($P = .002$), and presence of ≥ 2 tender joints ($P = .02$) were significantly associated with patient-provider discordance. No significant differences were observed between the groups in swollen joint counts or inflammatory markers. Among the comorbidities, fibromyalgia ($P < .001$) and depression ($P = .02$) showed significant association with discordance. However, excluding patients with fibromyalgia did not affect the association of pain VAS with positive discordance (mean pain VAS of 56 in the discordant group vs. 31 in the concordant group; $P < .001$). Current use of opioids (32% vs. 19%, $P = .009$), fibromyalgia medications

(17% vs. 7%, $P = .005$), antidepressants or anxiolytics (34% vs. 19%, $P = .003$), and sleep aids (17% vs. 8%, $P = .007$) was significantly higher in the discordant group. Both groups had similar treatment with conventional and biologic DMARDs, without significant differences in DMARD modification at the index visit.

Of 140 patients approached for the prospective substudy, 70 patients agreed to participate, including 50 patients from the discordant group and 20 from the concordant group. Four patients in the discordant group were among the 11 in the study population with lower discordance who were excluded, leaving 46 patients in the discordant group for analysis. In the discordant group, the disease of two patients was in remission, and 26 had LDA, 13 had MDA, and 5 had HDA. The discordant group reported higher median scores for pain VAS (49.0 vs. 25.0, $P = .002$), SF-MPQ-2 continuous pain (3.3 vs. 2.2, $P = .03$), neuropathic pain (2.0 vs. 1.2, $P = .045$), Fibromyalgia Survey WPI (7.0 vs. 4.5, $P = .008$), and polysymptomatic distress (11.5 vs. 7.5, $P = .007$) than the concordant group (Table 2). Of note, fatigue measures were not significantly different between the groups, either by Bristol Rheumatoid Arthritis Fatigue or PROMIS Fatigue Survey. Five patients (10.8%) in the discordant group had PHQ-9 scores ≥ 10, indicating moderate to severe clinical depression. An investigator (JMD) screened

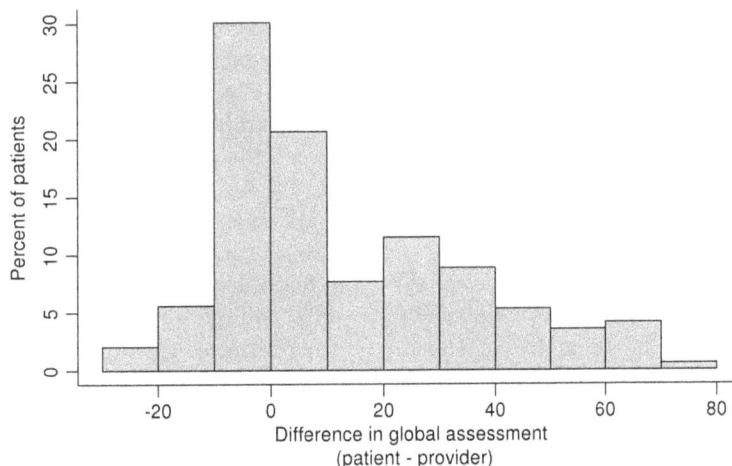

Fig. 1 Distribution of the continuous differences between the patient and provider global assessments of disease activity in the overall study population

Table 2 Comparison of patient-reported outcomes between the concordant and discordant groups in the prospective substudy

Patient-reported outcome	Concordant group (n = 20)	Discordant group[a] (n = 46)	P value
Pain VAS	25.0 (11.0–42.5)	49.0 (28.0–70.0)	.002
SF-MPQ-2 pain score			
Continuous	2.2 (1.8)	3.3 (2.0)	.03
Intermittent	1.8 (2.2)	1.8 (2.0)	.71
Neuropathic	1.2 (1.4)	2.0 (1.8)	.045
Affective	1.1 (1.4)	1.7 (2.0)	.06
Total	1.2 (0.4–2.7)	2.1 (1.2–2.9)	.09
Fibromyalgia Research Survey			
WPI	4.5 (2.5–7.0)	7.0 (5.0–10.0)	.008
SS score	3.5 (2.0–5.5)	4.5 (3.0–6.0)	.05
Polysymptomatic distress	7.5 (5.5–12.5)	11.5 (9.0–16.0)	.007
BRAF score	5.0 (3.8–5.5)	5.3 (4.3–6.7)	.10
PROMIS			
Fatigue	2.4 (1.4–3.4)	2.8 (2.0–3.8)	.22
Pain interference	1.7 (1.3–2.6)	2.2 (1.6–3.1)	.04
Sleep disturbance	2.0 (1.4–3.4)	2.8 (2.0–3.8)	.09
Ability to participate	3.9 (3.4–4.5)	3.5 (3.0–4.1)	.06
HAQ-II disability	0.4 (0.1–1.1)	1.0 (0.5–1.4)	.003
MAAS	4.6 (4.2–5.3)	5.1 (4.5–5.4)	.19
PHQ-9	2.5 (1.0–6.0)	4.0 (3.0–6.0)	.18
GAD-7	1.0 (0.0–1.5)	1.0 (0.0–3.0)	.12

Values are presented as median (interquartile range)

[a] Discordant group contains only those patients with patient global assessment greater than physician global assessmen

BRAF Bristol Rheumatoid Arthritis Fatigue, *GAD-7* Generalized Anxiety Disorder 7, *HAQ-II* Health Assessment Questionnaire II, *MAAS* Mindful Attention Awareness Scale, *PHQ-9* Patient Health Questionnaire 9, *PROMIS* Patient-Reported Outcome Measurement Information System, *SF-MPQ-2* Short-Form McGill Pain Questionnaire 2, *SS* Symptom Severity, *VAS* visual analog scale, *WPI* Widespread Pain Index

these five patients, and one patient consented to psychiatric evaluation on a nonurgent basis; the other patients chose to follow-up with their primary rheumatologist or primary care provider. None expressed suicidal ideation or required urgent evaluation.

To address the possibility of confounding of patient-reported outcome analyses by disease activity states, the next analysis separately compared individual patient-reported outcomes between discordant and concordant groups among patients with LDA versus MHDA (Table 3). Irrespective of disease activity category, the discordant group had higher median scores for pain VAS (for LDA, 37.0 vs. 18.5, $P = .006$; for MHDA, 66.0 vs. 36.0, $P = .02$) and higher median HAQ-II disability scores (for LDA, 0.9 vs. 0.2, $P = .001$; for MHDA, 1.2 vs. 0.9, $P = .10$). In the LDA category, the discordant group had impaired ability to function in activities and social roles according to the PROMIS ability to participate instrument (median, 3.5 vs. 4.3; $P = .02$) and higher PHQ-9 depression scores (median, 4.0 vs. 1.0, $P = .04$) compared with patients in the concordant group. In the MHDA category, patients in the discordant group had higher median scores for fibromyalgia WPI (8.0

vs. 4.0; $P = .005$) and polysymptomatic distress (13.5 vs. 7.5; $P = .01$).

In order to explore the different effects of depression and fibromyalgia on discordance depending on disease activity states, the analysis was also performed on the overall study population (Table 4). In the LDA category, a higher prevalence of depression in this analysis by provider diagnosis was evident in the discordant group (47% vs. 27%, $P = .006$), but in the MHDA category there was no difference in the prevalence of depression between the discordant and concordant groups (30% vs. 24%, $P = .46$). As compared to the abovementioned observations for the fibromyalgia WPI, a higher prevalence of fibromyalgia by provider diagnosis was observed in the discordant groups in both the LDA (15% vs. 3%, $P = .002$) and the MHDA (20% vs. 6%, $P = .015$) categories.

Multivariable logistic regression analysis in the total retrospective population showed that diagnoses of fibromyalgia (adjusted odds ratio (OR) 3.06, 95% confidence interval (CI) 1.87–8.00), depression (adjusted OR 1.79, 95% CI 1.02–3.15), and lack of erosions (adjusted OR 0.56, 95% CI 0.32–0.97) were independently associated

Table 3 Comparison of patient-reported outcomes between the groups according to clinical disease activity level

Measure	Remission/low disease activity[a]			Moderate-to-high disease activity[a]		
	Concordant group (n = 10)	Discordant group (n = 28)	P value	Concordant group (n = 10)	Discordant group (n = 18)	P value
Pain VAS	18.5 (3.0–26.0)	37.0 (24.0–56.0)	.006	36.0 (14.0–50.0)	66.0 (56.0–74.0)	.02
HAQ-II	0.2 (0.0–0.3)	0.9 (0.5–1.2)	.001	0.9 (0.4–1.2)	1.2 (0.7–1.2)	.10
SF-MPQ-2	0.7 (0.3–1.6)	1.4 (0.8–2.6)	.10	1.9 (1.0–2.7)	2.3 (1.8–3.9)	.18
WPI	5.0 (1.0–8.0)	6.0 (4.0–9.0)	.18	4.0 (3.0–7.0)	8.0 (6.0–10.0)	.005
SS score	2.5 (1.0–4.0)	4.0 (3.0–6.0)	.11	4.0 (2.0–6.0)	6.0 (3.0–8.0)	.16
PSD	8.0 (2.0–12.0)	9.0 (8.0–15.0)	.13	7.5 (6.0–13.0)	13.5 (10.0–16.0)	.01
BRAF score	4.5 (3.7–5.3)	5.2 (4.3–6.3)	.23	5.0 (4.0–6.0)	6.3 (4.3–7.0)	.28
PROMIS						
Pain interference	1.3 (1.1–1.8)	1.9 (1.5–2.4)	.05	2.2 (1.6–2.8)	2.9 (2.1–3.5)	.05
Ability to participate	4.3 (3.8–5.0)	3.5 (3.1–4.2)	.02	3.7 (3.1–4.0)	3.3 (2.6–4.0)	.43
Sleep disturbance	1.6 (1.3–2.3)	2.1 (1.8–2.9)	.06	2.3 (1.9–2.8)	2.5 (1.8–3.3)	.50
Fatigue	1.8 (1.0–3.4)	2.6 (2.0–3.5)	.10	2.9 (2.3–3.4)	3.1 (2.3–3.8)	.43
MAAS	5.0 (4.5–5.6)	5.1 (4.6–5.4)	.95	4.4 (4.1–4.9)	5.3 (4.5–5.5)	.07
PHQ-9	1.0 (0.0–5.0)	4.0 (2.0–6.0)	.04	4.0 (2.0–11.0)	4.0 (3.0–6.0)	>.99
GAD-7	0.0 (0.0–1.0)	1.0 (0.0–3.0)	.06	1.5 (0.0–4.0)	1.5 (1.0–6.0)	.71

Values are presented as median (interquartile range)

[a]Disease activity level was classified according to the Clinical Disease Activity Index

BRAF Bristol Rheumatoid Arthritis Fatigue, *FRS* Fibromyalgia Research Survey, *GAD-7* Generalized Anxiety Disorder 7, *HAQ-II* Health Assessment Questionnaire II, *MAAS* Mindful Attention Awareness Scale, *PHQ-9* Patient Health Questionnaire 9, *PROMIS* Patient-Reported Outcomes Measurement Information System, *PSD* polysymptomatic distress, *SF-MPQ-2* Short-Form McGill Pain Questionnaire 2, *SS* Symptom Severity, *VAS* visual analog score, *WPI* Widespread Pain Index

with patient-provider discordance (Table 5). The associations of body mass index and osteoarthritis with discordance did not reach statistical significance in the overall population. However, osteoarthritis was significantly associated with discordance in the LDA category (adjusted OR 3.36, 95% CI 1.35–8.34) but not in the MDHA category (adjusted OR 0.86, 95% CI 0.33–2.27). The addition of use of glucocorticoids, conventional or biologic DMARDs, opioids, fibromyalgia medications, and antidepressants or anxiolytics to this model did not reveal any significant associations. Pain VAS was not added to the final model for the purposes of this study due to colinearity with the patient global assessment as well as other variables in the model (e.g., fibromyalgia). Overall, the model showed strong performance, with a *C* statistic of 0.694.

Comparison of Ultrasound 7 scores between concordant and discordant groups was stratified by disease activity categories (Fig. 2). The ultrasound studies were performed for research purposes as part of the prospective substudy and were not available to the primary rheumatologist who completed the provider global assessment, so the Ultrasound 7 scores were independent of the determination of patient-provider discordance. No statistically significant differences were found in continuous scores for GS synovitis, PD synovitis, GS tenosynovitis, PD tenosynovitis, or GS erosions between the groups in the LDA or MHDA categories (*P* > .10 for all comparisons). Among patients with LDA, active GS synovitis (≥ 2) was detected in 60% of the concordant and discordant groups (*P* = .97), and active PD synovitis (≥ 2) was detected in 30% of the concordant group and

Table 4 Comparison of patient characteristics between the discordant and concordant groups according to clinical disease activity level in the overall retrospective study population[a]

Characteristic	Remission/low disease activity			Moderate-to-high disease activity		
	Concordant group (n = 157)	Discordant group (n = 53)	P value	Concordant group (n = 79)	Discordant group (n = 50)	P value
Age, years	64.9 (55.1–74.3)	66.3 (59.8–72.3)	.46	61.1 (55.1–71.5)	59.0 (50.3–71.0)	.23
Sex			.70			.15
Female	102 (65%)	36 (68%)		56 (71%)	41 (82%)	
Male	55 (35%)	17 (32%)		23 (29%)	9 (18%)	
Disease duration, years	7.0 (5.2–11.8)	7.9 (3.1–11.1)	.84	8.8 (2.2–11.6)	5.2 (1.6–7.8)	.47
Provider type			.60			.90
NP/PA	108 (69%)	39 (74%)		52 (66%)	31 (62%)	
Physician	37 (24%)	12 (23%)		24 (30%)	17 (34%)	
Fellow	12 (8%)	2 (4%)		3 (4%)	2 (4%)	
Comorbidities						
Fibromyalgia	5 (3%)	8 (15%)	.002	5 (6%)	10 (20%)	.018
Depression	42 (27%)	25 (47%)	.006	19 (24%)	15 (30%)	.46
Osteoarthritis	76 (48%)	39 (74%)	.001	45 (57%)	24 (48%)	.32
Sleep apnea	26 (17%)	10 (19%)	.70	21 (27%)	6 (12%)	.047
Obesity (BMI ≥ 30 kg/m^2)	50 (34%)	23 (47%)	.12	37 (48%)	20 (48%)	.96
BMI (kg/m^2)	27.6 (23.7–31.8)	29.0 (26.8–34.0)	.017	29.8 (25.8–35.4)	29.6 (26.1–38.3)	.75
Disease assessments						
Patient global (0–100)	10 (4–22)	50 (40–60)	<.001	49 (27–68)	66 (55–77)	< .001
Provider global (0–100)	10 (5–15)	10 (5–10)	.97	45 (30–60)	20 (15–30)	< .001
Pain (0–100 mm)	15 (5–28)	50 (37–66)	<.001	55 (32–76)	66 (57–80)	.007
Tender joint count ≥ 2	12 (8%)	9 (17%)	.05	63 (80%)	37 (74%)	.45
Swollen joint count ≥ 2	21 (31%)	17 (13%)	.98	61 (77%)	33 (66%)	.16
DAS28-CRP	1.9 (1.7–6.0)	2.6 (2.5–2.7)	.002	4.1 (3.6–5.0)	4.4 (3.4–5.0)	.98
CDAI	2.9 (1.1–5.5)	6.8 (5.5–8.7)	<.001	18.9 (13.6–30.8)	15.7 (12.0–21.5)	.026
Laboratory assessments						
CRP, mg/L	3.0 (2.9–7.7)	2.9 (2.9–6.6)	.58	4.1 (2.9–14.7)	5.4 (2.9–9.5)	.97
RF, positive	115 (76%)	29 (58%)	.017	58 (74%)	31 (65%)	.24
ACPA, positive	93 (69%)	27 (56%)	.10	53 (74%)	28 (62%)	.19
Radiographic joint erosions	96 (62%)	18 (35%)	.001	37 (47%)	21 (44%)	.69
Medication use						
Prednisone	62 (39%)	21 (40%)	.99	39 (49%)	28 (56%)	.46
Methotrexate	94 (60%)	40 (75%)	.041	54 (68%)	27 (54%)	.10
Biologics	52 (33%)	18 (34%)	.91	31 (39%)	24 (48%)	.33
Change of RA medications at index visit?	34 (22%)	6 (11%)	.10	35 (44%)	16 (32%)	.16
Opioid	10 (6%)	5 (9%)	.16	12 (15%)	11 (22%)	.32
Fibromyalgia medication	8 (5%)	6 (11%)	.12	8 (10%)	11 (22%)	.06
Sleep aid	12 (8%)	9 (17%)	.05	6 (8%)	9 (18%)	.07
Anti-depressant or anxiolytic	28 (18%)	21 (40%)	.001	17 (22%)	14 (28%)	.40

Values are median (interquartile range) or number (%)

[a]Discordant group contains only those with patient global assessment greater than physician global assessment

ACPA anti-cyclic citrullinated peptide antibody, *BMI* body mass index, *CDAI* Clinical Disease Activity Index, *CRP* C-reactive protein, *DAS28-CRP* Disease Activity Score in 28 joints using C-reactive protein, *NP* nurse practitioner, *PA* physician assistant, *RA* rheumatoid arthritis, *RF* rheumatoid factor

Table 5 Multivariable logistic regression model of patient-physician discordance compared with concordance in assessments of global disease activity

Characteristic	Odds ratio (95% CI)		
	Overall	Remission/low disease activity	Moderate-to-high disease activity
Fibromyalgia	3.06 (1.17–8.00)	4.26 (0.92–19.59)	2.56 (0.67–9.73)
Osteoarthritis	1.81 (0.98–3.36)	3.36 (1.35–8.34)	0.86 (0.33–2.27)
Depression	1.79 (1.02–3.15)	3.16 (1.43–6.98)	1.10 (0.43–2.82)
BMI, kg/m^2	1.03 (0.99–1.07)	1.07 (1.00–1.14)	1.00 (0.95–1.06)
Age, per year	1.00 (0.97–1.02)	1.00 (0.97–1.04)	0.99 (0.96–1.02)
Male sex	0.79 (0.43–1.45)	1.29 (0.56–2.98)	0.60 (0.22–1.63)
RF or anti-CCP antibody positivity	0.67 (0.35–1.28)	0.76 (0.30–1.89)	0.50 (0.18–1.36)
Radiographic joint erosion present	0.56 (0.32–0.97)	0.34 (0.16–0.74)	1.17 (0.50–2.76)

CI confidence interval, *anti-CCP* anticyclic citrullinated peptide, *BMI* body mass index, *RF* rheumatoid factor

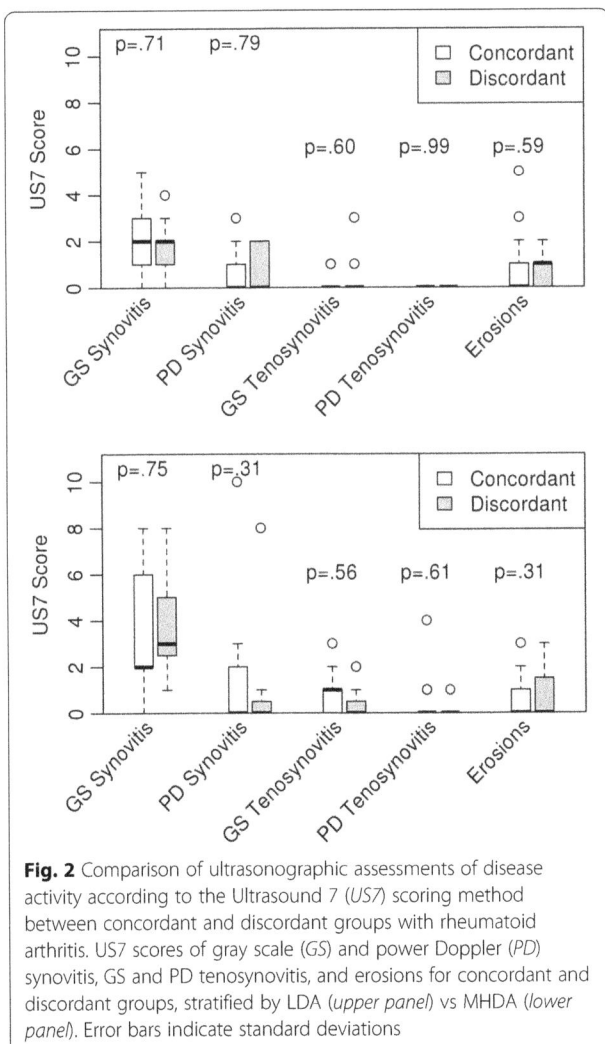

Fig. 2 Comparison of ultrasonographic assessments of disease activity according to the Ultrasound 7 (*US7*) scoring method between concordant and discordant groups with rheumatoid arthritis. US7 scores of gray scale (*GS*) and power Doppler (*PD*) synovitis, GS and PD tenosynovitis, and erosions for concordant and discordant groups, stratified by LDA (*upper panel*) vs MHDA (*lower panel*). Error bars indicate standard deviations

14% of the discordant group ($P = .27$). Among patients with MHDA in the concordant group vs. discordant group, active GS synovitis (≥ 2) was detected in 90% and 78% ($P = .42$) and active PD synovitis ($\geq$) was detected in 10% and 33% ($P = .17$).

To evaluate the potential for participation bias, the 70 participants in the prospective substudy were compared with 70 patients who declined to participate (Table 6). No significant differences were seen between participants and nonparticipants in discordance frequency, demographic characteristics, highest education level, provider type, or comorbidities. Participants were less likely than nonparticipants to have positive RF (53% vs. 76%, $P = .004$), anti-CCP antibodies (53% vs. 73%, $P = .02$), elevated CRP level (19% vs. 36%, $P = .04$), and radiographic joint erosions (35% vs. 54%, $P = .03$). However, no significant differences were found in pain, HAQ-II disability, clinical disease activity measures, or treatments between participants and nonparticipants.

Discussion

This study is among the first to perform a comprehensive clinical evaluation of the myriad potential correlates of patient-provider discordance—including several domains not previously assessed—in a real-world RA population. Overall, the prevalence of patient-provider discordance in this study was slightly less, at 33%, than the pooled estimate of 43% reported in a recent systematic review and meta-analysis [1]. The prevalence of discordance in which patients rate their disease as more severe than their providers (i.e., positive discordance) was 29%, which is nearly identical to studies by Barton et al. [3] and Khan et al. [2] at 29% and 30% of clinical encounters. In particular, fibromyalgia, depression, and nonerosive disease were independently associated with patient-provider discordance.

Barton et al. [3] have previously shown that positive discordance affects categorization of disease activity by

Table 6 Comparison of clinical characteristics between participants and patients who declined participation in the prospective substudy

Characteristic	Participants (n = 70)	Nonparticipants (n = 70)	P value
Study group			.70
Discordant	50 (71)	51 (73)	
Concordant, MHDA	10 (14)	7 (10)	
Concordant, LDA	10 (14)	12 (17)	
Age, years	63 (51–71)	59 (53–71)	.52
Sex			.56
Female	51 (73)	54 (77)	
Male	19 (27)	16 (23)	
Highest level of schooling completed			.46
Information missing	5	6	
Grade 8 or less	0 (0)	1 (2)	
Some high school but did not graduate	4 (6)	3 (5)	
High school graduation or GED	15 (23)	23 (36)	
Some college or 2-year degree	25 (38)	21 (33)	
4-year college degree	10 (15)	10 (16)	
Postgraduate studies	11 (17)	6 (9)	
Residence			.32
Minnesota	70 (100)	69 (99)	
Iowa	0 (0)	1 (1)	
Rochester, Minnesota	29 (41)	28 (41)	.92
Provider type			.38
Attending physician	20 (29)	18 (26)	
Fellow	1 (1)	4 (6)	
NP/PA	49 (70)	48 (69)	
Comorbidity			
BMI (kg/m^2)	29.7 (19.5–47.7)	28.9 (26.2–34.1)	.91
Degenerative joint disease	41 (59)	35 (50)	.31
Fibromyalgia	12 (17)	5 (7)	.07
Obstructive sleep apnea	9 (13)	10 (14)	.81
Depression	23 (33)	21 (30)	.72
Anxiety	6 (9)	7 (10)	.77
Disease activity assessment			
Tender joint count	0.5 (0.0–4.0)	1.0 (0.0–5.0)	.98
Swollen joint count	0 (0.0–4.0)	1.0 (0.0–4.0)	.53
HAQ-II disability index, 0–3	0.7 (0.3–1.1)	0.7 (0.0–1.3)	.75
Pain, 100 mm VAS	54 (23–68)	52 (25–70)	.87
Patient global assessment, 0–100	49 (29–60)	50 (30–70)	.25
Provider global assessment, 0–100	15 (0–80)	15 (0–100)	.71
DAS28-CRP	2.8 (2.4–3.5)	3.6 (2.5–4.6)	.33
CDAI	9.8 (5.7–17.7)	11.1 (6.0–17.4)	.69

Table 6 Comparison of clinical characteristics between participants and patients who declined participation in the prospective substudy *(Continued)*

CDAI Categories			.47
Remission	10 (14)	6 (9)	
LDA	28 (40)	26 (37)	
MDA	21 (30)	29 (41)	
HDA	11 (16)	9 (13)	
Laboratory testing			
Rheumatoid factor positivity	36 (53)	52 (76)	**.004**
Anti-CCP positivity	33 (53)	47 (73)	**.02**
ANA positivity	18 (31)	13 (23)	.35
CRP at index visit, mg/L	2.9 (1.6–46.1)	5.3 (2.9–11.0)	**.003**
Abnormal CRP concentration (≥ 8 mg/L)	11 (19)	20 (36)	**.04**
ESR at index visit, mm/h	9 (3–17)	10 (3,–21)	.50
Abnormal ESR (i.e., > 22 male and > 29 female)	6 (11)	11 (20)	.22
Radiographic erosion present	24 (35)	37 (54)	**.03**
Medication			
Prednisone	25 (36)	39 (56)	**.02**
Methotrexate	51 (73)	41 (59)	.08
Nonmethotrexate DMARD	27 (39)	25 (36)	.73
TNF inhibitor	18 (26)	19 (27)	.85
Any biologic	21 (30)	31 (44)	.08
Opioid	16 (23)	18 (26)	.31
Tramadol	7 (10)	12 (17)	.22
Gabapentin	9 (13)	4 (6)	.15
Pregabalin	1 (1)	0 (0)	.31
Duloxetine	2 (3)	2 (3)	> .99
Fibromyalgia medication	12 (17)	6 (9)	.13
NSAID	26 (37)	35 (50)	.13
Sleep aid	11 (16)	7 (10)	.31
Antidepressant or anxiolytic	18 (26)	22 (31)	.45
DMARD modification at index visit?			.10
No	59 (84)	51 (73)	
Yes	11 (16)	19 (27)	

Values are presented as median (interquartile range) or number (percentage) of patients

Significant results are indicated in bold typeface

ANA antinuclear antibodies, *anti-CCP* anticyclic citrullinated peptide, *BMI* body mass index, *CDAI* Clinical Disease Activity Index, *CRP* C-reactive protein, *DAS28-CRP* Disease Activity Score in 28 joints using C-reactive protein, *DMARD* disease-modifying antirheumatic drug, *ESR* erythrocyte sedimentation rate, *GED* general education development, *HAQ-II* Health Assessment Questionnaire II, *HDA* high disease activity, *LDA* low disease activity, *MDA* moderate disease activity, *MHDA* moderate-to-high disease activity, *NP* nurse practitioner, *NSAID* nonsteroidal anti-inflammatory drug, *PA* physician assistant, *TNF* tumor necrosis factor, *VAS* visual analog scale

composite measures, such that removal of the patient global assessment and calculation of the three-variable DAS28 led to shifting of patients from MHDA to LDA categories. The present study demonstrates that patients with positive discordance are less likely to be in remission and more likely to be in the LDA or MDA categories. Together, the findings underscore the difficulty in interpreting composite disease activity scores in the clinical setting of patient-provider discordance, considering the absence of meaningful correlation between discordance and inflammatory measures, as well as the uncertainties with implementation of current treat-to-target recommendations [23, 24].

Pain intensity is a key correlate of patient-provider discordance [1–3, 7, 25], but few studies have addressed specific characteristics or comorbidities related to pain etiologies. Based on the results of the SF-MPQ-2 analyses, continuous and neuropathic pain types are associated with patient-provider discordance in RA. The findings of this study are in agreement with Koop et al. [26], who reported neuropathic pain characteristics in patients with RA using the pain DETECT questionnaire.

Fibromyalgia prevalence ranges from 12% to 20% among RA patients, with an estimated incidence of 5 per 100 patient-years [27–30]. Ranzolin and colleagues [31] have shown that patients with RA and concomitant fibromyalgia have higher pain scores than RA patients without fibromyalgia, yet they have relatively low provider global assessments. Their study did not report patient global assessments. Khan et al. [2] reported in the Quantitative Standard Monitoring of Patients With Rheumatoid Arthritis study that 4.6% of the positive discordance group had investigator-reported fibromyalgia compared with 2.5% in the concordant group, which was statistically significant. The present finding of a 17% prevalence of fibromyalgia diagnosis by the treating physician in the discordant group is considerably higher than in the study by Khan et al. but certainly is consistent with the overall prevalence of fibromyalgia in RA, highlighting the clinical significance of previous data on fibromyalgia to patient-provider discordance. Previous studies have demonstrated that, among RA patients, fibromyalgia is associated with higher DAS28 and adverse scores for functional ability and health-related quality of life (HRQOL) [3, 30, 32, 33]. Data also show that patients with positive discordance may be overtreated with biologic therapies to which they are unlikely to respond [32]. Considering current concepts of centralized pain in patients with fibromyalgia, the data suggest that abnormal central pain processing may be the key driver of chronic widespread pain among patients with RA in the setting of positive patient-provider discordance and may also explain some inadequate responses to DMARD therapy [26, 34, 35].

Depression is also prevalent in RA patients and has been studied extensively in this population [36]. Barton et al. [3] showed that depression is strongly associated with patient-provider discordance. In their study, the frequency of depression as defined by a PHQ-9 score $\geq$ 10 among the population with positive discordance was 43%, which is similar to the frequency of clinical depression of 39% in the present study. Results of the multivariable analysis suggest that pain, fibromyalgia, and depression make complementary contributions to patient-provider discordance. Osteoarthritis and elevated body mass index appear also to make a small contribution to positive discordance, mainly in LDA states.

Indeed, comparison of patient-reported outcomes between the discordant and concordant groups separately in remission or with LDA versus MHDA suggests that depression and fibromyalgia have distinct roles in mediating patient-provider discordance. In LDA states, pain intensity and pain-related interference in activities and role functions, fibromyalgia, and depression are complementary mediators of positive discordance. In MHDA states, fibromyalgia as defined by the WPI and polysymptomatic distress are key determinants of discordance whereas depression has no effect. Interpretation of these findings must consider the differences in the definitions of fibromyalgia between the analyses shown in Table 3 (fibromyalgia WPI) and Table 4 (previous diagnosis of fibromyalgia). The findings suggest that the activity or severity of fibromyalgia is important, meaning that milder or partially treated fibromyalgia may be mediating discordance in LDA states and more active or severe fibromyalgia may be driving discordance in MHDA states. Wolfe [37] coined the term *fibromyalgianess*, noting that the distribution of polysymptomatic distress does not suggest a discrete entity but rather a continuous spectrum of illness. Perhaps the findings of the present study indicate interactions between higher inflammatory activity and abnormal pain processing in the development of complex, disease-related centralized pain and polysymptomatic distress [38, 39].

As suggested by Wolfe et al. [39], consideration should be given to disaggregation of domains within the patient global assessment to develop management pathways targeting optimal patient-centered outcomes. For example, high PHQ-9 scores in the present study identified several patients with undiagnosed depression. The findings suggest that routine measurement of patient-reported outcomes could help identify the central drivers of adverse health status apart from inflammatory disease activity and thereby could suggest potential interventions. Further research is necessary to develop a feasible, time-efficient set of patient-reported outcomes and determine how to integrate them into typical practice settings. In the meantime, rheumatologists may consider implementation of the tools reported in this study. The patient-reported outcome measures used in this study may be obtained at the following websites: for PROMIS, http://www.healthmeasures.net/explore-measurement-systems/

promis; PHQ-9, http://www.phqscreeners.com/select-screener; and for the fibromyalgia WPI and SS score, https://www.rheumatology.org/Practice-Quality/Clinical-Support/Criteria/ACR-Endorsed-Criteria.

Ultrasonography is a more sensitive measure of disease activity than clinical examination [40]. In the present study, although patients in the discordant group commonly had active synovitis, ultrasonography-defined synovitis did not discriminate the groups. Unrecognized disease activity does not appear to be a major factor in discordance. Nonetheless, this tool could be useful in evaluating disease activity and guiding disease-modifying therapy in patients with patient-provider discordance, considering that composite disease activity scores are less reliable in this clinical setting [41].

Limitations

Previous studies have emphasized differences between the patient global assessment of disease activity and the patient general health assessment [4, 42]. The question for the patient global assessment in the present study did not specifically ask about joint tenderness, swelling, or inflammation, but the wording was similar to previous studies [3, 43]. The cross-sectional design prevented assessment of the persistence of discordance over time, as well as causal associations. Future studies are necessary to understand the clinical factors leading to the development of discordance. Morning stiffness is an important symptom of RA but was not assessed in this study. The results show some evidence of selection bias in the prospective substudy, in which patients who chose to participate were somewhat less likely to have positivity for RF and anti-CCP antibodies and erosive disease than nonparticipants. However, participants and nonparticipants were otherwise similar for pain, disability, and clinical disease activity, so it is unlikely that this minor selection bias had a major impact on the patient-reported outcome and ultrasonography results. Speculatively, patients with seronegative RA may perceive greater uncertainty on the part of their providers, leading them to be more interested in participating in a study on patient-provider discordance. Discordance was not fully explained by the model used in this study, and in view of previous findings [43] it is an important limitation that patient education, health literacy, and patient-physician communication were not assessed in this study. Finally, several factors may limit the generalizability of the findings of this study, such as the site at an academic referral center with substantial clinical subspecialization, as well as the racial and ethnic homogeneity of the study population.

Conclusions

The contribution of this study is a comprehensive, patient-level description of the clinical phenotypes that are associated with patient-provider discordance. This study should inform the selection and testing of patient-

reported outcomes for routine evaluation of discordance. The findings should inform the development of a standardized approach to evaluation and management, as well as enhancement of patient-provider communication and shared decision making for RA patients in the scenario of discordance. At this time, it would be prudent for rheumatology care providers to diagnose and treat comorbidities, such as depression and fibromyalgia, using available pharmacologic and nonpharmacologic therapies and to monitor the impact on the health status of patients.

Abbreviations
ACR/EULAR: American College of Rheumatology/European League Against Rheumatism; anti-CCP: Anticyclic citrullinated peptide; CDAI: Clinical Disease Activity Index; CI: Confidence interval; DAS28: Disease Activity Score 28; DAS28-CRP: Disease Activity Score 28 using C-reactive protein; DMARD: Disease-modifying antirheumatic drug; GS: Gray scale; HAQ-II: Health Assessment Questionnaire-II; HDA: High disease activity; HRQOL: Health-related quality of life; LDA: Low disease activity; MDA: Moderate disease activity; MHDA: Moderate-to-high disease activity; OR: Odds ratio; PD: Power Doppler; PHQ-9: Patient Health Questionnaire 9; PROMIS: Patient-Reported Outcomes Measurement Information System; RA: Rheumatoid arthritis; RF: Rheumatoid factor; SF-MPQ-2: Short-Form McGill Pain Questionnaire 2; SS: Symptom Severity; VAS: Visual analog scale; WPI: Widespread Pain Index

Acknowledgements
The authors thank Jennifer Barton, MD, at Oregon Health and Science University in Portland, Oregon, for her thoughtful and constructive critique of the manuscript.

Funding
This study was supported by the Larry and Ruth Eaton Family Career Development Fund in Innovative Rheumatoid Arthritis Research and the CTSA Grant Number UL1 TR000135 from the National Center for Advancing Translational Science (NCATS). Its contents are solely the responsibility of the authors and do not necessarily represent the official views of the National Institutes of Health.

Authors' contributions
JMD and ALC conceived and designed this study, and JMD led the conduct of this study. DNC, ZK, TB, TGM, ELM, CJM, STP, DES, TLWM, KW, and JMD contributed to patient assessment and data collection. TB, KW, and JMD performed the ultrasound examinations. CSC performed the statistical analysis. DNC wrote the first draft of the manuscript, and JMD was a major contributor to writing and revising the manuscript. All authors contributed to data analysis and interpretation and reviewed and approved the final manuscript.

Competing interests
The authors declare that they have no competing interests.

Author details
[1]Division of Rheumatology, Mayo Clinic, 200 First St. SW, Rochester, MN 55905, USA. [2]Department of Physical Medicine and Rehabilitation, Mayo Clinic, 200 First St. SW, Rochester, MN 55905, USA. [3]Division of Biostatistics

and Informatics, Mayo Clinic, 200 First St. SW, Rochester, MN 55905, USA.
[4]Department of Emergency Medicine, Vanderbilt University Medical Center, Nashville, TN, USA.

References

1. Desthieux C, Hermet A, Granger B, Fautrel B, Gossec L. Patient-physician discordance in global assessment in rheumatoid arthritis: a systematic literature review with metaanalysis. Arthritis Care Res (Hoboken). 2016;68: 1767–73.
2. Khan NA, Spencer HJ, Abda E, Aggarwal A, Alten R, Ancuta C, et al. Determinants of discordance in patients' and physicians' rating of rheumatoid arthritis disease activity. Arthritis Care Res (Hoboken). 2012;64:206–14.
3. Barton JL, Imboden J, Graf J, Glidden D, Yelin EH, Schillinger D. Patient-physician discordance in assessments of global disease severity in rheumatoid arthritis. Arthritis Care Res (Hoboken). 2010;62:857–64.
4. Smolen JS, Strand V, Koenig AS, Szumski A, Kotak S, Jones TV. Discordance between patient and physician assessments of global disease activity in rheumatoid arthritis and association with work productivity. Arthritis Res Ther. 2016;18:114.
5. Kaneko Y, Kuwana M, Kondo H, Takeuchi T. Discordance in global assessments between patient and estimator in patients with newly diagnosed rheumatoid arthritis: associations with progressive joint destruction and functional impairment. J Rheumatol. 2014;41:1061–6.
6. Michelsen B, Kristianslund EK, Hammer HB, Fagerli KM, Lie E, Wierod A, et al. Discordance between tender and swollen joint count as well as patient's and evaluator's global assessment may reduce likelihood of remission in patients with rheumatoid arthritis and psoriatic arthritis: data from the prospective multicentre NOR-DMARD study. Ann Rheum Dis. 2016;76:708–11.
7. Studenic P, Radner H, Smolen JS, Aletaha D. Discrepancies between patients and physicians in their perceptions of rheumatoid arthritis disease activity. Arthritis Rheum. 2012;64:2814–23.
8. Aletaha D, Neogi T, Silman AJ, Funovits J, Felson DT, Bingham 3rd CO, et al. 2010 Rheumatoid arthritis classification criteria: an American College of Rheumatology/European League Against Rheumatism collaborative initiative. Arthritis Rheum. 2010;62:2569–81.
9. Prevoo ML, v 't Hof MA, Kuper HH, van Leeuwen MA, van de Putte LB, van Riel PL. Modified disease activity scores that include twenty-eight-joint counts: development and validation in a prospective longitudinal study of patients with rheumatoid arthritis. Arthritis Rheum. 1995;38:44–8.
10. Wells G, Becker JC, Teng J, Dougados M, Schiff M, Smolen J, et al. Validation of the 28-joint Disease Activity Score (DAS28) and European League Against Rheumatism response criteria based on C-reactive protein against disease progression in patients with rheumatoid arthritis, and comparison with the DAS28 based on erythrocyte sedimentation rate. Ann Rheum Dis. 2009;68:954–60.
11. Aletaha D, Smolen JS. The Simplified Disease Activity Index and Clinical Disease Activity Index to monitor patients in standard clinical care. Rheum Dis Clin North Am. 2009;35:759–72.
12. Dworkin RH, Turk DC, Revicki DA, Harding G, Coyne KS, Peirce-Sandner S, et al. Development and initial validation of an expanded and revised version of the Short-form McGill Pain Questionnaire (SF-MPQ-2). Pain. 2009;144:35–42.
13. Wolfe F, Clauw DJ, Fitzcharles MA, Goldenberg DL, Katz RS, Mease P, et al. The American College of Rheumatology preliminary diagnostic criteria for fibromyalgia and measurement of symptom severity. Arthritis Care Res (Hoboken). 2010;62:600–10.
14. Wolfe F, Walitt BT, Rasker JJ, Katz RS, Hauser W. The use of polysymptomatic distress categories in the evaluation of fibromyalgia (FM) and FM severity. J Rheumatol. 2015;42:1494–501.
15. Nicklin J, Cramp F, Kirwan J, Greenwood R, Urban M, Hewlett S. Measuring fatigue in rheumatoid arthritis: a cross-sectional study to evaluate the Bristol Rheumatoid Arthritis Fatigue Multi-Dimensional questionnaire, visual analog scales, and numerical rating scales. Arthritis Care Res (Hoboken). 2010;62:1559–68.
16. Kroenke K, Spitzer RL, Williams JB. The PHQ-9: validity of a brief depression severity measure. J Gen Intern Med. 2001;16:606–13.
17. Spitzer RL, Kroenke K, Williams JB, Lowe B. A brief measure for assessing generalized anxiety disorder: the GAD-7. Arch Intern Med. 2006;166:1092 7.
18. Brown KW, Ryan RM. The benefits of being present: mindfulness and its role in psychological well-being. J Pers Soc Psychol. 2003;84:822–48.
19. Wolfe F, Michaud K, Pincus T. Development and validation of the health assessment questionnaire II: a revised version of the health assessment questionnaire. Arthritis Rheum. 2004;50:3296–305.
20. Backhaus M, Ohrndorf S, Kellner H, Strunk J, Backhaus TM, Hartung W, et al. Evaluation of a novel 7-joint ultrasound score in daily rheumatologic practice: a pilot project. Arthritis Rheum. 2009;61:1194–201.
21. Backhaus TM, Ohrndorf S, Kellner H, Strunk J, Hartung W, Sattler H, et al. The US7 score is sensitive to change in a large cohort of patients with rheumatoid arthritis over 12 months of therapy. Ann Rheum Dis. 2013;72:1163–9.
22. Ohrndorf S, Fischer IU, Kellner H, Strunk J, Hartung W, Reiche B, et al. Reliability of the novel 7-joint ultrasound score: results from an inter- and intraobserver study performed by rheumatologists. Arthritis Care Res (Hoboken). 2012;64:1238–43.
23. Singh JA, Saag KG, Bridges Jr SL, Akl EA, Bannuru RR, Sullivan MC, et al. 2015 American College of Rheumatology guideline for the treatment of rheumatoid arthritis. Arthritis Rheumatol. 2016;68:1–26.
24. Smolen JS, Breedveld FC, Burmester GR, Bykerk V, Dougados M, Emery P, et al. Treating rheumatoid arthritis to target: 2014 update of the recommendations of an international task force. Ann Rheum Dis. 2016;75:3–15.
25. Nicolau G, Yogui MM, Vallochi TL, Gianini RJ, Laurindo IM, Novaes GS. Sources of discrepancy in patient and physician global assessments of rheumatoid arthritis disease activity. J Rheumatol. 2004;31:1293–6.
26. Koop SM, ten Klooster PM, Vonkeman HE, Steunebrink LM, van de Laar MA. Neuropathic-like pain features and cross-sectional associations in rheumatoid arthritis. Arthritis Res Ther. 2015;17:237.
27. Wolfe F, Hauser W, Hassett AL, Katz RS, Walitt BT. The development of fibromyalgia–I: examination of rates and predictors in patients with rheumatoid arthritis (RA). Pain. 2011;152:291–9.
28. Wolfe F, Michaud K. Severe rheumatoid arthritis (RA), worse outcomes, comorbid illness, and sociodemographic disadvantage characterize RA patients with fibromyalgia. J Rheumatol. 2004;31:695–700.
29. Naranjo A, Ojeda S, Francisco F, Erausquin C, Rua-Figueroa I, Rodriguez-Lozano C. Fibromyalgia in patients with rheumatoid arthritis is associated with higher scores of disability. Ann Rheum Dis. 2002;61:660–1.
30. Pollard LC, Kingsley GH, Choy EH, Scott DL. Fibromyalgic rheumatoid arthritis and disease assessment. Rheumatology (Oxford). 2010;49:924–8.
31. Ranzolin A, Brenol JC, Bredemeier M, Guarienti J, Rizzatti M, Feldman D, et al. Association of concomitant fibromyalgia with worse disease activity score in 28 joints, health assessment questionnaire, and short form 36 scores in patients with rheumatoid arthritis. Arthritis Rheum. 2009;61:794–800.
32. Lage-Hansen PR, Chrysidis S, Lage-Hansen M, Hougaard A, Ejstrup L, Amris K. Concomitant fibromyalgia in rheumatoid arthritis is associated with the more frequent use of biological therapy: a cross-sectional study. Scand J Rheumatol. 2015:1–4. [Epub ahead of print].
33. Leeb BF, Andel I, Sautner J, Nothnagl T, Rintelen B. The DAS28 in rheumatoid arthritis and fibromyalgia patients. Rheumatology (Oxford). 2004;43:1504–7.
34. Joharatnam N, McWilliams DF, Wilson D, Wheeler M, Pande I, Walsh DA. A cross-sectional study of pain sensitivity, disease-activity assessment, mental health, and fibromyalgia status in rheumatoid arthritis. Arthritis Res Ther. 2015;17:11.
35. Lee YC, Chibnik LB, Lu B, Wasan AD, Edwards RR, Fossel AH, et al. The relationship between disease activity, sleep, psychiatric distress and pain sensitivity in rheumatoid arthritis: a cross-sectional study. Arthritis Res Ther. 2009;11:R160.
36. Matchaba F, Rayner L, Steer S, Hotopf M. The prevalence of depression in rheumatoid arthritis: a systematic review and meta-analysis. Rheumatology (Oxford). 2013;52:2136–48.
37. Wolfe F. Fibromyalgianess. Arthritis Rheum. 2009;61:715–6.
38. Wolfe F, Walitt BT, Katz RS, Hauser W. Symptoms, the nature of fibromyalgia, and diagnostic and statistical manual 5 (DSM-5) defined mental illness in patients with rheumatoid arthritis and fibromyalgia. PLoS One. 2014;9:e88740.
39. Wolfe F, Michaud K, Busch RE, Katz RS, Rasker JJ, Shahouri SH, et al. Polysymptomatic distress in patients with rheumatoid arthritis: understanding disproportionate response and its spectrum. Arthritis Care Res (Hoboken). 2014;66:1465–71.

40. Ohrndorf S, Backhaus M. Musculoskeletal ultrasonography in patients with rheumatoid arthritis. Nat Rev Rheumatol. 2013;9:433–7.
41. Sokka T, Pincus T. Joint counts to assess rheumatoid arthritis for clinical research and usual clinical care: advantages and limitations. Rheum Dis Clin North Am. 2009;35:713–22.
42. Khan NA, Spencer HJ, Abda EA, Alten R, Pohl C, Ancuta C, et al. Patient's global assessment of disease activity and patient's assessment of general health for rheumatoid arthritis activity assessment: are they equivalent? Ann Rheum Dis. 2012;71:1942–9.
43. Hirsh JM, Boyle DJ, Collier DH, Oxenfeld AJ, Caplan L. Health literacy predicts the discrepancy between patient and provider global assessments of rheumatoid arthritis activity at a public urban rheumatology clinic. J Rheumatol. 2010;37:961–6.

5

Ultrasound of the hand is sufficient to detect subclinical inflammation in rheumatoid arthritis remission: a post hoc longitudinal study

Hilde Berner Hammer[1][*], Tore K. Kvien[1] and Lene Terslev[2]

Abstract

Background: Ultrasound (US) is a sensitive method for detecting joint/tendon inflammation in patients with rheumatoid arthritis (RA). Subclinical inflammation is often found in patients with RA in composite score remission. The purpose of the present study was to explore whether US of only the hands is sufficient to identify subclinical inflammation in patients with established RA in clinical remission.

Methods: A total of 209 patients with established RA (81% women, mean [SD] age 53.3 (13.2) years, disease duration 10.0 [8.8] years) were examined when initiating biologic disease-modifying anti-rheumatic drugs (bDMARDs) and after 6 months (184 patients) and 12 months (152 patients) of follow-up. They were assessed by US (greyscale [GS] and power Doppler [PD] of 36 joints and 4 tendons, scored 0–3) as well as clinical and laboratory examinations, and different disease activity composite scores were calculated. The presence of US synovitis (GS score ≥ 2, PD score ≥ 1 [PD1] and score ≥ 2 [PD2]) in composite score remission was explored.

Results: Remission at 6 and 12 months was achieved in 74 and 59 patients, respectively, for Disease Activity Score based on 28 joints (DAS28); in 37 and 38 patients, respectively, for Clinical Disease Activity Index; in 42 and 42 patients, respectively, for Simplified Disease Activity Index; and in 38 and 35 patients, respectively, for Boolean remission. The percentages of patients in DAS28 remission at 6 months with synovitis in hands/other regions were 73.0%/64.9% for GS, 64.9%/41.9% for PD1 and 32.4%/20.3% for PD2; at 12 months, the corresponding percentages were 61.0%/64.4% for GS, 62.7%/39.0% for PD1 and 44.1%/15.3% for PD2, respectively. PD activity was more often present in the hands ($p < 0.001$). In patients in various composite scores of remission, US only of the hands identified ≥ 90% of the patients having PD activity in any of the assessed joints/tendons.

Conclusions: A high percentage of patients had US synovitis despite being in clinical remission. US examination performed only of the hands captured ≥ 90% of patients with subclinical inflammation and could be feasible for assessing bDMARD-treated patients with RA in remission.

Keywords: Rheumatoid arthritis, Ultrasound, Inflammation, Synovium, Hand, Biologic therapies

* Correspondence: hbham@online.no
[1]Department of Rheumatology, Diakonhjemmet Hospital, Box 23 Vinderen, 0319 Oslo, Norway
Full list of author information is available at the end of the article

Background

With the treat-to-target strategy (T2T), the updated treatment recommendations for rheumatoid arthritis (RA) in 2016 are aimed at remission within 3–6 months, though low disease activity may be an acceptable target in patients with RA with long-standing disease [1]. The current treatment strategy for patients with RA includes tight control with monotherapy or combination therapy using disease-modifying anti-rheumatic drugs (DMARDs). The aim of this strategy is to obtain rapid disease control, thereby preventing pain and joint destruction. Several clinical definitions of remission are proposed, mainly using composite scores where Boolean remission is the strictest [2–5].

Ultrasound (US) has been used as an instrument for monitoring disease activity in RA, where a synovial hypertrophy score ≥ 2 by greyscale (GS) and a power Doppler (PD) score ≥ 1 may be a sign of inflammatory activity. Recent studies have indicated that the presence of Doppler activity with a score of 1 may be seen in normal joints, suggesting a higher PD cut-off of ≥ 2 as a sign of pathology, though a certain cut-off between normality and pathology still needs to be determined [6–9].

Several reduced US joint sets have been proposed for optimising clinical utility, ranging from US assessment of 6- to 12-joint counts either unilaterally or bilaterally, all including hands and feet with or without tendon assessment [10–12]. The reduced scores have all been developed to retain as much information as possible from the more elaborate joint counts that may include up to 78 joints [10–12].

Though recent studies have shown that the added value of US assessments in a T2T strategy may be limited in very early RA if tight clinical control is applied [13, 14], several studies have shown that Doppler activity in patients in composite score remission predicts flare and radiographic progression, both at the patient and at the joint level [15–17]. It has also been found that, despite composite score remission, US joint inflammation is still frequent [18]. Hence, the most optimal situation is when patients are both in composite score and PD score remission, because this is found to cause a very low degree of radiographic progression [13].

A comprehensive US assessment is time-consuming, and clinical as well as US experience has shown that the hands are frequently involved in patients with established RA. Some of the proposed reduced joint sets have included tendons [12, 19], and the presence of tenosynovitis has been suggested to be related to flare in patients with RA in remission [20] and may thus be important in US assessments [21, 22].

The objective of the present study was to explore, in a post hoc analysis, the presence of GS and PD pathology in a high number of joints/tendons and to assess the frequency of US pathology in hands compared with other joints/tendons in patients with established RA in remission according to different composite scores. An additional objective was to explore whether PD assessment of the hands only is sensitive enough to detect subclinical inflammatory activity in patients with RA in composite score remission.

Methods

The present cohort has previously been explored for the development of a reduced score set of joints and tendons for RA monitoring [12, 19]. Patients with RA fulfilling the American College of Rheumatology (ACR) 1987 criteria [23] were included in the study when initiating or changing biologic disease-modifying anti-rheumatic drug (bDMARD) treatment in the period from January 2010 to June 2013 (Australian New Zealand Clinical Trials Registry, ACTRN12610000284066).

Clinical examinations

The patients were assessed at baseline and after 6 and 12 months by two trained study nurses with long experience in evaluation of tender and swollen joints, and the study nurses were blinded to the US findings. Patient and assessor global visual analogue scale (VAS) scores, as well as laboratory examinations (erythrocyte sedimentation rate [ESR] and C-reactive protein [CRP]), were assessed. The Disease Activity Score based on 28 joint counts with erythrocyte sedimentation rate (DAS28[ESR]) [2], Clinical Disease Activity Index (CDAI) [3] and Simplified Disease Activity Index (SDAI) [4] scores were calculated.

US examinations

US examinations (blinded for the results of the clinical assessments) were performed as described previously [19]. In short, the same experienced sonographer (HBH) performed the US assessments throughout the study using a Siemens Antares Excellence version (Siemens Medical Solutions, Malvern, PA, USA) equipped with a 5- to 13-MHz linear probe, with 11.4 MHz used for GS assessments. PD settings were optimised for inflammatory flow with pulse repetition frequency 391 Hz, Doppler frequency 7.3 MHz and gain just below the level of noise [24]. The same US machine with the same settings for all joints and tendons was used throughout the study, with no software upgrades. US was performed on 36 joints and 4 tendons for signs of synovitis and tenosynovitis, including bilateral evaluation of the hands (metacarpophalangeal [MCP] joint 1–5 and proximal interphalangeal [PIP] joints 2 and 3, wrist [scoring radio-carpal, mid-carpal and radio-ulnar joints separately] and the extensor carpi ulnaris [ECU] tendon) as well as of other regions (elbow, knee, talocrural and metatarsophalangeal [MTP] joints 1–5, and the tibialis posterior [TP] tendon). Each joint/tendon was scored semi-quantitatively on a 0–3 scale for GS and PD as described previously [12, 19] and according to the US atlas by Hammer et al. [25] using the Outcome Measures in Rheumatology definitions for synovitis and tenosynovitis [26, 27]. The sonographer in the present study (HBH) had previously demonstrated a high intra-observer reliability for scoring of joints and tendons [19, 25].

GS synovial hypertrophy score ≥ 2 was defined as pathology, and for PD activity, two scores were explored: PD ≥ 1 and PD ≥ 2. The study was approved by the Regional Committee for Medical and Health Research Ethics South East (REK), and the patients gave written consent according to the Declaration of Helsinki (REK number 2009/1254).

Statistics

Patients with at least one joint/tendon with GS score ≥ 2 or PD scores ≥ 1 or ≥ 2 in individual joints/tendons or groups of joints/tendons at baseline and at 6 and 12 months were identified. To explore the value of examining PD only of the hands (i.e., wrist, MCP joints 1–5, PIP joints 2–3, ECU tendon bilaterally), patients were identified with PD pathology detected in at least one joint/tendon in the hands and/or in at least one joint/tendon in the other sites. The percentages of patients with PD scores ≥ 1 or ≥ 2 in the hands and/or other sites were calculated for the whole cohort as well as for those in composite score remission. Remission criteria were used for DAS28 (<2.6), CDAI (≤2.8), SDAI (≤3.3) and ACR/European League Against Rheumatism Boolean remission (patient's global VAS 0–10, tender and swollen joint counts and CRP [mg/dl] all ≤ 1) [2–5]. The Mann-Whitney U test was used to explore differences in frequencies of joint/tendon involvement. Missing data during follow-up (<5% missing values) were handled by use of the last observation carried forward. All tests for significance were two-sided, and $p < 0.05$ was considered significant.

Results

Patient characteristics and treatment

A total of 209 patients (81% women, mean [SD] age 53.3 [13.2] years, disease duration 10.0 [8.8] years, 79.2% anti-cyclic citrullinated peptide-positive and 68.6% positive for rheumatoid factor) were included [19]; 184 (87.1%) completed 6 months of follow-up; and 152 (72.7%) completed 12 months of follow-up. At baseline, the mean (SD) values of the composite scores were DAS28 4.55 (1.45), SDAI 21.2 (12.5) and CDAI 20.0 (11.8), whereas the sum US scores were 30.0 (18.9) for GS and 14.2 (13.6) for PD.

The patients initiated (and continued throughout the study) treatment with one of the following as their first (44.6%), second (30.1%), third (17.1%) or fourth to seventh (8.3%) bDMARD: etanercept (34.9%), rituximab (20.6%), certolizumab (11.0%), infliximab (10.0%), tocilizumab (8.6%), adalimumab (6.7%), golimumab (5.3%) and abatacept (2.9%). In addition, 83.6% were on synthetic DMARDs (90.6% of them used methotrexate), and 55% were on prednisolone with a mean (SD) dose of 8.0 (5.3) mg.

Presence of US pathology in the whole cohort

Most of the US pathologies in the cohort were found in the joints of the hands and in MTP joints at both follow-up visits. Table 1 shows the percentages of patients with GS scores ≥ 2 as well as PD scores ≥ 1 or ≥ 2 in different joints and in groups of joints and tendons at baseline and at 6 and 12 months. The tendons were involved less frequently than the small joints but more often than the large joints. At baseline, there were significantly more patients with PD activity in at least one joint/tendon in the hands than in all the other joints/tendons ($p < 0.001$). Focussing only on the hands, we observed significantly more patients with PD activity in MCP joints and wrist joints than in the ECU tendon ($p < 0.001$), but we found no statistically significant difference between the presence of PD in MCP and wrist joints at any of the follow-up assessments.

In the total cohort, GS scores ≥ 2 only in joints other than the hands were found in 9.9% of the patients at 6 months and in 12.6% at 12 months. At the joint level, GS scores ≥ 2 only in joints other than the hands were explained by MTP joint involvement in 15 of 18 patients at 6 months and in 19 of 20 patients at 12 months.

Table 2 illustrates the percentages of patients in the cohort at 6 and 12 months having PD activity in at least on joint/tendon only in the hands versus PD in at least one joint/tendon in any of the other areas, showing that not more than 4-9% of the patients were missed having PD pathology when only assessing the hands.

Presence of US pathology in patients in remission with different composite scores

At 6 and 12 months, respectively, remission was found for DAS28 in 74 (40.7%)/59 (38.8%) patients, for CDAI in 37 (20.3%)/38 (25.0%) patients, for SDAI in 42 (23.1%)/42 (27.6%) patients and for Boolean in 38 (20.9%)/35 (23.0%) patients. Table 3 shows the percentages of patients in remission (based on composite scores) still having US pathology. Independent of type of composite score applied in the cohort, GS and PD pathology was present in a high proportion of patients.

Of patients in remission based on composite score, ≥ 90.5% had PD activity (≥1 or ≥ 2) detected by assessing only the hands bilaterally (wrist [radio-carpal, midcarpal, radio-ulnar joints], MCP joints 1–5, PIP joints 2–3 and ECU tendon) at 6- and 12-month follow-up (Table 4).

Table 1 Patients with greyscale or power Doppler pathology in different joint/tendon regions at baseline and after 6 and 12 months

	Baseline (n = 209)			6 months (n = 184)			12 months (n = 152)		
	GS ≥ 2	PD ≥ 1	PD ≥ 2	GS ≥ 2	PD ≥ 1	PD ≥ 2	GS ≥ 2	PD ≥ 1	PD ≥ 2
Wrists (RC, MC, RU)	62.0	69.8	37.6	45.8	56.5	26.0	43.9	53.5	18.1
ECU	29.8	31.3	20.2	16.5	20.9	11.5	16.4	15.1	10.7
MCP 1–5	67.9	65.1	54.5	63.2	48.4	29.1	49.7	45.9	31.4
PIP 2–3	46.6	32.4	26.5	29.7	18.1	13.7	31.4	17.6	11.9
Elbow	20.2	19.7	12.0	15.5	11.0	3.9	13.8	9.4	5.0
Knee	18.1	9.8	2.9	6.2	1.7	1.1	5.1	3.2	0.0
Ankle	10.5	3.8	1.0	6.0	0.5	0.0	3.8	1.9	0.0
TP	27.4	32.2	21.2	18.7	20.9	13.2	10.1	11.9	5.7
MTP 1–5	78.5	56.5	38.0	65.1	37.8	16.4	61.7	28.9	12.1

Abbreviations: RC Radio-carpal joint, *MC* Mid-carpal joint, *RU* Radio-ulnar joint, *ECU* Extensor carpi ulnaris tendon, *MCP* Metacarpophalangeal joint, *PIP* Proximal interphalangeal joint, *TP* Tibialis posterior tendon, *MTP* Metatarsophalangeal joint

Discussion

To improve the implementation of US as a clinical tool for evaluating inflammation, several reduced joint counts have been proposed to increase feasibility. They all include as a minimum the hands and feet [10–12]. The results of the present study support these findings because both regions appeared to be the most frequently inflamed joint regions, despite clinical remission. However, as reflected in the DAS28 assessment of clinical disease activity, the inclusion of the feet may prove difficult in a busy clinic. The objective of the present study was therefore to explore whether US examination of only the hands could be sufficient for detecting representative subclinical signs of inflammatory activity at the patient level. We found that > 90% of the patients with subclinical inflammation were identified by the presence of PD activity in the hands.

It has previously been established that US is more sensitive than clinical examination for the detection of subclinical disease, both at the time of diagnosis and in states of remission [28, 29]. The present study supports the existing literature by showing that, in patients fulfilling different clinical remission criteria, independent of the type of composite score applied, a high percentage still have US pathology at both 6 and 12 months [15, 18, 28]. Establishing subclinical inflammation has been shown to be important because US-detected inflammation (especially Doppler activity) in patients with RA during remission predicted erosive progression over time and was the best predictor of flare [15–17]. In addition, it has been demonstrated that the presence of Doppler activity is the best predictor for unsuccessful tapering of biologic treatment [30]. The importance of maintaining remission and avoiding flare is underlined by the increased likelihood of radiographic progression seen in patients with short-term remission compared with those achieving long-term remission. Furthermore, flare has also been shown to be associated with increased functional disability, pain and morning stiffness over time [31, 32].

In the present study, we chose a GS score ≥ 2 to define synovial hypertrophy. This cut-off was chosen because a GS score of 1 has been found to be a frequent finding in healthy persons [9, 33, 34] and appears less responsive to treatment in patients with RA [33]. In our cohort, US examination of only the hands captured the majority of patient with a GS score ≥ 2, and most of the pathology not detected was found in the MTP joints. Because the clinical experience is that GS score ≥ 2 is a frequent finding in MTP joints during follow-up of patients with RA, and because this degree of GS pathology also was found in MTP joints in healthy persons [9], the present study

Table 2 Percentages of patients with PD activity at 6 and 12 months

	6 Months (n = 184)	12 Months (n = 152)
No joints with PD ≥ 1/≥ 2	16.5/44.0	21.4/50.9
PD ≥ 1/≥ 2 in hands as well as in other regions	40.1/18.7	37.1/14.5
PD ≥ 1/≥ 2 in hands but not in other regions	36.8/28.6	37.7/29.6
No PD ≥ 1/≥ 2 in hands but PD ≥ 1/≥ 2 in other regions	6.6/8.8	3.8/5.0

Abbreviations: PD ≥ 1/≥ 2 Power Doppler score ≥ 1/≥ 2 in the wrist (radio-carpal, mid-carpal and radio-ulnar joints), *ECU* Extensor carpi ulnaris tendon, *MCP* Metacarpophalangeal joint, *PIP* Proximal interphalangeal joint, *MTP* Metatarsophalangeal joint, *TP* Tibialis posterior tendon, *n* Number of patients
PD activity is based on scores ≥ 1 or ≥ 2 detected in at least one joint/tendon in the hands (wrist, MCP joints 1–5, PIP joints 2–3, ECU tendon bilaterally) versus other regions (elbow, knee, ankle, MTP joints 1–5, TP bilaterally)

Table 3 Patients in remission based on composite scores at 6- and 12-month follow-up

Remission	Hands (%)			Other regions (%)		
	GS ≥ 2	PD ≥ 1	PD ≥ 2	GS ≥ 2	PD ≥ 1	PD ≥ 2
6 months						
DAS28 (n = 74)	73.0	64.9	32.4	64.9	41.9	20.3
CDAI (n = 37)	62.2	62.2	27.0	62.2	35.1	16.2
SDAI (n = 42)	61.9	64.3	26.2	66.7	35.7	19.0
Boolean (n = 38)	68.4	63.2	26.3	71.1	31.6	13.2
12 months						
DAS28 (n = 59)	61.0	62.7	28.8	64.4	39.0	15.3
CDAI (n = 38)	47.4	57.9	15.8	50.0	34.2	13.2
SDAI (n = 42)	50.0	59.5	16.7	52.4	31.0	11.9
Boolean (n = 35)	42.9	54.3	17.1	54.3	31.4	14.3

Abbreviations: GS ≥ 2 Greyscale score ≥ 2, *PD ≥ 1* Power Doppler score ≥ 1, *PD ≥ 2* Power Doppler score ≥ 2, *DAS28* Disease Activity Score based on 28 joints), *CDAI* Clinical Disease Activity Index, *SDAI* Simplified Disease Activity Index
Data represent percentages of patients still having ultrasound pathology in at least one joint/tendon in the hands (wrist [radio-carpal, mid-carpal, radio-ulnar], metacarpophalangeal joints 1–5, proximal interphalangeal joints 2–3, extensor carpi ulnaris tendon bilaterally) versus other regions (elbow, knee, ankle, metatarsophalangeal joints 1–5, tibialis posterior tendon bilaterally)

was not focused on the GS pathology in patients in clinical remission.

Two different cut-offs for PD activity were explored in the present study (PD ≥ 1 and PD ≥ 2) because both cut-offs have been shown to predict relapse or erosive progression [15, 30, 35]. However, we found the percentage of patients with the two cut-offs to be almost similar for the identification of patients with subclinical inflammation at both 6 and 12 months.

There is no consensus on the inclusion of tendons in US assessments of patients with RA. However, the ECU tendon was included in reduced joint scores [12], and in the present study this tendon was found to have PD activity more frequently than the large joints during follow-up. This supports a previous study where PD tenosynovitis in the hands was associated with shorter remission duration [20].

The present study was focussed on how to make US more feasible in daily clinical practise for detecting inflammation in patients in composite score remission. This topic was previously explored by Naredo et al. [36], who found GS and PD pathology in a high percentage of patients in remission by examining 44 joints, and they suggested assessing wrist, MCP, ankle and MTP joints to detect subclinical inflammation. In a recent study [37], 38 joints were assessed for subclinical inflammation, and PD ≥ 2 was found in at least one joint in 60% of patients in clinical remission. By reducing assessment to six joints (bilateral wrists and MCP joints 2–3), the researchers identified 75% of the patients with PD ≥ 2 [37], thus supporting our present findings based on assessing only the hands to explore subclinical inflammation. The six joints were explored post hoc in our present cohort, and PD ≥ 1 was found in 89% of all patients at 6 and 12 months, and PD ≥ 2 was found in 77% at 6 months and in 71% at 12 months. Among patients in remission (depending on the different composite scores), PD ≥ 1 was found in 55–60%/40–53% and PD ≥ 2 was found in 18–23%/5–17% at 6/12 months, respectively, which were lower than found by use of the present, more extended hand examination (Table 3).

In a previous study exploring patients with RA in clinical remission for the presence of US inflammation in the MCP joints, more than half of the joints had GS synovitis, and almost one-third had PD activity [38]. An important additional result was the presence of PD activity in half of the joints with US-detected erosion, supporting the association between US bone erosion and the persistence of subclinical inflammation. This finding strengthens our suggestion of performing US examination of the finger joints in patients with RA in clinical remission. However, researchers in future studies should continue to explore the optimal joints for a feasible US assessment to detect subclinical inflammation.

The limitations of the present study are the inclusion of only patients with established RA, as well as only patients initiating bDMARDs. Thus, whether the results

Table 4 Patients in composite score remission at 6 and 12 months with power Doppler activity in at least 1 joint/tendon of 36 joints/4 tendons

Remission	6 months			12 months		
	No. of patients	PD ≥ 1 (%)	PD ≥ 2 (%)	No. of patients	PD ≥ 1 (%)	PD ≥ 2 (%)
DAS28	74	91.9	91.9	59	94.9	96.6
CDAI	37	94.6	91.9	38	97.4	94.7
SDAI	42	92.9	90.5	42	97.6	95.2
Boolean	38	94.7	94.7	35	97.1	94.3

Abbreviations: DAS28 Disease Activity Score based on 28 joints with erythrocyte sedimentation rate, *SDAI* Simplified Disease Activity Index, *CDAI* Clinical Disease Activity Index, *PD* Power Doppler
Percentage of patients where ultrasound assessments performed only of the hands (wrist (radiocarpal, midcarpal, radioulnar), metacarpophalangeal 1-5, proximal interphalangeal 2-3, extensor carpi ulnaris tendon bilaterally) would capture PD activity (≥1 or ≥ 2)

are also representative of patients with recent-onset RA and receiving synthetic DMARD treatment should be explored in further studies. In addition, this was a single-centre study, which may limit the generalisability of the US findings. However, a standard US scoring system was used, and the experienced sonographer had shown high reliability for US scoring [25].

Conclusions

The present study shows that, in patients with established RA on bDMARD treatment and in composite score clinical remission, US examination of only the hands is sufficient to detect > 90% of patients with subclinical inflammation. This suggests that US of the hands is a relevant clinical tool for this patient group during follow-up.

Abbreviations

ACR: American College of Rheumatology; bDMARD: Biologic disease-modifying anti-rheumatic drug; CDAI: Clinical Disease Activity Index; CRP: C-reactive protein; DAS28(ESR): Disease Activity Score based on 28 joints with erythrocyte sedimentation rate; DMARD: Disease-modifying anti-rheumatic drug; ECU: Extensor carpi ulnaris; ESR: Erythrocyte sedimentation rate; GS: Greyscale; MC: Mid-carpal joint; MCP: Metacarpophalangeal; MTP: Metatarsophalangeal; PD: Power Doppler; PIP: Proximal interphalangeal; RA: Rheumatoid arthritis; RC: Radio-carpal; RU: Radio-ulnar; SDAI: Simplified Disease Activity Index; T2T: Treat-to-target strategy; TP: Tibialis posterior; US: Ultrasound; VAS: Visual analogue scale

Acknowledgements

Anne Katrine Kongtorp and Britt Birketvedt, study nurses, performed important assessments, including the clinical examinations in the study.

Funding

This work was supported by AbbVie in the form of study grants to the Department of Rheumatology, Diakonhjemmet Hospital, Oslo, Norway (to HBH). LT is supported by the Danish Rheumatism Association.

Authors' contributions

HBH made substantial contributions to study conception and design, acquisition of data, and analysis and interpretation of data; was involved in drafting the manuscript and revising it critically for important intellectual content; and gave final approval of the version to be published. TKK and LT made substantial contributions to analysis and interpretation of data, were involved in drafting the manuscript and revising it critically for important intellectual content, and gave final approval of the version to be published. All authors participated sufficiently in the work to take public responsibility for appropriate portions of the content and agreed to be accountable for all aspects of the work in ensuring that questions related to the accuracy or integrity of any part of the work are appropriately investigated and resolved. All authors read and approved the final manuscript.

Competing interests

HBH has received fees for speaking and/or consulting from AbbVie, Pfizer, UCB, Roche, MSD, Bristol-Myers Squibb and Novartis. TKK has received fees for speaking and/or consulting from AbbVie, Bristol-Myers Squibb, Boehringer Ingelheim, Celgene, Celltrion, Eli Lilly, Hospira, Merck-Serono, MSD, Novartis, Orion Pharma, Pfizer, Roche, Sandoz and UCB and has received research funding via Diakonhjemmet Hospital from AbbVie, Bristol-Myers Squibb, MSD, Pfizer, Roche and UCB. LT has received speaker's fees from AbbVie, Bristol-Myers Squibb, Pfizer, UCB, Roche, Janssen, Novartis and MSD.

Author details

[1]Department of Rheumatology, Diakonhjemmet Hospital, Box 23 Vinderen, 0319 Oslo, Norway. [2]Centre for Rheumatology and Spinal Diseases, Copenhagen University Hospital Rigshospitalet, Copenhagen, Denmark.

References

1. Smolen JS, Breedveld FC, Burmester GR, Bykerk V, Dougados M, Emery P, et al. Treating rheumatoid arthritis to target: 2014 update of the recommendations of an international task force. Ann Rheum Dis. 2016;75:3–15.
2. Prevoo ML, Hof MA v 't, Kuper HH, van Leeuwen MA, van de Putte LB, Van Riel PL. Modified disease activity scores that include twenty-eight-joint counts: development and validation in a prospective longitudinal study of patients with rheumatoid arthritis. Arthritis Rheum. 1995;38:44–8.
3. Aletaha D, Nell VP, Stamm T, Uffmann M, Pflugbeil S, Machold K, et al. Acute phase reactants add little to composite disease activity indices for rheumatoid arthritis: validation of a clinical activity score. Arthritis Res Ther. 2005;7:R796–806.
4. Smolen JS, Breedveld FC, Schiff MH, Kalden JR, Emery P, Eberl G. A simplified disease activity index for rheumatoid arthritis for use in clinical practice. Rheumatology (Oxford). 2003;42:244–57.
5. Felson DT, Smolen JS, Wells G, Zhang B, van Tuyl LH, Funovits J, et al. American College of Rheumatology/European League against Rheumatism provisional definition of remission in rheumatoid arthritis for clinical trials. Ann Rheum Dis. 2011;70:404–13.
6. Millot F, Clavel G, Etchepare F, Gandjbakhch F, Grados F, Saraux A, et al. Musculoskeletal ultrasonography in healthy subjects and ultrasound criteria for early arthritis (the ESPOIR cohort). J Rheumatol. 2011;38:613–20.
7. Terslev L, Torp-Pedersen S, Qvistgaard E, von der Recke P, Bliddal H. Doppler ultrasound findings in healthy wrists and finger joints. Ann Rheum Dis. 2004;63:644–8.
8. Kitchen J, Kane D. Greyscale and power Doppler ultrasonographic evaluation of normal synovial joints: correlation with pro- and anti-inflammatory cytokines and angiogenic factors. Rheumatology. 2015;54:458–62.
9. Padovano I, Costantino F, Breban M, D'Agostino MA. Prevalence of ultrasound synovial inflammatory findings in healthy subjects. Ann Rheum Dis. 2016;75:1819–23.
10. Hammer HB, Kvien TK. Comparisons of 7- to 78-joint ultrasonography scores: all different joint combinations show equal response to adalimumab treatment in patients with rheumatoid arthritis. Arthritis Res Ther. 2011;13:R78.
11. Perricone C, Ceccarelli F, Modesti M, Vavala C, Di Franco M, Valesini G, et al. The 6-joint ultrasonographic assessment: a valid, sensitive-to-change and feasible method for evaluating joint inflammation in RA. Rheumatology (Oxford). 2012;51:866–73.
12. Aga AB, Hammer HB, Olsen IC, Uhlig T, Kvien TK, van der Heijde D, et al. First step in the development of an ultrasound joint inflammation score for rheumatoid arthritis using a data-driven approach. Ann Rheum Dis. 2016;75: 1444–51.
13. Haavardsholm EA, Aga AB, Olsen IC, Lillegraven S, Hammer HB, Uhlig T, et al. Ultrasound in management of rheumatoid arthritis: ARCTIC randomised controlled strategy trial. BMJ. 2016;354:i4205.
14. Dale J, Stirling A, Zhang R, Purves D, Foley J, Sambrook M, et al. Targeting ultrasound remission in early rheumatoid arthritis: the results of the TaSER study, a randomised clinical trial. Ann Rheum Dis. 2016;75:1043–50.
15. Brown AK, Conaghan PG, Karim Z, Quinn MA, Ikeda K, Peterfy CG, et al. An explanation for the apparent dissociation between clinical remission and continued structural deterioration in rheumatoid arthritis. Arthritis Rheum. 2008;58:2958–67.
16. Scirè CA, Montecucco C, Codullo V, Epis O, Todoerti M, Caporali R. Ultrasonographic evaluation of joint involvement in early rheumatoid arthritis in clinical remission: power Doppler signal predicts short-term relapse. Rheumatology (Oxford). 2009;48:1092–7.
17. Saleem B, Brown AK, Quinn M, Karim Z, Hensor EM, Conaghan P, et al. Can flare be predicted in DMARD treated RA patients in remission, and is it important? A cohort study. Ann Rheum Dis. 2012;71:1316–21.
18. Saleem B, Brown AK, Keen H, Nizam S, Freeston J, Wakefield R, et al. Should imaging be a component of rheumatoid arthritis remission criteria? A comparison between traditional and modified composite remission scores and imaging assessments. Ann Rheum Dis. 2011;70:792–8.
19. Hammer HB, Kvien TK, Terslev L. Tenosynovitis in rheumatoid arthritis patients on biologic treatment: involvement and sensitivity to change compared to joint inflammation. Clin Exp Rheum. 2017 May 15. [Epub ahead of print]. PMID: 28516887

20. Bellis E, Scirè CA, Carrara G, Adinolfi A, Batticciotto A, Bortoluzzi A, et al. Ultrasound-detected tenosynovitis independently associates with patient-reported flare in patients with rheumatoid arthritis in clinical remission: results from the observational study STARTER of the Italian Society for Rheumatology. Rheumatology (Oxford). 2016;55:1826–36.

21. Hammer HB, Kvien TK. Ultrasonography shows significant improvement in wrist and ankle tenosynovitis in rheumatoid arthritis patients treated with adalimumab. Scand J Rheumatol. 2011;40:178–82.

22. Ammitzbøll-Danielsen M, Østergaard M, Naredo E, Terslev L. Validity and sensitivity to change of the semi-quantitative OMERACT ultrasound scoring system for tenosynovitis in patients with rheumatoid arthritis. Rheumatology. 2016;55:2156–66.

23. Arnett FC, Edworthy SM, Bloch DA, McShane DJ, Fries JF, Cooper NS, et al. The American Rheumatism Association 1987 revised criteria for the classification of rheumatoid arthritis. Arthritis Rheum. 1988;31:315–24.

24. Torp-Pedersen ST, Terslev L. Settings and artefacts relevant in colour/power Doppler ultrasound in rheumatology. Ann Rheum Dis. 2008;67:143–9.

25. Hammer HB, Bolton-King P, Bakkeheim V, Berg TH, Sundt E, Kongtorp AK, et al. Examination of intra and interrater reliability with a new ultrasonographic reference atlas for scoring of synovitis in patients with rheumatoid arthritis. Ann Rheum Dis. 2011;70:1995–8.

26. Wakefield RJ, Balint PV, Szkudlarek M, Filippucci E, Backhaus M, D'Agostino MA, et al. Musculoskeletal ultrasound including definitions for ultrasonographic pathology. J Rheumatol. 2005;32:2485–7.

27. Naredo E, D'Agostino MA, Wakefield RJ, Möller I, Balint PV, Filippucci E, et al. Reliability of a consensus-based ultrasound score for tenosynovitis in rheumatoid arthritis. Ann Rheum Dis. 2013;72:1328–34.

28. Brown AK, Quinn MA, Karim Z, Conaghan PG, Peterfy CG, Hensor E, et al. Presence of significant synovitis in rheumatoid arthritis patients with disease-modifying antirheumatic drug-induced clinical remission: evidence from an imaging study may explain structural progression. Arthritis Rheum. 2006;54:3761–73.

29. Wakefield RJ, Green MJ, Marzo-Ortega H, Conaghan PG, Gibbon WW, McGonagle D, et al. Should oligoarthritis be reclassified? Ultrasound reveals a high prevalence of subclinical disease. Ann Rheum Dis. 2004;63:382–5.

30. Naredo E, Valor L, De la Torre I, Montoro M, Bello N, Martínez-Barrio J, et al. Predictive value of Doppler ultrasound-detected synovitis in relation to failed tapering of biologic therapy in patients with rheumatoid arthritis. Rheumatology (Oxford). 2015;54:1408–14.

31. Molenaar ET, Voskuyl AE, Dinant HJ, Bezemer PD, Boers M, Dijkmans BA. Progression of radiologic damage in patients with rheumatoid arthritis in clinical remission. Arthritis Rheum. 2004;50:36–42.

32. Markusse IM, Dirven L, Gerards AH, van Groenendael JH, Ronday HK, Kerstens PJ, et al. Disease flares in rheumatoid arthritis are associated with joint damage progression and disability: 10-year results from the BeSt study. Arthritis Res Ther. 2015;17:232.

33. Witt M, Mueller F, Nigg A, Reindl C, Leipe J, Proft F, et al. Relevance of grade 1 gray-scale ultrasound findings in wrists and small joints to the assessment of subclinical synovitis in rheumatoid arthritis. Arthritis Rheum. 2013;65:1694–701.

34. Ellegaard K, Torp-Pedersen S, Holm CC, Danneskiold-Samsøe B, Bliddal H. Ultrasound in finger joints: findings in normal subjects and pitfalls in the diagnosis of synovial disease. Ultraschall Med. 2007;28(4):401–8.

35. Iwamoto T, Ikeda K, Hosokawa J, Yamagata M, Tanaka S, Norimoto A, et al. Prediction of relapse after discontinuation of biologic agents by ultrasonographic assessment in patients with rheumatoid arthritis in clinical remission: high predictive values of total gray-scale and power Doppler scores that represent residual synovial inflammation before discontinuation. Arthritis Care Res (Hoboken). 2014;66:1576–81.

36. Naredo E, Valor L, De la Torre I, Martínez-Barrio J, Hinojosa M, Aramburu F, et al. Ultrasound joint inflammation in rheumatoid arthritis in clinical remission: how many and which joints should be assessed? Arthritis Care Res (Hoboken). 2013;65:512–7.

37. Aydin SZ, Gunal EK, Ozata M, Keskin H, Ozturk AB, Emery P, et al. Six-joint ultrasound in rheumatoid arthritis: a feasible approach for implementing ultrasound in remission. Clin Exp Rheum. 2017 Jun 16. [Epub ahead of print]. PMID: 28628469.

38. Vreju FA, Filippucci E, Gutierrez M, Di Geso L, Ciapetti A, Ciurea ME, et al. Subclinical ultrasound synovitis in a particular joint is associated with ultrasound evidence of bone erosions in that same joint in rheumatoid patients in clinical remission. Clin Exp Rheumatol. 2016;34:673–8.

6

Whole blood microRNA expression pattern differentiates patients with rheumatoid arthritis, their seropositive first-degree relatives, and healthy unrelated control subjects

Vidyanand Anaparti[1,2,3] (iD), Irene Smolik[1,3,4], Xiaobo Meng[1,2,3], Victor Spicer[2], Neeloffer Mookherjee[1,2,5] and Hani El-Gabalawy[1,2,3,4,5*]

Abstract

Background: Epigenetic mechanisms can integrate gene-environment interactions that mediate disease transition from preclinical to clinically overt rheumatoid arthritis (RA). To better understand their role, we evaluated microRNA (miRNA, miR) expression profile in indigenous North American patients with RA who were positive for anticitrullinated protein antibodies; their autoantibody-positive, asymptomatic first-degree relatives (FDRs); and disease-free healthy control subjects (HCs).

Methods: Total RNA was isolated from whole blood samples obtained from HC ($n = 12$), patients with RA ($n = 18$), and FDRs ($n = 12$). Expression of 35 selected relevant miRNAs, as well as associated downstream messenger RNA (mRNA) targets of miR-103a-3p, was determined by qRT-PCR.

Results: Whole blood expression profiling identified significantly differential miRNA expression in patients with RA (13 miRNAs) and FDRs (10 miRNAs) compared with HCs. Among these, expression of miR-103a-3p, miR-155, miR-146a-5p, and miR-26b-3p was significantly upregulated, whereas miR-346 was significantly downregulated, in both study groups. Expression of miR-103a-3p was consistently elevated in FDRs at two time points 1 year apart. We also confirmed increased miR-103a-3p expression in peripheral blood mononuclear cells from patients with RA compared with HCs. Predicted target analyses of differentially expressed miRNAs in patients with RA and FDRs showed overlapping biological networks. Consistent with these curated networks, mRNA expression of *DICER1*, *AGO1*, *CREB1*, *DAPK1*, and *TP53* was downregulated significantly with miR-103a-3p expression in FDRs.

Conclusions: We highlight systematically altered circulating miRNA expression in at-risk FDRs prior to RA onset, a profile they shared with patients with RA. Prominently consistent miR-103a-3p expression indicates its utility as a prognostic biomarker for preclinical RA while highlighting biological pathways important for transition to clinically detectable disease.

Keywords: MicroRNA, Rheumatoid arthritis, Epigenetics, miRNA, miR-103a-3p, Whole blood, miR-103a

* Correspondence: hani.elgabalawy@umanitoba.ca
[1]Department of Internal Medicine, Rady Faculty of Health Sciences, University of Manitoba, Room 799, 715 McDermot Avenue, Winnipeg, MB R3E 3P4, Canada
[2]Manitoba Centre for Proteomics and Systems Biology, University of Manitoba, Winnipeg, MB, Canada
Full list of author information is available at the end of the article

Background

Rheumatoid arthritis (RA) is a chronic autoimmune disease that results from a complex interplay between genetics, environmental factors, and the immune system. Retrospective studies of RA onset based on archival serum samples have indicated that rheumatoid factor (RF) and anticitrullinated protein antibodies (ACPA) are detectable months to years prior to clinical disease onset, and they exhibit a progressive increase in titer as disease onset approaches. In the case of ACPA, this phenomenon is believed to relate to expansion of an autoantigen repertoire targeted by the ACPA, a process that has been termed *epitope spreading* [1–3].

We previously demonstrated a high prevalence of RA in an indigenous North American (INA) population in Manitoba, Canada, an observation that is consistent with those in other INA populations [4]. In this population, RA is characterized by familial disease aggregation and early age of disease onset [5, 6]. A high proportion of these INA patients with RA are genetically predisposed by having shared epitope encoding HLA-DRB1 alleles, particularly *1402 and *0404 [7]. The disease is primarily seropositive, and it is severe and disabling, with frequent large joint involvement. In studying the first-degree relatives (FDRs) of INA patients with RA, we have demonstrated frequent RF and ACPA seropositivity, and we have shown that the serum cytokine profile of the FDRs resembles that of their affected relatives more so than that of control subjects with no family history of autoimmune disease [6–8]. Thus, this population is ideally suited for studying the onset of RA in high-risk individuals and the potential role that genetic, environmental, and epigenetic factors play in the process.

MicroRNAs (miRNAs, miRs) are conserved, small, noncoding, single-stranded RNAs (~18–25 nucleotides) that play a role in posttranscriptional gene regulation. miRNAs bind to the 3′-untranslated region (3′-UTR) of target messenger RNA (mRNA) and induce gene silencing by either promoting mRNA degradation or transcript destabilization, resulting in suppression of target protein synthesis [9, 10]. In RA, proinflammatory cytokines (e.g., tumor necrosis factor-α, interleukin [IL]-1β, and IL-17) alter the expression of multiple miRNAs (e.g., miR-155, miR-146a, miR-26b, miR-16, and miR-21) in peripheral blood mononuclear cells (PBMCs), synovial fibroblasts, T lymphocytes, and synovial tissues derived from patients with RA [11–13]. In turn, miRNAs regulate inflammatory and signaling pathways influencing cellular differentiation and bone homeostasis within the synovial microenvironment [11]. Consequently, miRNAs play a central role in the regulation of inflammatory processes, synovial proliferation, and osteoclastogenesis, thus affecting the disease activity in RA [12–14]. Therefore, miRNAs may serve as a critical epigenetic component in the breakdown of immune tolerance and progression toward RA disease onset.

There is limited knowledge on the role of miRNAs in RA pathogenesis, particularly during the preclinical phase of the disease. To define mechanisms underpinning the progression of autoimmunity toward disease onset in at-risk individuals, we sought to evaluate miRNA expression profiles in blood samples derived from INA patients with RA, their seropositive FDRs, and healthy control subjects (HCs). This is the first study to demonstrate unique and reproducible differences in miRNA expression patterns in whole blood between these groups. Furthermore, we demonstrated that miR-103a-3p is uniquely upregulated in both patients with RA and FDRs. The observed miRNA patterns and the molecular networks they represent are of value in defining new mechanisms involved in RA onset while being potentially useful as biomarkers for predicting onset of preclinical RA.

Methods

Study design

INA study participants were recruited from Cree, Ojibway, and Oji-Cree communities in central Canada [5, 6]. The biomedical research ethics board of the University of Manitoba approved the overall design of the study and the consent forms (ethics, 2005:093; protocol, HS14453). Specific research agreements with the study communities were developed and approved by the community leadership. The conduct of the study was guided by the principles of community-based participatory research, a cornerstone of the Canadian Institutes of Health Research guidelines for Aboriginal health research (http://www.cihr-irsc.gc.ca/e/29134.html). As such, community leadership provided input into the initial development of the project, as well as ongoing input through advisory board meetings. Local healthcare providers were trained in study methodology and standard operating procedures. Regular knowledge translation activities such as newsletters and local radio appearances by study investigators provided the communities with updates regarding progress and significance. The study participants provided informed consent after the study was explained to them in detail, with the help of an INA translator from their community where necessary. The following three groups were included in this study: (1) ACPA-positive patients with RA, (2) their unaffected ACPA-positive FDRs, and (3) HCs negative for ACPA and RF. The demographics of the study groups are summarized in Table 1. RA diagnosis was made on the basis of fulfilling the 2010 American College of Rheumatology/European League Against Rheumatism classification criteria. None of the FDRs or HCs demonstrated clinical evidence of synovitis, as determined by a rheumatologist (HEG).

Table 1 Clinical characteristics of the study population

	Healthy control subjects ($n = 12$)	ACPA+/patients with RA ($n = 18$)	ACPA+/FDRs ($n = 12$)
Age, years, median (range)	40 (23–66)	46.6 (29–70)	33.65 (28–60)
Sex, female/male	10/2	14/4	12/1
Disease duration, years, median (range)	NA	12.02 (0–35.6)	NA
CRP titer, median (range)	3.35 (1.07 –9.25)	6.91 (2–42.6)	2.595 (1.01–15.9)
RF titer, IU/ml, median (range)ml	<20	321 (20–1540)	34.9 (20–570)
Anti-CCP titer, median (range)	1 (0.4–2.0)	201 (19–289)	114 (7–365)
BMI, kg/m^2, median (range)	29.54 (19.9–34.4)	27.37 (20.4–39.6)	26.09 (19.6–40.7)

Abbreviations: ACPA Anticitrullinated protein antibodies, *BMI* Body mass index, *Anti-CCP* Anticyclic citrullinated protein antibodies, *CRP* C-reactive protein, *FDR* First-degree relative, *RA* Rheumatoid arthritis, *RF* Rheumatoid factor, *NA* Not applicable
All values are reported as median (range) unless otherwise indicated

Sample collection

Venous blood was collected into PAXgene® Blood RNA tubes (PreAnalytiX, Hombrechtikon, Switzerland), processed as per the manufacturer's instructions, and used to isolate total RNA. PBMCs were isolated using SepMate®-50 tubes (STEMCELL Technologies, Vancouver, BC, Canada) as per the manufacturer's protocol. Briefly, venous blood was drawn into ethylenediaminetetraacetic acid-coated tubes and diluted 1:1 with incomplete Gibco RPMI medium (Life Technologies, Carlsbad, CA, USA), layered onto SepMate®-50 tubes with Histopaque Plus (Sigma-Aldrich, St. Louis, MO, USA), and centrifuged at $1000 \times g$ for 10 minutes at room temperature. Buffy coat was separated, and cells were washed in RPMI 1640 medium prior to RNA isolation.

Immunoassays

Serum C-reactive protein (CRP) levels were monitored in serum by using a human high-sensitivity C-reactive protein (hs-CRP) enzyme-linked immunosorbent assay kit (Biomatik, Cambridge, ON, Canada) as per the manufacturer's instructions. The concentration of ACPA was monitored in serum using the BioPlex® 2200 anticyclic citrullinated protein antibodies reagent kit (Bio-Rad Laboratories, Hercules, CA, USA).

Total RNA extraction and qRT-PCR

Total RNA was isolated from whole blood and PBMCs using the Ambion *mir*VANA miRNA isolation kit (catalogue number AM1561; Life Technologies, Carlsbad, CA, USA) as per the manufacturer's instructions. RNA quality was determined using Bioanalyzer with the RNA 6000 Nano Kit (Agilent Technologies, Santa Clara, CA, USA). Total RNA with absorbance at 260 and 280 nm ≥ 2.0 and RNA integrity number ≥ 7.0 was used for monitoring miRNA expression using a two-step qRT-PCR protocol as previously described [15]. Briefly, we used the Applied Biosystems TaqMan® MicroRNA Reverse Transcription Kit (Life Technologies) with miRNA-specific stem-loop primers for reverse transcription (Additional file 1:

Table S1). Specific amplification of miRNA targets was performed using TaqMan® Universal Master Mix II and target-specific TaqMan® MicroRNA Assay Mix in the ABI PRISM 7300 Real-Time PCR System (all from Life Technologies). For mRNA amplification, first-strand complementary DNA was synthesized from total RNA (1 µg) using SuperScript® VILO™ MasterMix (Life Technologies) as per the manufacturer's instructions. Target mRNA was amplified using Applied Biosystems® *Power* SYBR® Green Master Mix (Life Technologies) as per the manufacturer's instructions. Primers used for mRNA amplification of miR-103a-3p are listed in Additional file 1: Table S2.

Data analysis and statistics

Candidate endogenous control miRNAs for data normalization were selected on the basis of prior literature (RNU48, RNU44, U6 snRNA, RNU6B, and miR-16). Expression of these selected miRNAs was assessed for stable expression across samples in whole blood and PBMCs obtained from HCs, patients with RA, and FDRs. RefFinder, a web-based comprehensive gene analysis platform that integrates geNorm, NormFinder, BestKeeper, and comparative cycle threshold (ΔC_t) methods, was used to identify the miRNA candidates suitable as endogenous controls for data normalization. On the basis of this approach, RNU48 and RNU6B were identified as optimum reference miRNAs for normalization across all samples in this study [16]. Reference C_t values for data normalization were determined by calculating the average C_t value of RNU48 and RNU6B [reference C_t = mean (C_t {RNU48} – C_t (RNU6B)] and used for each sample. Raw C_t values for each target miRNA were then normalized with reference C_t values to obtain ΔC_t values for each sample [ΔC_t (target miRNA) = C_t (target) – reference C_t]. ΔC_t values of each miRNA were further corrected using a global mean normalization strategy to obtain normalized ΔC_t values [normalized ΔC_t = ΔC_t (target miRNA) – mean ΔC_t] for all assessed miRNAs [17–19]. Relative fold changes were calculated using the

$\Delta\Delta C_t$ method [20]. Of the 35 miRNAs analyzed, 33 showed detectable expression ($C_t \leq 35$) (Table 2) and were considered for further analyses. Target mRNA expression was determined in samples after normalization using 18S ribosomal RNA as an endogenous control [20], and relative fold changes were calculated using the $\Delta\Delta C_t$ method.

GraphPad Prism version 5.0 was used for miRNA analysis and generating volcano plots, scatterplots, and bar graphs. Empirical cumulative distribution plots (based on the Kolmogorov-Smirnov [KS] test) and ROC curves were generated using MS Excel (Microsoft, Redmond, WA, USA) and Prism (GraphPad Prism, La Jolla, CA, USA) software, respectively. The KS test is a nonparametric

Table 2 Fold change expression of microRNAs

miRNA	RA vs HC			FDR vs HC		FDR vs RA	
	P Value	Fold change	Rank	P Value	Fold change	P Value	Fold change
hsa-miR-103a-3p	**0.0064**	**3.96**	**1**	**0.0238**	**7.68**	0.1223	1.97
hsa-miR-155	**0.0002**	**2.47**	**2**	**0.0115**	**1.98**	0.3627	−1.25
hsa-miR-29b	0.0648	1.91	3	0.8636	−1.55	0.0754	−2.96
hsa-miR-132	**0.0016**	**1.90**	**4**	0.0687	1.37	0.2530	−1.39
hsa-miR-26b-3p	**0.0010**	**1.88**	**5**	**0.0024**	**2.28**	0.2530	1.21
hsa-miR-152	**0.0038**	**1.83**	**6**	0.1309	1.97	0.4981	1.08
hsa-miR-19a	0.0732	1.73	**7**	**0.0205**	**1.55**	0.9662	−1.11
hsa-Let-7a	0.0569	1.73	**7**	0.2086	1.17	0.2358	−1.47
hsa-miR-19b	**0.0260**	**1.67**	**9**	0.1169	1.34	0.4091	−1.24
hsa-miR-146a-5p	**0.0083**	**1.54**	**10**	**0.0031**	**1.99**	0.3408	1.29
hsa-miR-451	**0.0076**	**1.53**	**11**	**0.0127**	**1.56**	0.7031	1.02
RNU44	**0.0120**	**1.52**	**12**	**0.0162**	**1.30**	0.9157	−1.17
hsa-miR-125a-5p	**0.0272**	**1.30**	**13**	0.0553	1.50	0.7508	1.15
hsa-miR-222	0.0796	1.29	14	0.2154	1.20	0.4587	−1.07
hsa-miR-107	0.0576	1.28	15	0.2481	−1.02	0.4587	−1.31
hsa-miR-29c	0.2428	1.28	16	0.1457	1.11	0.8159	−1.15
hsa-Let-7e	0.0502	1.27	17	0.5837	−1.20	0.0987	−1.53
hsa-miR-21	**0.0261**	**1.24**	**18**	0.0924	1.22	0.7832	−1.16
hsa-miR-223	**0.0115**	**1.22**	**19**	0.5487	1.03	0.5115	−1.82
hsa-miR-26b-5p	0.1191	1.21	20	0.6744	−1.45	**0.0277**	**−1.76**
hsa-miR-323-3p	0.1123	1.17	21	0.2033	1.12	0.9831	−1.04
hsa-miR-26a	0.1849	1.14	22	0.1159	1.33	0.8822	1.16
hsa-miR-29a	0.1031	1.14	23	0.6174	−1.29	0.1124	1.46
hsa-miR-15a	0.5594	1.11	24	0.8292	−1.56	0.1223	−1.72
hsa-miR-150	0.6104	1.10	25	0.41	1.20	0.7669	1.09
hsa-miR-34a*	0.1065	1.06	26	**0.0495**	**−1.84**	**0.0262**	**−1.94**
hsa-miR-221	0.1842	1.06	27	0.9914	−1.37	0.2356	−1.45
hsa-miR-24	0.2956	−1.05	28	0.8651	1.03	0.9831	1.04
hsa-miR-18a	0.7615	−1.07	29	0.7639	−1.85	0.1124	−1.72
U6	0.8069	−1.11	30	**0.0001**	**−1.59**	0.0625	−1.43
hsa-miR-125a-3p	0.1654	−1.20	31	0.6178	−1.10	0.4847	1.10
hsa-miR-16	0.9950	−3.94	32	0.8276	−1.24	0.2802	−1.23
hsa-miR-346	**0.0001**	**−8.70**	**33**	**0.0001**	**−20.00**	0.0338	−2.32

Abbreviations: FDR First-degree relative, HC Healthy control subjects, miRNA or miR MicroRNA, RA Rheumatoid arthritis
miRNA profiling was analyzed in the whole blood total RNA samples obtained from HC, patients with RA, and FDRs using TaqMan probes. P values were obtained using the Mann-Whitney U test, and median fold change values were used to classify miRNAs rankwise. Columns highlighted in bold represent miRNAs that show significant differential expression after Benjamini-Hochberg correction for multiple comparison analyses (Q < 0.04). RA vs HC indicates miRNA expression in patients with RA compared with HCs. FDR vs HC indicates miRNA expression in FDRs compared with HCs. FDR vs RA indicates miRNA expression in FDRs compared with patients with RA. hsa-miR-34a* represents hsa-miR-34a-3p

statistical method that does not assume normal distribution [21]. Differences between the datasets were represented as KS scores (in the range of –1 and 1) corresponding to maximum degree of separation between the cumulative distributions of the datasets being compared and directly proportional to relative expression levels. KS scores > 0.5 were considered significant. Heat maps were generated with unsupervised hierarchical clustering using the TIGR multiple experiment viewer. Ingenuity Pathway Analysis ([IPA] www.ingenuity.com; QIAGEN Bioinformatics, Redwood City, CA, USA) was used for biomolecular network analyses and to predict mRNAs targeted by the differentially expressed miRNAs identified in this study. The Mann-Whitney U test, the Kruskal-Wallis test with Dunn's post hoc method, or Spearman's rank correlation coefficient analysis was used for statistical analysis as required, and P values < 0.05 were considered significant. Differentially expressed miRNAs were determined after adjusting P values with Benjamini-Hochberg correction for multiple comparisons [22].

Results

Study population

Participants were age-matched, ethnically homogeneous individuals, and approximately 80% of them were women (Table 1). As expected, patients with RA demonstrated higher hs-CRP levels (mean ± SD 10.05 ± 10.02 μg/ml) than HCs (mean ± SD 4.03 ± 2.31 μg/ml) and FDR (mean ± SD 4.18 ± 3.09 μg/ml). Patients with RA in the study were on disease-modifying antirheumatic drugs and had an established disease profile that was either inactive or moderately active, as indicated by their Disease Activity Score in 28 joints (Table 1 and Additional file 1: Table S3).

Whole blood miRNA expression profile was altered in patients with RA and FDRs

Using targeted TaqMan® miRNA assay probes (Life Technologies), we analyzed the expression of 33 selected miRNAs. The miRNAs were selected on the basis of their relevance to RA as described in the literature (Additional file 1: Table S1). Overall, our analysis indicated that RA and FDR groups exhibited uniquely similar miRNA expression patterns compared with HC in whole blood samples (Table 2 and Fig. 1; Additional file 1: Table S4), but there were notable differences between these three groups. Whereas expression of 13 miRNAs was significantly different in patients with RA, 10 miRNAs were differentially expressed in FDRs, compared with HCs. Notably, the expression of miR-103a-3p was increased in both patients with RA (~3.96-fold) and FDR (~7.68-fold), whereas the expression of miR-346 was decreased in both groups (~8.7-fold and ~ 20-fold, respectively). Finally, in comparing patients with RA with FDRs, miR-34a*, miR-26b-5p, and miR-346 differed significantly in their expression levels.

Unsupervised hierarchical clustering (Fig. 1a) of all 33 detectable miRNAs in patients with RA and FDRs was performed to generate a tree clearly separating miRNAs into two major clusters. Volcano scatter plots further demonstrated that miR-103a-3p and miR-346 were the most upregulated (upper right corner of the plot) and downregulated (upper left corner of the plot), respectively (Fig. 1b). These findings suggested that miR-103a-3p was uniquely upregulated in both patients with RA and their FDRs compared with HCs. On this basis, we undertook further analyses to examine the performance of miR-103a-3p as a biomarker in this population.

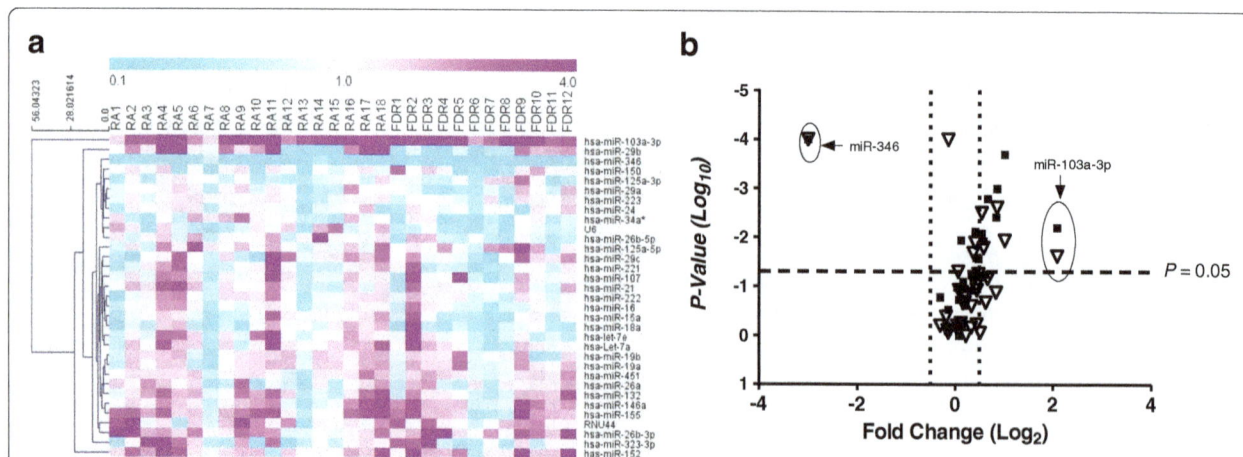

Fig. 1 a Unsupervised hierarchical clustering generated using fold change expression values of microRNAs (miRNAs, miRs) analyzed in patients with rheumatoid arthritis (RA) and first-degree relatives (FDRs) compared with healthy control subjects. Color scheme: *Violet* = increased expression; *cyan* = decreased expression; and *white* = unchanged. **b** Volcano plot showing expression of 33 miRNAs in the whole blood of patients with RA (*closed squares*) and FDRs (*open triangles*). The miRNAs that are significantly altered in both groups are located above the *horizontal dashed line* corresponding to $P \leq 0.05$

Performance of miR-103a-3p as a biomarker

Empirical cumulative distribution plots, together with ROC analysis, showed that miR-103a-3p can effectively distinguish between HCs, patients with RA, and FDRs ($P < 0.0001$; 0.01% false discovery rate). The calculated KS distance between HCs and patients with RA based on miR-103a-3p expression was 0.59 (at $\Delta C_t = 22.29$), whereas FDRs were separated by 0.75 (at $\Delta C_t = 21.32$) from HCs and by 0.49 (at $\Delta C_t = 20.89$) from patients with RA (Fig. 2a). We determined the sensitivity and specificity of miR-103a-3p expression using KS distance as a cutoff point (Fig. 2b). At 95% CI, the AUC of the ROC plot was 0. 8072 for ACPA-positive patients with RA ($P < 0.0001$; 92% specificity and 67% sensitivity), whereas FDRs showed AUCs of 0.9350 ($P < 0.0001$; 92% specificity and 83% sensitivity) compared with HCs and 0.7507 ($P < 0.001$; 71% specificity and 78% sensitivity) compared with patients with RA. These analyses suggest that elevated whole blood levels of miR-103a-3p may serve as a robust biomarker in ACPA-positive individuals at risk for developing future RA.

Elevated whole blood miR-103a-3p expression levels are stable feature in FDRs

FDRs, as a group, showed a ~ 7.6-fold increase in miR-103a-3p expression compared with HCs and a ~ 1.96-fold increase compared with patients with RA (Fig. 3a). We then sought to determine whether the increased miR-103a-3p expression levels were stable over time in specific individuals. Whole blood was collected from six HCs and two FDRs at two independent time points (~1 year apart), and miR-103a-3p expression was compared at the two time points. These experiments demonstrated that at both time points, the expression of miR-103a-3p was higher in FDRs (as indicated by lower ΔC_t values) compared with HCs (Fig. 3b). This suggests that there is sustained upregulation of miR-103a-3p in FDRs compared with HCs. We observed limited variability in miR-103a-3p expression related to time between sampling, sample acquisition, and sample storage (data not shown). The delineation of the relative contributions of various cellular subsets in whole blood to the observed increase in miR-103a-3p requires further experiments where individual cellular subsets are fractioned and tested.

Pairwise miR-103a-3p target correlation analysis distinctly segregates FDRs

Biomolecular interaction between the differentially expressed miRNAs (Table 2) with their respective annotated transcript targets was analyzed using the IPA bioinformatics tool. The biomolecular network revealed that tumor protein 53 (TP53) and Argonaute 2 (AGO2) were the two major hubs within the network that were proposed to regulate the expression of most of the differentially expressed miRNAs identified in this study (Additional file 1: Figure S1). The curated functional pathways (log P value > 2.0 by Fisher's exact test; threshold value = 0.05) predicted to be regulated by the miRNAs identified in this study included metabolic and physiological processes such as cellular growth, development,

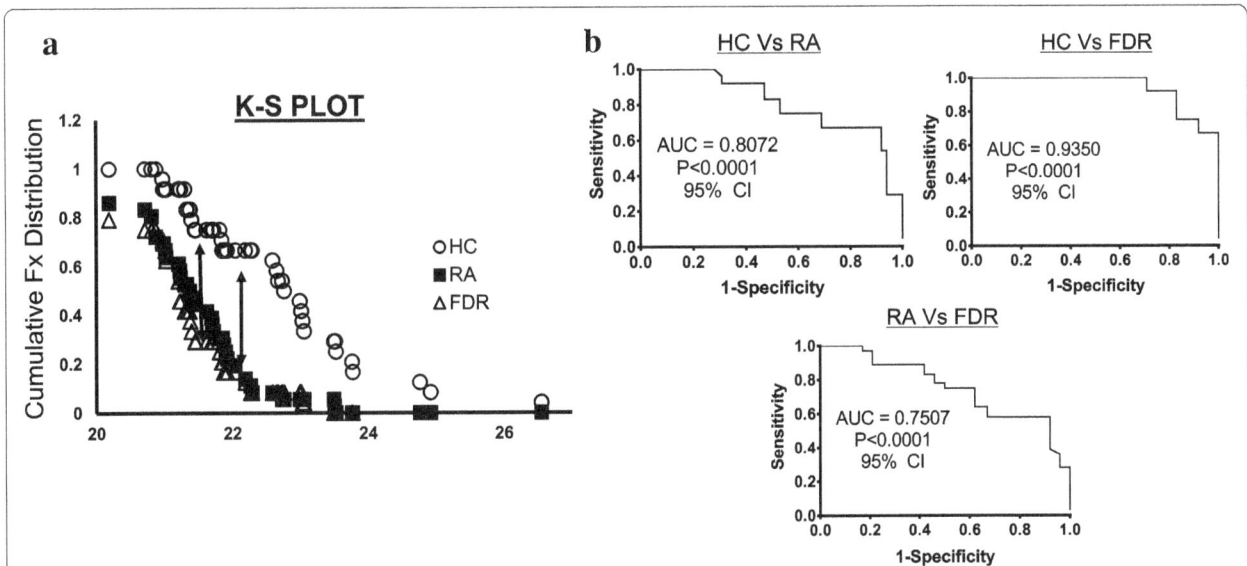

Fig. 2 a Kolmogorov-Smirnov (K-S) plots showing cumulative distribution of microRNA (miR) miR-103a-3p expression for healthy control subjects (HCs; *open circles*), patients with rheumatoid arthritis (RA; *closed squares*), and first-degree relatives (FDRs; *open triangles*). The distance between two distribution plots is represented by *double arrows*. K-S distance ≥ 0.5 was considered significant. **b** ROC curves (representing 1-specificity vs sensitivity values) for HCs, patients with RA, and FDRs, calculated using expression values of miR-103a-3p

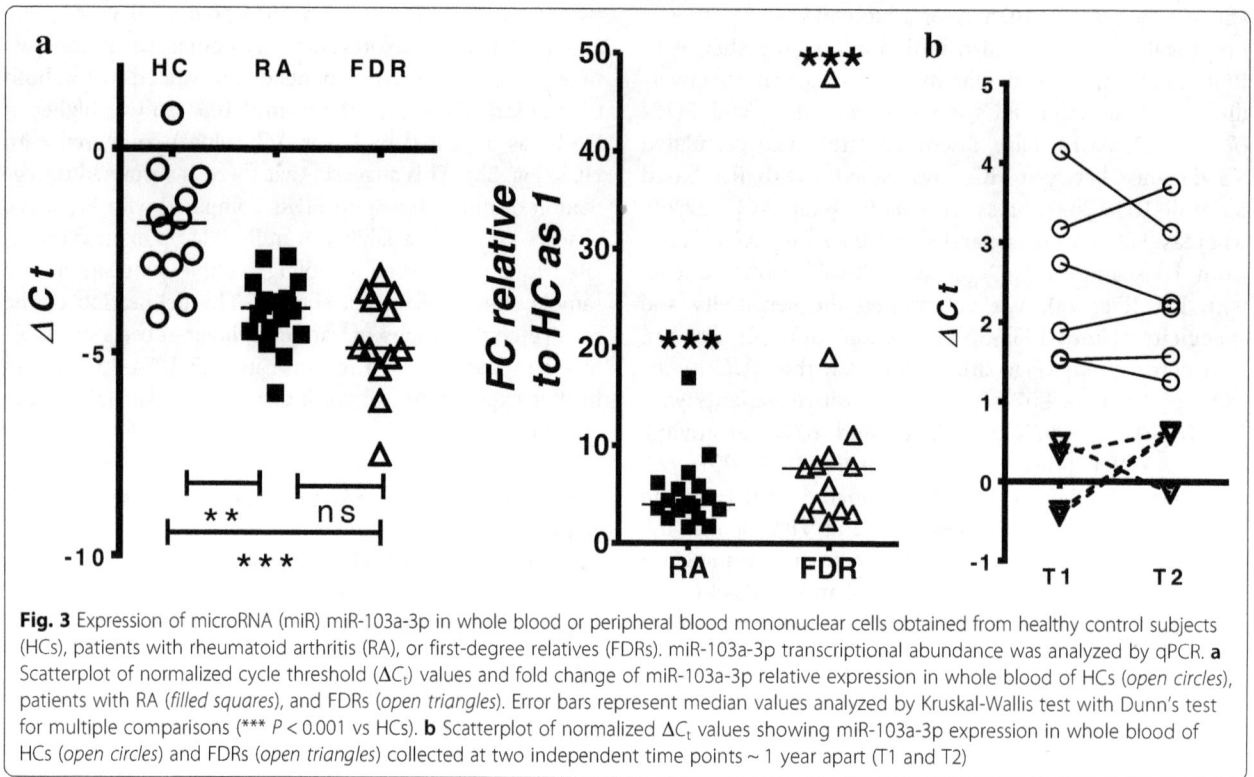

Fig. 3 Expression of microRNA (miR) miR-103a-3p in whole blood or peripheral blood mononuclear cells obtained from healthy control subjects (HCs), patients with rheumatoid arthritis (RA), or first-degree relatives (FDRs). miR-103a-3p transcriptional abundance was analyzed by qPCR. **a** Scatterplot of normalized cycle threshold (ΔC_t) values and fold change of miR-103a-3p relative expression in whole blood of HCs (*open circles*), patients with RA (*filled squares*), and FDRs (*open triangles*). Error bars represent median values analyzed by Kruskal-Wallis test with Dunn's test for multiple comparisons (*** $P < 0.001$ vs HCs). **b** Scatterplot of normalized ΔC_t values showing miR-103a-3p expression in whole blood of HCs (*open circles*) and FDRs (*open triangles*) collected at two independent time points ~ 1 year apart (T1 and T2)

proliferation, and cell death and are overrepresented in chronic diseases (Additional file 1: Table S5).

Consistent with curated network analysis, available literature suggests that miR-103a-3p expression is regulated by *TP53* and *AGO2* [23–29]. Furthermore, miR-103a-3p binds to 3'-UTRs of *CCNE*, *CDK1*, *DICER1*, *AGO1*, *GPD1*, *ID2*, *CREB1*, *TIMP3*, *DAPK1*, *KLF4*, and *PTEN* and regulates diverse physiological functions, including vascular inflammation, glucose metabolism, adipogenesis, endothelial cell activation, tumor metastasis, cellular apoptosis, and oxidative stress. Therefore, we monitored the expression of all the above-mentioned mRNAs by qRT-PCR (Fig. 4 and Additional file 1: Table S6). Compared with HCs, whole blood expression of Argonaute 1 (AGO1), cyclic AMP-responsive element-binding protein 1 (CREB1), death-associated protein kinase 1 (DAPK1), and TP53 was significantly down-regulated in FDRs. DICER1 mRNA expression showed a similar trend, albeit statistically nonsignificant. No significant change was observed in whole blood of patients with RA compared with HCs, except for AGO1. Additionally, Spearman's correlation analysis with Benjamini-Hochberg correction for multiple comparisons (Additional file 1: Table S6) did not demonstrate any statistical significance between miR-103a-3p and any of its target mRNA expression levels. This suggests that regulation of miR-103a-3p and its targets is complex and warrants further investigation.

Discussion

In the present study, we examined the expression pattern of a wide spectrum of miRNAs in whole blood samples from a cohort of INA patients with RA, their ACPA-positive unaffected FDRs, and unaffected INA control subjects with no clinical or serological evidence of autoimmunity. We demonstrated distinct differences

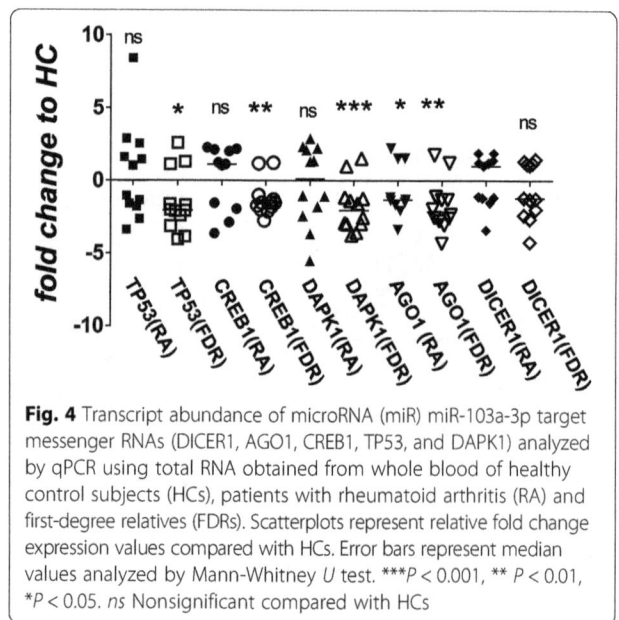

Fig. 4 Transcript abundance of microRNA (miR) miR-103a-3p target messenger RNAs (DICER1, AGO1, CREB1, TP53, and DAPK1) analyzed by qPCR using total RNA obtained from whole blood of healthy control subjects (HCs), patients with rheumatoid arthritis (RA) and first-degree relatives (FDRs). Scatterplots represent relative fold change expression values compared with HCs. Error bars represent median values analyzed by Mann-Whitney U test. ***$P < 0.001$, ** $P < 0.01$, *$P < 0.05$. *ns* Nonsignificant compared with HCs

between all three groups, and to our knowledge, we are the first to demonstrate that miR-103a-3p is overexpressed in patients with RA and FDRs compared with HCs. Although aberrant miRNA expression patterns in the peripheral blood of patients with RA has been widely reported [13, 30], aberrant expression in ACPA-positive unaffected individuals has not been reported previously. This study provides an impetus for evaluating the whole blood miRNA profile, particularly miR-103a-3p expression, as a potential biomarker for predicting imminent disease in individuals at risk for developing RA. It also points to specific biological pathways that may be involved in the transition to clinically detectable disease.

We elected to examine miRNA profiles using whole blood samples collected in PAXgene® RNA tubes for several reasons. First and foremost is the ease with which these samples are collected and stored, along with the remarkable resistance of the miRNA to endogenous ribonuclease activity, as well as stability to extreme pH, temperature, and storage conditions [31, 32]. An alternative approach that is being widely investigated in a spectrum of chronic diseases is testing miRNA levels in serum or plasma [33, 34]. Although this latter cell-free approach has the advantage of potentially harnessing large archival serum/plasma sample repositories, it suffers from limitations in providing a complete and unbiased miRNA profile of the circulating peripheral blood compartment of an individual. This relates to factors such as preprocessing of samples, cellular contamination, and inconsistency in miRNA levels in serum vs plasma [35, 36].

One major advantage of using whole blood to determine miRNA levels is that this approach retains the rich compositional architecture of the circulating blood, thus providing the most unbiased representation of this space. Although this approach may be ideally suited for biomarker discovery, its primary disadvantage is the inability to define the cellular subsets that are contributing to the observed miRNA profiles. Combined with the marked cellular compositional heterogeneity of whole blood, the generation of mechanistic hypotheses is challenging. To address this challenge, most of the previous studies of circulating miRNA expression in RA have been focused on PBMCs and their subsets [13]. However, attempts to correlate PBMC expression patterns with those evident in whole blood have produced conflicting results [15]. For instance, Atarod et al. demonstrated discordant expression of miR-146a-5p and miR-155 expression between PBMCs and whole blood [37]. These findings contradict the findings of our previous study [15], which demonstrated more concordance between whole blood and PBMC expression patterns. These differences may be attributable to total RNA isolation methodology used in each of these sample types. Alternatively, this discordance can also be attributed

to blood cell counts and red blood cell hemolysis [38]. We acknowledge the absence of such information pertaining to our study participants.

Previous studies on miRNA expression in RA, including our own, have been focused on differences in miR-146a and miR-155 expression between patients with RA and unaffected control subjects, both tending to be increased in RA PBMCs and synovial tissues [13, 15, 39]. In the present study, we compared the expression levels of these two miRNAs in whole blood and PBMCs and found that the levels were concordantly elevated not only in patients with RA as previously documented but also, surprisingly, in ACPA-positive FDRs with no clinical evidence of arthritis. Moreover, as shown in Fig. 1, the overall miRNA expression patterns in patients with RA and ACPA-positive FDRs were relatively similar to those of unaffected control subjects. These observations suggest that the similarity between patients with RA and unaffected ACPA-positive FDRs in the peripheral blood miRNA profile is more likely to relate to autoimmune than to inflammatory mechanisms. Moreover, we demonstrated that these patterns are relatively stable over a short time frame. It will be of interest to determine how the miRNA patterns evolve as individuals at risk for developing RA transition to clinically detectable synovitis. It will also be of interest to determine whether these RA-associated patterns are retained in patients with RA who have achieved clinical remission.

The large difference in miR-103a-3p expression that discriminated both patients with RA and FDRs from unaffected, population-based control subjects is noteworthy and, to our knowledge, not previously reported. Located within the intronic regions of pantothenate kinase enzymes, miR-103a-3p is a member of the miR-15/107 cluster and regulates lipid, cholesterol, and fatty acid metabolism; adipocyte differentiation; and insulin signaling [40–42]. However, the potential role that these biological functions play in RA pathogenesis remains largely unknown. Some studies have suggested that miR-103 upregulation is associated with obesity and insulin resistance in liver and adipose tissue, as well as with atherosclerosis [24, 43, 44]. Interestingly, the indigenous First Nations population as a whole, including the cohort we have studied, demonstrates a strikingly high prevalence of obesity, type 2 diabetes, and cardiovascular disease [45, 46].

To identify potential gene targets of miR-103a-3p and delineate the biological functions that they regulate, we performed computational predictive analysis using IPA. On the basis of the curated IPA target network analysis, we identified TP53 and AGO2 as central nodes in miRNA patterns detected in patients with RA and ACPA-positive unaffected FDRs. AGO2 is an integral component of RNA-induced silencing complex (RISC) that cleaves double-stranded immature miRNAs to single-stranded mature forms, a reaction catalyzed by an

RNase III-type enzyme called Dicer [9]. Altered TP53 expression has been observed in lymphocytes and synovial tissues from patients with RA and is associated with synovial proliferation and increased proinflammatory IL-6 secretion in the synovium [47, 48]. Interestingly, miR-103a-3p associates with AGO2 within RISC and is known to suppress Dicer [24, 49]. TP53 also regulates miR-103 expression via targeting components of miRNA biogenesis, including DICER1 and AGO2 [50]. Together, our observations point to miR-103a-3p-associated miRNA target reorganization in patients with RA and ACPA-positive FDRs at risk for developing RA. It is notable that the regulatory networks of miRNAs, including miR-103a-3p and its target mRNAs, are extremely complex and known to control physiological processes at multiple levels [51]. Considering that miRNAs are involved in an intricate network of feedback and feedforward regulatory loops, it is likely that the target mRNAs monitored in our study may modulate the expression of other miRNAs [52, 53]. In this regard, further research is warranted to investigate the interaction network between miR-103a-3p and its target mRNAs in different cohorts, especially FDRs, to examine biological processes prior to onset of RA.

Conclusions

We present evidence that the miRNA signature detectable in the peripheral blood of ACPA-positive individuals with no clinical evidence of RA resembles that of seropositive patients with RA and that this pattern differs considerably from that seen in unaffected seronegative controls. The substantial elevation of miR-103a-3p levels compared with unaffected control subjects is particularly discriminating and, in conjunction with phenomena such as the epitope spreading of the ACPA response, may serve as a potential biomarker for imminent RA in at-risk individuals. Longitudinal studies will be needed to determine how this miRNA signature evolves as individuals develop clinical disease and detectable synovitis. This in turn will provide new insights into the biological mechanisms underlying this important transition point.

Additional file

Additional file 1: Table S1. Details of miRNAs included in the study. **Table S2.** Primers for mRNA targets of miR-103a-3p. Primers were designed using the PrimerQuest tool (Integrated DNA Technologies, Coralville, IA, USA) and the Universal ProbeLibrary system (Roche Life Sciences, Indianapolis, IN, USA) and verified by Primer-BLAST (National Center for Biotechnology Information, Bethesda, MD, USA). 18S ribosomal RNA, F Forward, R Reverse. **Table S3.** Clinical features of ACPA-positive patients with RA. **Table S4.** Differentially expressed miRNAs in probands and FDRs: significantly upregulated (↑) and downregulated (↓) or unaltered miRNAs. # Only miRNAs differentially expressed in FDRs compared with patients with RA. **Figure S1.** IPA target analysis. IPA network showing curated molecular interactions between differentially expressed miRNAs and their experimentally

validated target genes. **Table S5.** Summary of findings derived from IPA regarding gene targets of differentially expressed miRNAs: top molecular and cellular functions, physiological system development and function, diseases and disorders, and networks regulated by significantly modulated miRNAs and their gene targets (P < 0.05 by Fisher's exact test). **Table S6.** Spearman's rank correlation coefficient values and corresponding P values for miR-103a-3p and target mRNAs. ΔC_t values of miR-103a-3p Vs target mRNAs from HC, patients with RA, and FDRs were combined for this correlation analysis. Q values represent adjusted P values after applying the Benjamini-Hochberg correction for multiple comparisons. (DOCX 836 kb)

Abbreviations
ACPA: Anticitrullinated protein antibodies; AGO1: Argonaute 1; AGO2: Argonaute 2; Anti-CCP: Anticyclic citrullinated protein antibodies; CCNE1: Cyclin E1; CDK1: Cyclin-dependent kinase 1; CIHR: Canadian Institutes of Health Research; CREB1: Cyclic AMP-responsive element-binding protein 1; CRP: C-reactive protein; ΔC_t: Cycle threshold method; DAPK1: Death-associated protein kinase 1; DICER1: Dicer 1, ribonuclease III; FDR: First-degree relative; GPD1: Glycerol-3-phosphate dehydrogenase 1; HC: Healthy control subjects; hs-CRP: High-sensitivity C-reactive protein; ID2: Inhibitor of DNA binding 2; IL: Interleukin; INA: Indigenous North American; IPA: Ingenuity Pathway Analysis; KLF4: Kruppel-like factor 4; KS: Kolmogorov-Smirnov; miRNA or miR: MicroRNA; mRNA: Messenger RNA; PBMC: Peripheral blood mononuclear cell; PTEN: Phosphatase and tensin homolog; RA: Rheumatoid arthritis; RF: Rheumatoid factor; RISC: RNA-induced silencing complex; TIMP3: Tissue inhibitor of metalloproteinase 3; TP53: Tumor protein 53; UTR: Untranslated region

Acknowledgements
We acknowledge the contribution of study participants from indigenous communities who donated blood for our study. We also recognize Chief and Band Councils of Norway House and St. Theresa Point Manitoba for their invaluable cooperation, as well as Dr. Hemsekhar Mahadevappa for his valuable scientific input.

Funding
This study was supported by individual grants to HEG from the Canadian Institutes of Health Research (CIHR). VA is a recipient of a Research Manitoba Postdoctoral Fellowship.

Authors' contributions
VA, NM, and HEG conceived of the research concept. VA designed and performed the experiments, analyzed data, and prepared figures. IS and XM assisted in patient recruitment, sample collection, and sample storage. VS assisted in data analysis. VA, NM, and HEG drafted, revised, and edited the manuscript. All authors read and approved the final manuscript.

Ethics approval and consent to participate
The biomedical research ethics board of the University of Manitoba approved the overall design of the study and consent forms (ethics, 2005:093; protocol, HS14453). Specific research agreements with the study communities were developed and approved by the community leadership. The conduct of the study was guided by the principles of community-based participatory research, a cornerstone of the Canadian Institutes of Health Research guidelines for aboriginal health research (http://www.cihr-irsc.gc.ca/e/29134.html). As such, community leadership provided input into the initial development of the project as well as ongoing input through advisory board meetings. Local healthcare providers were trained in study methodology and standard operating procedures. Regular knowledge translation activities such as newsletters and local radio appearances by study investigators provided the communities with updates regarding progress and significance. The study participants provided informed consent after the study was explained to them in detail, with the help of an INA translator from their community where necessary.

Competing interests
The authors declare that they have no competing interests.

Author details
[1]Department of Internal Medicine, Rady Faculty of Health Sciences, University of Manitoba, Room 799, 715 McDermot Avenue, Winnipeg, MB R3E 3P4, Canada. [2]Manitoba Centre for Proteomics and Systems Biology, University of Manitoba, Winnipeg, MB, Canada. [3]Rheumatic Diseases Unit, University of Manitoba, Winnipeg, MB, Canada. [4]Division of Rheumatology, Faculty of Health Sciences, University of Manitoba, Winnipeg, MB, Canada. [5]Department of Immunology, Rady Faculty of Health Sciences, University of Manitoba, Winnipeg, MB, Canada.

References
1. Nielen MM, van Schaardenburg D, Reesink HW, van de Stadt RJ, van der Horst-Bruinsma IE, de Koning MH, Habibuw MR, Vandenbroucke JP, Dijkmans BA. Specific autoantibodies precede the symptoms of rheumatoid arthritis: a study of serial measurements in blood donors. Arthritis Rheum. 2004;50(2):380–6.
2. Sokolove J, Bromberg R, Deane KD, Lahey LJ, Derber LA, Chandra PE, Edison JD, Gilliland WR, Tibshirani RJ, Norris JM, et al. Autoantibody epitope spreading in the pre-clinical phase predicts progression to rheumatoid arthritis. PLoS One. 2012;7(5), e35296.
3. van de Stadt LA, de Koning MH, van de Stadt RJ, Wolbink G, Dijkmans BA, Hamann D, van Schaardenburg D. Development of the anti-citrullinated protein antibody repertoire prior to the onset of rheumatoid arthritis. Arthritis Rheum. 2011;63(11):3226–33.
4. Ferucci ED, Schumacher MC, Lanier AP, Murtaugh MA, Edwards S, Helzer LJ, Tom-Orme L, Slattery ML. Arthritis prevalence and associations in American Indian and Alaska Native people. Arthritis Rheum. 2008;59(8):1128–36.
5. El-Gabalawy HS, Robinson DB, Hart D, Elias B, Markland J, Peschken CA, Smolik I, Montes-Aldana G, Schroeder M, Fritzler MJ, et al. Immunogenetic risks of anti-cyclical citrullinated peptide antibodies in a North American Native population with rheumatoid arthritis and their first-degree relatives. J Rheumatol. 2009;36(6):1130–5.
6. El-Gabalawy HS, Robinson DB, Smolik I, Hart D, Elias B, Wong K, Peschken CA, Hitchon CA, Li X, Bernstein CN, et al. Familial clustering of the serum cytokine profile in the relatives of rheumatoid arthritis patients. Arthritis Rheum. 2012;64(6):1720–9.
7. El-Gabalawy HS, Robinson DB, Daha NA, Oen KG, Smolik I, Elias B, Hart D, Bernstein CN, Sun Y, Lu Y, et al. Non-HLA genes modulate the risk of rheumatoid arthritis associated with HLA-DRB1 in a susceptible North American Native population. Genes Immun. 2011;12(7):568–74.
8. Peschken CA, Hitchon CA, Robinson DB, Smolik I, Barnabe CR, Prematilake S, El-Gabalawy HS. Rheumatoid arthritis in a North American Native population: longitudinal followup and comparison with a white population. J Rheumatol. 2010;37(8):1589–95.
9. Bartel DP. MicroRNAs: genomics, biogenesis, mechanism, and function. Cell. 2004;116(2):281–97.
10. Gulyaeva LF, Kushlinskiy NE. Regulatory mechanisms of microRNA expression. J Transl Med. 2016;14(1):143.
11. Maeda Y, Farina NH, Matzelle MM, Fanning PJ, Lian JB, Gravallese EM. Synovium-derived microRNAs regulate bone pathways in rheumatoid arthritis. J Bone Miner Res. 2017;32(3):461–72.
12. Wittmann J, Jack HM. microRNAs in rheumatoid arthritis: midget RNAs with a giant impact. Ann Rheum Dis. 2011;70 Suppl 1:i92–6.
13. Churov AV, Oleinik EK, Knip M. MicroRNAs in rheumatoid arthritis: altered expression and diagnostic potential. Autoimmun Rev. 2015;14(11):1029–37.
14. Chen XM, Huang QC, Yang SL, Chu YL, Yan YH, Han L, Huang Y, Huang RY. Role of micro RNAs in the pathogenesis of rheumatoid arthritis: novel perspectives based on review of the literature. Medicine (Baltimore). 2015; 94(31), e1326.
15. Mookherjee N, El-Gabalawy HS. High degree of correlation between whole blood and PBMC expression levels of miR-155 and miR-146a in healthy controls and rheumatoid arthritis patients. J Immunol Methods. 2013;400–401:106–10.
16. Xie F, Xiao P, Chen D, Xu L, Zhang B. miRDeepFinder: a miRNA analysis tool for deep sequencing of plant small RNAs. Plant Mol Biol. 2012;80(1):75–84.
17. D'Haene B, Mestdagh P, Hellemans J, Vandesompele J. miRNA expression profiling: from reference genes to global mean normalization. Methods Mol Biol. 2012;822:261–72.
18. Mestdagh P, Van Vlierberghe P, De Weer A, Muth D, Westermann F, Speleman F, Vandesompele J. A novel and universal method for microRNA RT-qPCR data normalization. Genome Biol. 2009;10(6):R64.
19. Carlsen AL, Schetter AJ, Nielsen CT, Lood C, Knudsen S, Voss A, Harris CC, Hellmark T, Segelmark M, Jacobsen S, et al. Circulating microRNA expression profiles associated with systemic lupus erythematosus. Arthritis Rheum. 2013;65(5):1324–34.
20. Pfaffl MW. A new mathematical model for relative quantification in real-time RT-PCR. Nucleic Acids Res. 2001;29(9), e45.
21. Hathout Y, Brody E, Clemens PR, Cripe L, DeLisle RK, Furlong P, Gordish-Dressman H, Hache L, Henricson E, Hoffman EP, et al. Large-scale serum protein biomarker discovery in Duchenne muscular dystrophy. Proc Natl Acad Sci U S A. 2015;112(23):7153–8.
22. Benjamini Y, Hochberg Y. Controlling the false discovery rate: a practical and powerful approach to multiple testing. J R Stat Soc Series B Stat Methodol. 1995;57(1):289–300.
23. Liao Y, Lonnerdal B. Global microRNA characterization reveals that miR-103 is involved in IGF-1 stimulated mouse intestinal cell proliferation. PLoS One. 2010;5(9), e12976.
24. Hartmann P, Zhou Z, Natarelli L, Wei Y, Nazari-Jahantigh M, Zhu M, Grommes J, Steffens S, Weber C, Schober A. Endothelial Dicer promotes atherosclerosis and vascular inflammation by miRNA-103-mediated suppression of KLF4. Nat Commun. 2016;7:10521.
25. Yu D, Zhou H, Xun Q, Xu X, Ling J, Hu Y. microRNA-103 regulates the growth and invasion of endometrial cancer cells through the downregulation of tissue inhibitor of metalloproteinase 3. Oncol Lett. 2012;3(6):1221–6.
26. Annibali D, Gioia U, Savino M, Laneve P, Caffarelli E, Nasi S. A new module in neural differentiation control: two microRNAs upregulated by retinoic acid, miR-9 and -103, target the differentiation inhibitor ID2. PLoS One. 2012;7(7), e40269.
27. Kiriakidou M, Nelson PT, Kouranov A, Fitziev P, Bouyioukos C, Mourelatos Z, Hatzigeorgiou A. A combined computational-experimental approach predicts human microRNA targets. Genes Dev. 2004;18(10):1165–78.
28. Chen HY, Lin YM, Chung HC, Lang YD, Lin CJ, Huang J, Wang WC, Lin FM, Chen Z, Huang HD, et al. miR-103/107 promote metastasis of colorectal cancer by targeting the metastasis suppressors DAPK and KLF4. Cancer Res. 2012;72(14):3631–41.
29. Chou CH, Chang NW, Shrestha S, Hsu SD, Lin YL, Lee WH, Yang CD, Hong HC, Wei TY, Tu SJ, et al. miRTarBase 2016: updates to the experimentally validated miRNA-target interactions database. Nucleic Acids Res. 2016; 44(D1):D239–47.
30. Lai NS, Yu HC, Yu CL, Koo M, Huang HB, Lu MC. Anti-citrullinated protein antibodies suppress let-7a expression in monocytes from patients with rheumatoid arthritis and facilitate the inflammatory responses in rheumatoid arthritis. Immunobiology. 2015;220(12):1351–8.
31. Koberle V, Pleli T, Schmithals C, Augusto Alonso E, Haupenthal J, Bonig H, Peveling-Oberhag J, Biondi RM, Zeuzem S, Kronenberger B, et al. Differential stability of cell-free circulating microRNAs: implications for their utilization as biomarkers. PLoS One. 2013;8(9), e75184.
32. Malentacchi F, Pizzamiglio S, Wyrich R, Verderio P, Ciniselli C, Pazzagli M, Gelmini S. Effects of transport and storage conditions on gene expression in blood samples. Biopreserv Biobank. 2016;14(2):122–8.
33. Witwer KW. Circulating microRNA biomarker studies: pitfalls and potential solutions. Clin Chem. 2015;61(1):56–63.
34. Grasedieck S, Sorrentino A, Langer C, Buske C, Dohner H, Mertens D, Kuchenbauer F. Circulating microRNAs in hematological diseases: principles, challenges, and perspectives. Blood. 2013;121(25):4977–84.
35. Keller A, Meese E. Can circulating miRNAs live up to the promise of being minimal invasive biomarkers in clinical settings? Wiley Interdiscip Rev RNA. 2016;7(2):148–56.
36. Moldovan L, Batte KE, Trgovcich J, Wisler J, Marsh CB, Piper M. Methodological challenges in utilizing miRNAs as circulating biomarkers. J Cell Mol Med. 2014;18(3):371–90.
37. Atarod S, Smith H, Dickinson A, Wang XN. MicroRNA levels quantified in whole blood varies from PBMCs. F1000Res. 2015;3:183.
38. Pritchard CC, Kroh E, Wood B, Arroyo JD, Dougherty KJ, Miyaji MM, Tait JF, Tewari M. Blood cell origin of circulating microRNAs: a cautionary note for cancer biomarker studies. Cancer Prev Res (Phila). 2012;5(3):492–7.

39. Ammari M, Jorgensen C, Apparailly F. Impact of microRNAs on the understanding and treatment of rheumatoid arthritis. Curr Opin Rheumatol. 2013;25(2):225–33.

40. Finnerty JR, Wang WX, Hebert SS, Wilfred BR, Mao G, Nelson PT. The miR-15/107 group of microRNA genes: evolutionary biology, cellular functions, and roles in human diseases. J Mol Biol. 2010;402(3):491–509.

41. Rottiers V, Naar AM. MicroRNAs in metabolism and metabolic disorders. Nat Rev Mol Cell Biol. 2012;13(4):239–50.

42. Vienberg S, Geiger J, Madsen S, Dalgaard LT. MicroRNAs in metabolism. Acta Physiol (Oxf). 2017;219(2):346–61.

43. Trajkovski M, Hausser J, Soutschek J, Bhat B, Akin A, Zavolan M, Heim MH, Stoffel M. MicroRNAs 103 and 107 regulate insulin sensitivity. Nature. 2011; 474(7353):649–53.

44. Martello G, Rosato A, Ferrari F, Manfrin A, Cordenonsi M, Dupont S, Enzo E, Guzzardo V, Rondina M, Spruce T, et al. A MicroRNA targeting dicer for metastasis control. Cell. 2010;141(7):1195–207.

45. Lu MC, Yan ST, Yin WY, Koo M, Lai NS. Risk of rheumatoid arthritis in patients with type 2 diabetes: a nationwide population-based case-control study. PLoS One. 2014;9(7), e101528.

46. Riediger ND, Lix LM, Lukianchuk V, Bruce S. Trends in diabetes and cardiometabolic conditions in a Canadian First Nation community, 2002-2003 to 2011-2012. Prev Chronic Dis. 2014;11, E198.

47. Maas K, Westfall M, Pietenpol J, Olsen NJ, Aune T. Reduced p53 in peripheral blood mononuclear cells from patients with rheumatoid arthritis is associated with loss of radiation-induced apoptosis. Arthritis Rheum. 2005;52(4):1047–57.

48. Sun Y, Cheung HS. p53, proto-oncogene and rheumatoid arthritis. Semin Arthritis Rheum. 2002;31(5):299–310.

49. Azuma-Mukai A, Oguri H, Mituyama T, Qian ZR, Asai K, Siomi H, Siomi MC. Characterization of endogenous human Argonautes and their miRNA partners in RNA silencing. Proc Natl Acad Sci U S A. 2008;105(23):7964–9.

50. Boominathan L. The tumor suppressors p53, p63, and p73 are regulators of microRNA processing complex. PLoS One. 2010;5(5), e10615.

51. Peter ME. Targeting of mRNAs by multiple miRNAs: the next step. Oncogene. 2010;29(15):2161–4.

52. Hendrickson DG, Hogan DJ, Herschlag D, Ferrell JE, Brown PO. Systematic identification of mRNAs recruited to argonaute 2 by specific microRNAs and corresponding changes in transcript abundance. PLoS One. 2008;3(5), e2126.

53. Krell J, Stebbing J, Carissimi C, Dabrowska AF, de Giorgio A, Frampton AE, Harding V, Fulci V, Macino G, Colombo T, et al. TP53 regulates miRNA association with AGO2 to remodel the miRNA-mRNA interaction network. Genome Res. 2016;26(3):331–41.

7

Resistin upregulates chemokine production by fibroblast-like synoviocytes from patients with rheumatoid arthritis

Hiroshi Sato[1,2], Sei Muraoka[2], Natsuko Kusunoki[2], Shotaro Masuoka[1,2], Soichi Yamada[1,2], Hideaki Ogasawara[3], Toshio Imai[3], Yoshikiyo Akasaka[4], Naobumi Tochigi[5], Hiroshi Takahashi[6], Kazuaki Tsuchiya[6], Shinichi Kawai[7] and Toshihiro Nanki[1,2]*

Abstract

Background: Adipokines are bioactive hormones secreted by adipose tissues. Resistin, an adipokine, plays important roles in the regulation of insulin resistance and inflammation. Resistin levels are known to be increased in the serum and synovial fluid of rheumatoid arthritis (RA) patients. However, the pathogenic role of resistin in RA has not yet been elucidated.

Methods: The expression of resistin and adenylate cyclase-associated protein 1 (CAP1), a receptor for resistin, was examined immunohistochemically in synovial tissue. CAP1 expression in in vitro cultured fibroblast-like synoviocytes (FLSs) was assessed with a reverse transcription-polymerase chain reaction (PCR) and western blotting. The gene expression of resistin-stimulated FLSs was evaluated by RNA sequencing (RNA-Seq) and quantitative real-time PCR. Concentrations of chemokine (C-X-C motif) ligand (CXCL) 8, chemokine (C-C motif) ligand (CCL) 2, interleukin (IL)-1β, IL-6 and IL-32 in culture supernatants were measured by enzyme-linked immunosorbent assay. Small interfering RNA (siRNA) for CAP1 was transfected into FLSs in order to examine inhibitory effects.

Results: The expression of resistin and CAP1 in synovial tissue was stronger in RA than in osteoarthritis (OA). Resistin was expressed by macrophages in the RA synovium, while CAP1 was expressed by macrophages, FLSs and endothelial cells. In vitro cultured RA FLSs also expressed CAP1. RNA-Seq revealed that the expression levels of 18 molecules were more than twofold higher in resistin-stimulated FLSs than in unstimulated FLSs. Seven chemokines, CXCL1, CXCL2, CXCL3, CXCL5, CXCL6, CXCL8, and CCL2, were included among the 18 molecules. Increases induced in the expression of CXCL1, CXCL8, and CCL2 by the resistin stimulation were confirmed by real-time PCR. The stimulation with resistin increased the protein levels of CXCL8 and CCL2 produced by RA FLSs, and the upregulated expression of CXCL8 was inhibited by the abrogation of CAP1 by siRNA for CAP1. Production of IL-6 by FLSs was also increased by resistin. Expression of IL-1β and IL-32 was not detected by ELISA.

Conclusions: Resistin contributes to the pathogenesis of RA by increasing chemokine production by FLSs via CAP1 in synovial tissue.

Keywords: Resistin, Adenylate cyclase-associated protein 1, Rheumatoid arthritis, Chemokine, Fibroblast-like synoviocytes, RNA sequencing

* Correspondence: toshihiro.nanki@med.toho-u.ac.jp
[1]Department of Internal Medicine, Graduate School of Medicine, Toho University, Tokyo, Japan
[2]Division of Rheumatology, Department of Internal Medicine, Toho University School of Medicine, 6-11-1 Omori-Nishi, Ota-ku, Tokyo 143-8541, Japan
Full list of author information is available at the end of the article

Background

Adipokines are bioactive hormones secreted by adipose tissues. More than 600 adipokines have been identified to date (e.g. adiponectin, leptin, tumor necrosis factor α, interleukin (IL)-1, IL-6, apelin, visfatin, and resistin) [1, 2]. Resistin was discovered as a protein secreted by differentiated 3T3-L1 cells, and its expression was found to be downregulated by treatment with thiazolidinedione rosiglitazone [3]. In mice, resistin is mainly expressed by mature adipocytes in white adipose tissue. In contrast, resistin in humans is mainly expressed by monocytes and macrophages and less so by adipocytes [4]. Therefore, resistin may contribute not only to insulin resistance, but also inflammation.

Rheumatoid arthritis (RA) is characterized by chronic polyarthritis. Inflammatory mediators, such as cytokines and chemokines, contribute to the pathogenesis of RA. The immunomodulatory properties of adipokines in RA have been evaluated [5]. Adiponectin enhances the production of proinflammatory factors (IL-6 and chemokine (C-X-C motif) ligand (CXCL) 8), vascular endothelial growth factor, and matrix metalloproteinases (MMPs) by fibroblast-like synoviocytes (FLSs) [6–8]. Previous meta-analyses revealed that serum resistin levels are higher in patients with RA than in healthy controls [9]. Furthermore, we previously demonstrated that the serum level of resistin is positively associated with serum C-reactive protein levels in patients with RA [10], while another group showed that the concentration of resistin is elevated in the synovial fluid in RA [11]. However, the pathogenic role of resistin in RA has not yet been elucidated.

In the present study, we examined the stimulatory effects of resistin on FLSs from patients with RA using RNA sequencing (RNA-Seq). We found that the expression of chemokines was increased in resistin-stimulated FLSs.

Methods

Samples

Synovial tissues were obtained from patients with RA and with osteoarthritis (OA) who underwent total knee or hip replacement. FLSs were prepared from synovial tissues as described previously [12]. FLSs from RA synovial tissues were also obtained from the Japanese Collection of Research Bioresources Cell Bank. The experimental protocol was approved in advance by the Ethics Committees of Toho Medical Center Omori Hospital (M16020) and the Ethics Committees of the Faculty of Medicine, Toho University (27060, 2703024007).

Immunohistochemical assessment

Synovial tissues were fixed with freshly prepared 4% (v/v) paraformaldehyde in Tris-buffered saline. Sections (3 μm) were immersed in ethanol containing 3% (v/v) H_2O_2 for 30 min to block endogenous peroxidase activity. Sections were incubated with protein block serum-free (Agilent Technologies) for 30 min to block non-specific binding. Sections were subsequently incubated at 4 °C overnight with a rabbit anti-resistin polyclonal antibody (pAb) (Bioss Antibodies), rabbit anti-adenylyl cyclase-associated protein 1 (CAP1) monoclonal antibody (mAb) (EPR8339(B); Abcam), or isotype control (Agilent Technologies) as a primary antibody. Expression was detected using an EnVision + kit™ (Agilent Technologies) and counterstained with hematoxylin.

Non-specific binding was blocked with protein block serum-free for immunofluorescence double staining, and sections were incubated at 4 °C overnight with rabbit anti-resistin pAb or CAP1 mAb. Samples were subsequently incubated at room temperature with biotinylated anti-rabbit IgG for 40 min followed by Fluorescein Avidin D (Vector laboratories) for 20 min. Samples were incubated with mouse anti-CD68 mAb (KP1; Abcam), mouse anti-cadherin-11 mAb (16A; Acris Antibodies), or mouse anti-von Willebrand factor (vWF) mAb (F8/86; Agilent Technologies) and then with a Texas Red® horse anti-mouse IgG antibody at room temperature for 20 min. A nuclear stain was performed with 4′, 6-diamidino-2-phenylindole. Slides were examined using the BX61 (Olympus). To determine the percentages of CAP1-expressing cells, the number of CAP1-positive cells in the lining layer, and in the CD68-positive or cadherin-11-positive cells was counted under fluorescence microscope.

RNA extraction

FLSs were seeded in Roswell Park Memorial Institute (RPMI) 1640 medium containing 10% fetal bovine serum (FBS) in 10-cm dishes (1×10^6 cells/dish), and were then incubated with 1000 ng/ml resistin (PeproTech) for 18 h. Total RNA was isolated from FLSs using TRIzol® (Invitrogen) according to the manufacturer's instructions. RNA samples were digested with an RNase-free DNase set (Qiagen) to remove genomic DNA and further purified using the RNeasy kit (Qiagen). The quality of RNA samples was examined by the Agilent 2100 Bioanalyzer (Agilent Technologies) using RNA 6000 NanoChips. RNA samples with an RNA integrity number higher than 7 were used in further analyses, including a RNA-Seq and real-time polymerase chain reaction (PCR).

RNA-Seq transcriptome analysis

The RNA-Seq library was prepared using the SureSelect Strand-Specific RNA Library Prep Kit (Agilent Technologies) in accordance with the manufacturer's instructions optimized to Illumina Multiplexed Sequencing. After purification of the amplified libraries, the DNA quality of products was assessed using the 2100 Bioanalyzer DNA 1000 Assay. Paired-end sequencing of the

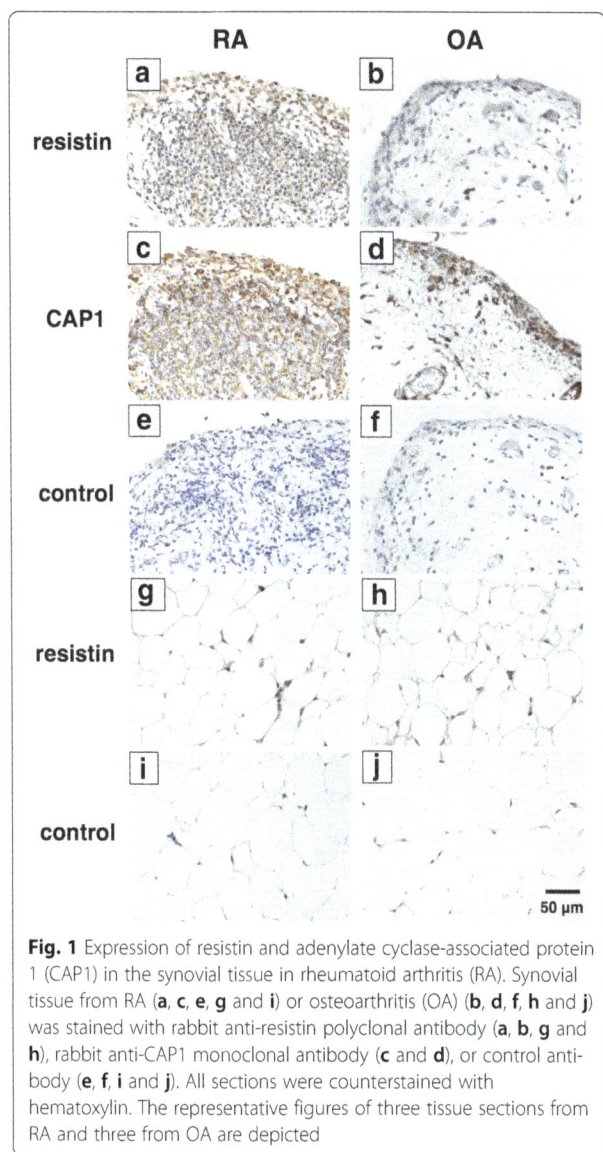

Fig. 1 Expression of resistin and adenylate cyclase-associated protein 1 (CAP1) in the synovial tissue in rheumatoid arthritis (RA). Synovial tissue from RA (**a**, **c**, **e**, **g** and **i**) or osteoarthritis (OA) (**b**, **d**, **f**, **h** and **j**) was stained with rabbit anti-resistin polyclonal antibody (**a**, **b**, **g** and **h**), rabbit anti-CAP1 monoclonal antibody (**c** and **d**), or control antibody (**e**, **f**, **i** and **j**). All sections were counterstained with hematoxylin. The representative figures of three tissue sections from RA and three from OA are depicted

RNA-seq libraries was performed using an Illumina MiSeq system (Illumina; 2×75 bases paired-end run). FASTQ files were imported into CLC Genomics Workbench v9.01 software (CLC bio) for post-processing and data analysis. Sequences were trimmed based on the FASTQC report and mapped onto annotated human genes with support from reference human genome (hg19). Data were normalized by total reads per million and analyzed for differential gene expression empirical analysis of differential gene expression subroutine based on reads per kilobase of transcript per million reads mapped (RPKM).

Quantitative real-time PCR
Total RNA samples were reverse transcribed into cDNA using random primers and an RNA PCR Kit (AMV) Ver.3.0 (Takara Bio Inc.). CXCL1, CXCL8, and chemokine (C-C motif) ligand (CCL) 2 levels were measured using the Power SYBR Green PCR Master Mix (Applied Biosystems). The following primers were used for analyses: 5′-TGC AGG GAA TTC ACC CCA AG-3′ and 5′-CAG GGC CTC CTT CAG GAA CA-3′ for CXCL1; 5′-ACT CCA AAC CTT TCC ACC CCA-3′ and 5′-TTT CCT TGG GGT CCA GAC AGA-3′ for CXCL8; 5′-CTT CTG TGC CTG CTG CTC AT-3′ and 5′-CGG AGT TTG GGT TTG CTT GTC-3′ for CCL2; 5′-GAA GGT GAA GGT CGG AGT CA-3′ and 5′-GAG GTC AAT GAA GGG GTC AT-3′ for glyceraldehyde-3-phosphate dehydrogenase (GAPDH). The Prism 7500 Fast Real-time PCR system (Applied Biosystems) was used for analyses, and the mRNA levels of the genes tested were represented as relative values to the expression level of GAPDH.

Reverse transcription (RT)-PCR
Total RNA was extracted with an RNeasy Mini kit (Qiagen) from the cultured FLSs of patients with RA. RT was performed using a SuperScript first-strand synthesis system for RT-PCR according to the recommendations of the manufacturer (Invitrogen) with 1 μg of total RNA from FLSs. Equal amounts of each RT product were amplified by PCR with HotStarTaq® DNA polymerase (Qiagen). The primer sequences and numbers of base pairs (bp) were as follows: for CAP1 (118 bp), 5′-AGG CAT TTG ACT CGC TGC TTG and 5′- TCG CTC CAA CTT CAA ACC TGT G; and for GAPDH (598 bp), 5′- CCA CCC ATG GCA AAT TCC ATG GCA and 5′-TCT AGA CGG CAG GTC AGG TCC ACC. After initial denaturation at 95 °C for 15 min, PCR involved amplification for 32 cycles at 95 °C for 30 s, at 56 °C for 30 s, and at 72 °C for 45 s, followed by elongation at 72 °C for 5 min. Amplified DNA fragments were resolved by electrophoresis on a 2% agarose gel, and were detected under ultraviolet light using LAS-3000 (Fujifilm) after staining the gel with ethidium bromide.

Western blot analysis
The western blotting procedure was previously described [13]. Membranes were incubated with rabbit anti-CAP1 mAb (EPR8339(B); Abcam) or rabbit anti-GAPDH pAb (Santa Cruz Biotechnology), with a dilution of 1:1000 (CAP1) and 1:100 (GAPDH), the secondary antibody (horseradish peroxidase-conjugated goat anti-rabbit antibody) was added (at a dilution of 1:2000), and an incubation was performed for 3 h using the iBind Flex Western System (Thermo Fisher Scientific). Protein bands were detected with the enhanced Novex® ECL Chemiluminescent Substrate Reagent Kit (Invitrogen) using LAS-3000 (Fujifilm).

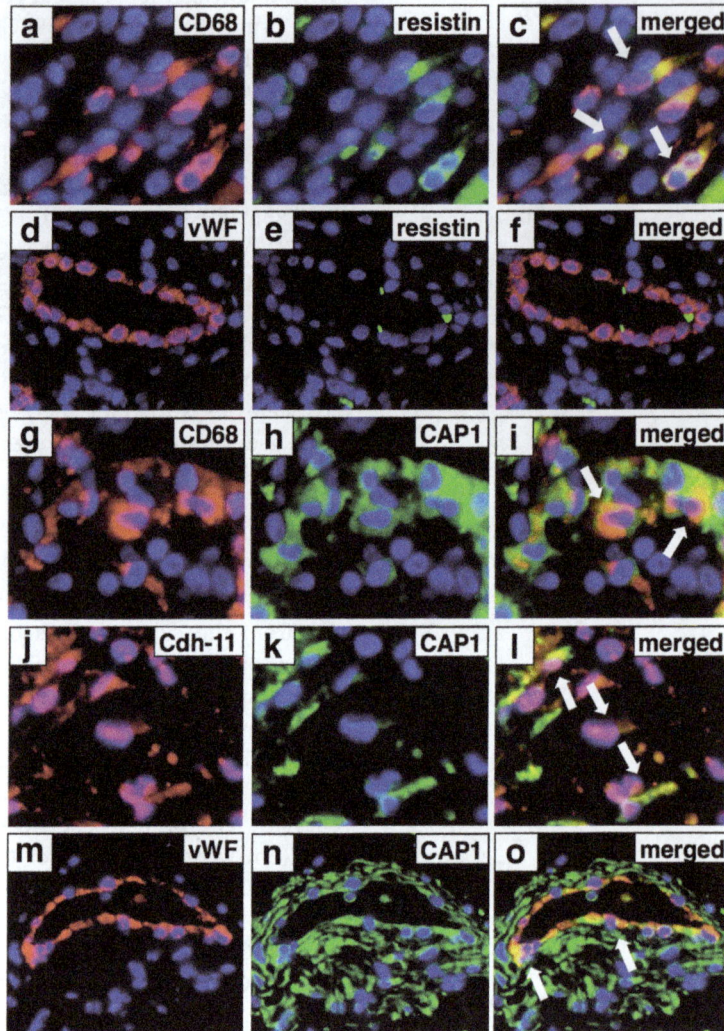

Fig. 2 Resistin-expressing and adenylate cyclase-associated protein 1 (CAP1)-expressing cells in synovial tissues in rheumatoid arthritis (RA). Sections of synovial tissue from RA were double-stained with resistin, and CD68 or von Willebrand factor (vWF) (CD68 (**a**); resistin (**b**); merge of **a** with **b** (**c**); vWF (**d**); resistin (**e**); merge of **d** with **e** (**f**)), and CAP1, and CD68, cadherin-11 or vWF (CD68 (**g**); CAP1 (**h**); merge of **g** with **h** (**i**); cadherin-11 (**j**); CAP1 (**k**); merge of **j** with **k** (**l**); vWF (**m**); CAP1 (**n**); merge of **m** with **n** (**o**)). Arrows indicate double-positive cells in the merged image. Cdh-11, cadherin-11

Enzyme-linked immunosorbent assay (ELISA)

FLSs were cultured overnight in 96-well plates (2×10^4 cells/well) and then incubated with recombinant human resistin (0, 10, 100, or 1000 ng/ml; PeproTech) at 37 °C for 24 h in RPMI1640 medium containing 1% FBS. Concentrations of CXCL8, CCL2, IL-1β, IL-6, and IL-32 in culture supernatants were assessed using the ELISA kit (R&D Systems), according to the instructions of the manufacturer.

Signaling pathway of resistin via CAP1

Stealth RNAi™ small interfering RNA (siRNA) targeting CAP1 and negative control siRNA were purchased from Thermo Fisher Scientific. Lipofectamine® RNAiMAX reagent (Thermo Fisher Scientific) was used to formulate transfecting siRNAs. FLSs were transfected with siRNA at 37 °C for 48 h, and cells were then treated with resistin (PeproTech) for another 24 h. CXCL8 concentrations in the culture supernatant were assessed by ELISA.

Statistical analysis

Results are expressed as the mean +/- standard error (SE). Statistical analyses were performed using StatFlex software (ver. 6; ARTEC). The production of CXCL8, CCL2, and IL-6 was analyzed by analysis of variance using Dunnett's test. The paired t test was applied to compare CXCL8 production between control siRNA-transfected and CAP1 siRNA-transfected cells. In all analyses, $p < 0.05$ was considered to indicate significance.

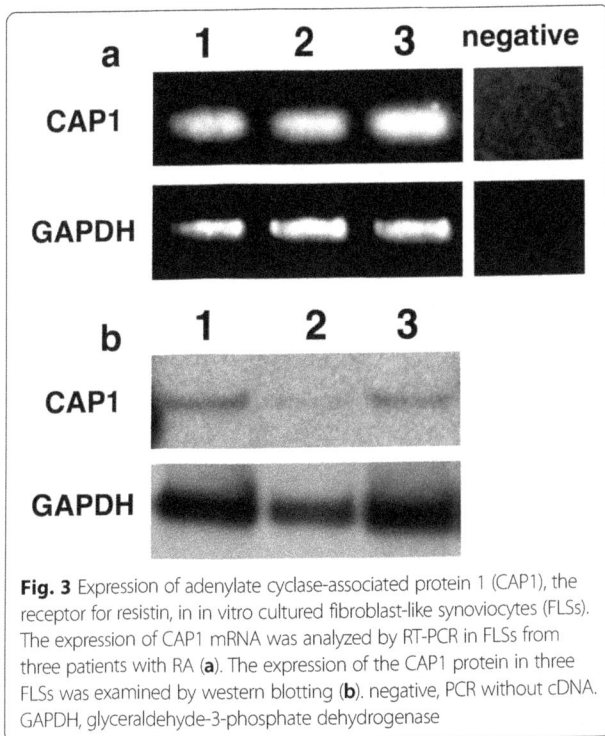

Fig. 3 Expression of adenylate cyclase-associated protein 1 (CAP1), the receptor for resistin, in in vitro cultured fibroblast-like synoviocytes (FLSs). The expression of CAP1 mRNA was analyzed by RT-PCR in FLSs from three patients with RA (**a**). The expression of the CAP1 protein in three FLSs was examined by western blotting (**b**). negative, PCR without cDNA. GAPDH, glyceraldehyde-3-phosphate dehydrogenase

Results

Expression of resistin and CAP1 in synovial tissues of RA

We immunohistochemically investigated the expression of resistin and CAP1 in synovial tissues harvested from patients with RA and with OA. Resistin was strongly expressed in the synovial lining and sub-lining cells of synovial tissue in RA (Fig. 1a), while resistin expression was minimal in the synovium in OA (Fig. 1b). On the other hand, the expression of CAP1 was observed in the lining and sub-lining cells of the synovium in RA (Fig. 1c), while CAP1 was expressed in the lining cells of the synovium in OA (Fig. 1d). In fat tissue around the synovial tissue, resisitin was weakly expressed in RA and OA (Fig. 1g and h).

We performed double immunohistochemical assessment to identify resistin-expressing and CAP1-expressing cells in the synovium in RA. As shown in Fig. 2, resistin was expressed by CD68[+] macrophages (Fig. 2a-c). However, resistin was not expressed by vWF[+] endothelial cells (Fig. 2d-f). CAP1 was expressed by CD68[+] macrophages (Fig. 2g-i) and also by cadherin-11[+] FLSs (Fig. 2j-l) and vWF[+] endothelial cells (Fig. 2m-o) in synovial tissues in RA. The percentage of CAP1-positive cells was 94% (187/200) in the lining layer. The frequency of CAP1-positive cells in CD68[+] cells was 97%

Table 1 Increased gene expression by resistin-stimulated RA FLSs

Gene	Description	Fold change (resistin/not stimulated)				RPKM						Ensembl gene ID
						Lot 1		Lot 2		Lot 3		
		Lot 1	Lot 2	Lot 3	Mean	Non	RS	Non	RS	Non	RS	
CXCL5	C-X-C motif chemokine ligand 5	3.51	31.88	3.40	12.93	0.088	0.310	0.151	4.822	0.245	0.832	ENSG00000163735
CXCL6	C-X-C motif chemokine ligand 6	7.76	20.32	3.76	10.61	0.205	1.594	0.106	2.144	0.821	3.089	ENSG00000124875
IL34	Interleukin 34	17.56	5.63	2.37	8.52	0.033	0.588	0.172	0.967	0.309	0.732	ENSG00000157368
CXCL1	C-X-C motif chemokine ligand 1	3.13	18.39	3.63	8.39	2.538	7.952	1.066	19.609	3.991	14.506	ENSG00000163739
CXCL8	C-X-C motif chemokine ligand 8	5.07	10.25	4.21	6.51	0.592	3.002	1.384	14.183	1.152	4.853	ENSG00000169429
BIRC3	Baculoviral IAP repeat containing 3	3.44	7.06	6.42	5.64	0.230	0.789	0.195	1.376	0.129	0.828	ENSG00000023445
IL1B	Interleukin 1 beta	2.20	10.47	4.12	5.59	0.097	0.212	0.149	1.558	0.134	0.550	ENSG00000125538
AFP	Alpha fetoprotein	4.39	6.56	2.57	4.51	0.023	0.101	0.024	0.155	0.106	0.272	ENSG00000081051
SOD2	Superoxide dismutase 2	3.27	5.33	3.63	4.08	4.587	15.002	4.327	23.048	5.692	20.663	ENSG00000112096
CCL2	C-C motif chemokine ligand 2	2.31	5.80	2.89	3.66	20.170	46.526	23.381	135.522	16.826	48.585	ENSG00000108691
ANXA8L1	Annexin A8 like 1	2.63	3.19	4.94	3.59	0.035	0.093	0.180	0.575	0.032	0.160	ENSG00000264230
SLC5A2	Solute carrier family 5 member 2	3.51	2.11	4.94	3.52	0.017	0.059	0.069	0.145	0.015	0.076	ENSG00000140675
CXCL3	C-X-C motif chemokine ligand 3	3.95	3.09	2.63	3.23	0.270	1.065	0.346	1.071	0.466	1.228	ENSG00000163734
ZNF296	Zinc finger protein 296	2.05	3.75	2.96	2.92	0.129	0.263	0.088	0.330	0.119	0.352	ENSG00000170684
ICAM1	Intercellular adhesion molecule 1	2.29	3.56	2.43	2.76	2.380	5.455	2.590	9.227	1.935	4.705	ENSG00000090339
IL32	Interleukin 32	3.25	2.33	2.39	2.66	0.690	2.245	3.020	7.042	1.061	2.539	ENSG00000008517
LY75	Lymphocyte antigen 75	2.63	2.81	2.30	2.58	0.016	0.042	0.024	0.069	0.044	0.101	ENSG00000054219
CXCL2	C-X-C motif chemokine ligand 2	2.07	2.29	2.33	2.23	0.698	1.444	0.819	1.872	1.011	2.361	ENSG00000081041

FLSs fibroblast-like synoviocytes, *RA* rheumatoid arthritis, *RPKM* reads per kilobase of transcript per million reads mapped, *RS* resistin-stimulated, *Non* non-stimulated. FLSs from synovial tissue in RA were incubated with 1000 ng/ml resistin for 18 h. mRNA expression was analyzed by next-generation sequencing. Genes with expression levels that were more than twofold higher in resistin-stimulated FLSs than in unstimulated FLSs are shown

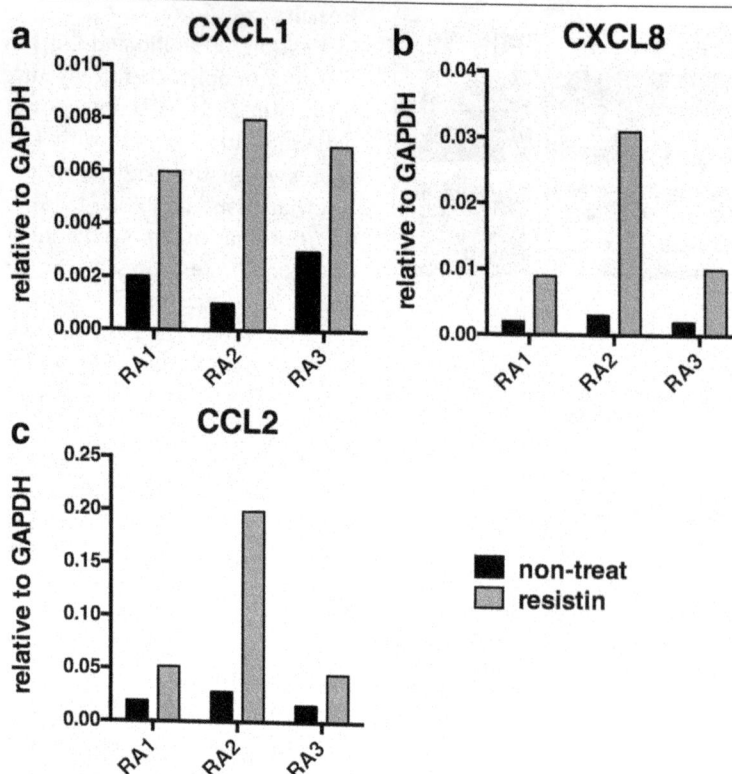

Fig. 4 Increased chemokine expression by fibroblast-like synoviocytes (FLSs) from patients with rheumatoid arthritis (RA) with resistin stimulation. FLSs were incubated with 1000 ng/ml resistin for 18 h. The mRNA expression of CXCL1 (**a**), CXCL8 (**b**), and CCL2 (**c**) by FLSs from three patients with RA was measured using quantitative real-time reverse transcription PCR. GAPDH, glyceraldehyde-3-phosphate dehydrogenase

(97/100) in the lining layer and 95% (95/100) in the sub-lining layer. The percentage of CAP1-positive cells in cadherin-11$^+$ cells was 95% (95/100) in the lining layer and 81% (81/100) in the sub-lining layer.

CAP1 expression in cultured FLSs established from synovial tissue in RA was evaluated with RT-PCR and western blotting. The mRNA and protein expression of CAP1 was also observed in in vitro cultured FLSs (Fig. 3).

Stimulatory effects of resistin on FLSs in RA

We examined the stimulatory effects of resistin on FLSs in vitro. FLSs were incubated with 1000 ng/ml resistin for 18 h. Total RNA was extracted from the cells, and complementary DNA (cDNA) was synthesized. The nucleotide sequence of cDNA was analyzed by next-generation sequencing and expression levels were compared between unstimulated and resistin-stimulated FLSs. As shown in Table 1, the expression levels of 18 molecules were more than twofold higher in all three lots of resistin-stimulated FLSs than in unstimulated FLSs. Seven chemokines, CXCL1, CXCL2, CXCL3, CXCL5, CXCL6, CXCL8, and CCL2 were included among the 18 molecules.

We also analyzed CXCL1, CXCL8, and CCL2 expression by quantitative real-time RT-PCR using three lots of FLSs from patients with RA. The expression of CXCL1, CXCL8, and CCL2 increased in all three lots of FLSs following the resistin stimulation (Fig. 4).

Chemokine production by the resistin-CAP1 pathway

We examined the protein levels of chemokine expression by resistin-stimulated FLSs in vitro. FLSs were incubated with various concentrations of resistin for 24 h. The concentrations of CXCL8 and CCL2, which were observed as upregulated chemokines by RNA-seq and real-time RT-PCR, were assessed in culture supernatants using ELISA kits. The CXCL8 level was significantly increased by the stimulation with resistin (Fig. 5a). CCL2 expression was dose-dependently increased by resistin (Fig. 5b). We also analyzed expression of IL-1β and IL-32, which were identified as upregulated cytokines by RNA-seq (Table 1), and IL-6, which was identified as a slightly upregulated cytokine by RNA-seq (fold change 1.969, 3.721, and 1.997 in each lot). IL-1β and IL-32 were not detected by ELISA with or without stimulation with resistin. The concentration of IL-6 was increased by resistin (Fig. 5c).

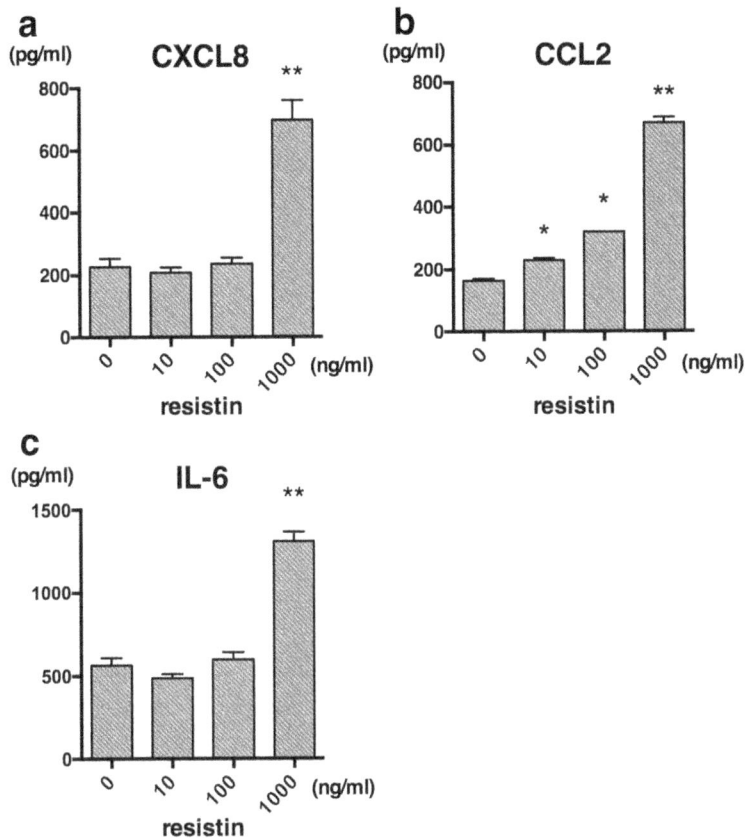

Fig. 5 CXCL8, CCL2 and IL-6 expression by resistin-stimulated fibroblast-like synoviocytes (FLSs) from patients with rheumatoid arthritis (RA). FLSs from patients with RA were incubated with resistin (10–1000 ng/ml) for 24 h, and the concentrations of CXCL8 (**a**), CCL2 (**b**), and IL-6 (**c**) in the culture supernatant were measured by ELISA. Data are the mean +/- SE for one of three independent experiments analyzed in triplicate: *$p < 0.05$, **$p < 0.01$, versus no stimulation

In order to verify the involvement of CAP1 in the resistin stimulation, siRNA for CAP1 was transfected into RA FLSs. The FLSs were pretreated with CAP1 siRNA or control siRNA. The transfection of CAP1 siRNA significantly decreased CAP1 expression from that with the transfection of control siRNA (Fig. 6a). Resistin-induced CXCL8 production by FLSs was significantly inhibited by the abrogation of CAP1 by siRNA (Fig. 6b). These results indicate that the resistin-CAP1 pathway contributes to chemokine production by RA FLSs.

Discussion

The purpose of the present study was to elucidate the role of resistin in the pathogenesis of RA. We found that the expression of resistin was increased in synovial tissue in RA, and stimulation with resistin enhanced the production of various chemokines by FLSs via CAP1. These results suggest that resistin contributes to inflammatory cell infiltration into synovial tissue in RA through chemokine production by FLSs.

We previously reported that serum resistin levels are associated with C-reactive protein levels [10]. In the present study, we showed that resistin was strongly

expressed in macrophages in synovial tissue in RA, which is consistent with previous findings [11]. A recent study reported that CAP1 is a functional receptor for resistin in THP-1 cells [14]. We found that CAP1 is more abundantly expressed in synovial tissue in RA than in OA. CAP1 is expressed by macrophages, FLSs and endothelial cells in synovial tissue in RA, and in in vitro cultured FLSs. These results suggest that resistin, an adipokine, stimulates CAP1-expressing macrophages, FLSs and endothelial cells in synovial tissue in RA. CAP1 expression in HP-AEpiC cells is decreased by treatment with matrix metalloproteinase 9 (MMP-9) [15]. On the other hand, we examined CAP1 expression on FLSs treated with TNF-α, IL-1β and resistin. These stimulations did not alter CAP1 expression significantly (data not shown). Regulation of CAP1 expression in the RA synovial cells has not been elucidated.

Toll-like receptor 4 (TLR4), decorin and receptor tyrosine kinase like orphan receptor 1 (ROR1) were reported as putative receptors for resistin [16–18]. Lee et al. [14] identified CAP1 as a functional receptor for resistin on monocytes. Abrogation of CAP1 inhibited production of inflammatory cytokines and cellular migration by

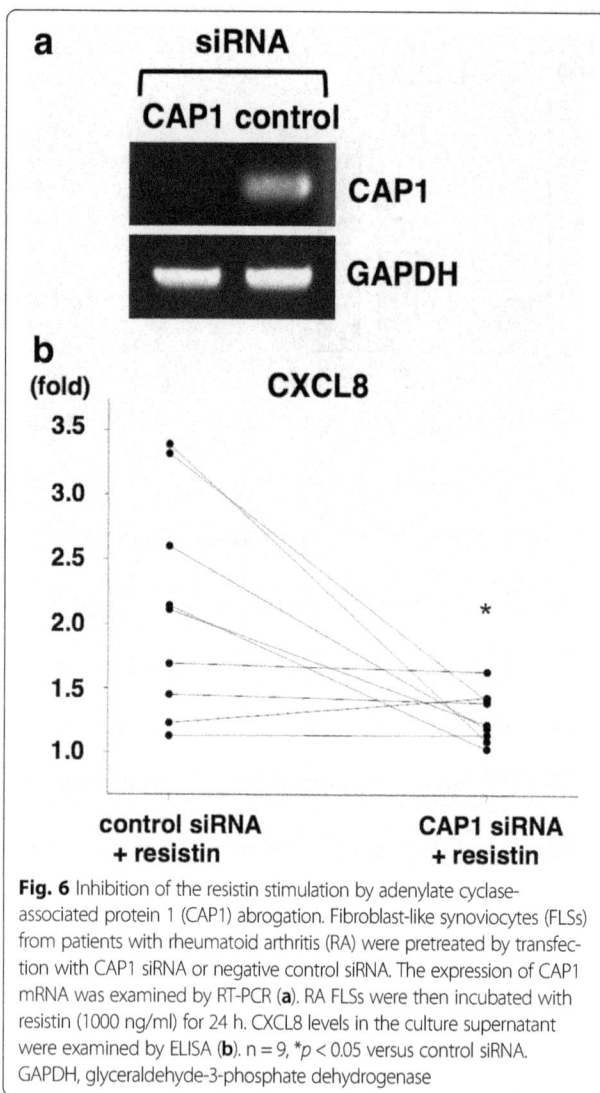

Fig. 6 Inhibition of the resistin stimulation by adenylate cyclase-associated protein 1 (CAP1) abrogation. Fibroblast-like synoviocytes (FLSs) from patients with rheumatoid arthritis (RA) were pretreated by transfection with CAP1 siRNA or negative control siRNA. The expression of CAP1 mRNA was examined by RT-PCR (**a**). RA FLSs were then incubated with resistin (1000 ng/ml) for 24 h. CXCL8 levels in the culture supernatant were examined by ELISA (**b**). n = 9, *$p < 0.05$ versus control siRNA. GAPDH, glyceraldehyde-3-phosphate dehydrogenase

chemokines could promote angiogenesis [20]. Chemokines upregulated by resistin stimulation in the present study were mostly ELR^+ C-X-C motif chemokines. Therefore, resistin may be involved in angiogenesis and inflammatory cell accumulation, in the synovial tissue in RA via ELR^+ C-X-C motif chemokine production.

In the present study, we also demonstrated that stimulation with resistin increased CXCL8 and CCL2 production by FLSs. Abrogation of CAP1 inhibited the resistin-enhanced CXCL8 production. These results indicate that CAP1 is a functional receptor for resistin on FLSs. CXCL8 has been reported to induce angiogenesis and exerts chemotactic effects on neutrophils and dendritic cells [21, 22]. Furthermore, the inhibition of CXCL8 has been reported to suppress $CD14^+$ monocyte-osteoclast differentiation in anti-cyclic citrullinated peptide antibody-positive RA [23]. CXCL8 is strongly expressed in the synovial tissue of patients with RA with a high level of disease activity [24]. Therefore, CXCL8 may be involved in angiogenesis, inflammatory cell migration, and osteoclast differentiation in synovial tissue in RA. CCL2 is also strongly expressed in the synovial tissue [25] and synovial fluid of patients with RA [26]. CCL2 induces the migration and infiltration of monocytes and macrophages [27]. In addition, stimulation with CCL2 enhances the production of IL-6 and CXCL8 by FLSs [28]. CCL2 may be involved in monocyte/macrophage migration and inflammatory molecule production in the synovium in RA. CXCL1 is also increased in the serum, synovial fluid, and synovial tissue of patients with RA [29], and is produced by synovial neutrophils, macrophages, and FLSs [29, 30]. CXCL2 is produced by FLSs in the synovium in RA [31]. CXCL1 and CXCL2 are involved in the migration of neutrophils, proliferation of FLSs, and angiogenesis. CXCL5 is increased in synovial fluid and synovial tissue in RA, and is involved in neutrophil infiltration and angiogenesis [32]. Taken together, resistin contributes to the pathogenesis of RA via chemokine production by FLSs, which may be involved in angiogenesis, inflammatory cell migration, production of inflammatory molecules, and osteoclastogenesis.

In addition, stimulation with resistin upregulated production of IL-6 by RA FLSs. IL-6 might also contribute to chronic inflammation in RA. Increased IL-6 may induce chemokine production by FLSs. However, it is also possible that chemokines upregulated by resistin induced IL-6 production [28].

In the present study, we examined the stimulatory effects of resistin on FLSs. However, macrophages and endothelial cells in the synovial tissue in RA also expressed CAP1. Therefore, further studies are needed

stimulation with resistin. However, abrogation of TLR4, decorin and ROR1 had little effect on the resistin stimulation. Based on the results, we thought that CAP1 is a functional receptor for resistin. However, the function of TLR4, decorin and ROR1 for resistin on FLSs has not been clarified yet. We have found that at least TLR4 was expressed on FLSs. Therefore, further study is needed to show the function of the three putative receptors against resistin stimulation on FLSs.

Using RNA-seq, we found that the stimulation with resistin enhanced the expression of 18 genes by FLSs in vitro. Seven chemokines, CXCL1, CXCL2, CXCL3, CXCL5, CXCL6, CXCL8, and CCL2, were included. Furthermore, six out of the seven chemokines were C-X-C motif chemokines. Several C-X-C motif chemokines (CXCL1, CXCL2, CXCL3, CXCL5, CXCL6, CXCL7, and CXCL8) contain an ELR motif (Glu-Leu-Arg) at the NH2 terminus [19]. These ELR^+ C-X-C motif in order to elucidate the effects of resistin on macrophages and endothelial cells in RA. We also need to compare resistin and CAP1 expression between early and late RA, and also analyze the effect of treatment to resistin and CAP1 expression to reveal the role of the resistin-CAP1 pathway in the pathogenesis of RA.

Conclusion

The present results suggest that resistin expressed in synovial tissue in RA contributes to RA pathogenesis by enhancing chemokine production by FLSs in synovial tissue.

Abbreviations

bp: Base pairs; CAP1: Adenylate cyclase-associated protein 1; CCL: Chemokine (C-C motif) ligand; CXCL: Chemokine (C-X-C motif) ligand; ELISA: Enzyme-linked immunosorbent assay; FBS: Fetal bovine serum; FLSs: Fibroblast-like synoviocytes; GAPDH: Glyceraldehyde-3-phosphate dehydrogenase; IL: Interleukin; mAb: Monoclonal antibody; MMP: Matrix metalloproteinase; OA: Osteoarthritis; pAb: Polyclonal antibody; PCR: Polymerase chain reaction; RA: Rheumatoid arthritis; RNA-Seq: RNA sequencing; ROR1: Receptor tyrosine kinase like orphan receptor 1; RPKM: Reads per kilobase of transcript per million reads mapped; RPMI: Roswell Park Memorial Institute; RT: Reverse transcription; SE: Standard error; siRNA: Small interfering RNA; TLR4: Toll-like receptor 4; TNF: Tumor necrosis factor; vWF: von Willebrand factor

Acknowledgements
We thank Sonoko Sakurai for her secretarial assistance and Kayo Tsuburaya for her excellent assistance with immunohistochemical analysis.

Funding
This study was supported by Project Research Grants (27-17 and 28-36) from Toho University School of Medicine to HS, a Research Promotion Grant from Toho University Graduate School of Medicine (No. 17-01) to TN, the Program for the Strategic Research Foundation for Private Universities (S1411015) from the Ministry of Education, Culture, Sports, Science, and Technology, Japan to TN, and the Private University Research Branding Project from the Ministry of Education, Culture, Sports, Science, and Technology, Japan to TN.

Authors' contributions
HS participated in the design of the study, performed the experiments and statistical analyses, and drafted the manuscript. SMu participated in the design of the study, assisted in technical support and data interpretation, and revised the manuscript. NK, HO, and YA performed the experiments, and helped in the preparation of the manuscript. SMa, SY, and TI assisted in performing the experiments, and revised the manuscript. NT, HT, and KT provided samples, assisted in performing the experiments, and revised the manuscript. SK conceived the study, participated in its design, and revised the manuscript. TN conceived the study, participated in its design and coordination, and helped to draft the manuscript. All authors read and approved the final manuscript for publication.

Competing interests
The authors declare that they have no competing interests.

Author details
[1]Department of Internal Medicine, Graduate School of Medicine, Toho University, Tokyo, Japan. [2]Division of Rheumatology, Department of Internal Medicine, Toho University School of Medicine, 6-11-1 Omori-Nishi, Ota-ku, Tokyo 143-8541, Japan. [3]KAN Research Institute Inc, 6-8-2 Minatojima-minamimachi, Chuo-Ku, Kobe 650-0047, Japan. [4]Unit of Regenerative Diseases Research, Division of Research Promotion and Development, Advanced Medical Research Center, Toho University Graduate School of Medicine, Tokyo, Japan. [5]Department of Surgical Pathology, Toho University School of Medicine, Tokyo, Japan. [6]Department of Orthopedic Surgery, Toho University School of Medicine, Tokyo, Japan. [7]Department of Inflammation and Pain Control Research, Toho University School of Medicine, Tokyo, Japan.

References
1. Van de Voorde J, Pauwels B, Boydens C, Decaluwe K. Adipocytokines in relation to cardiovascular disease. Metabolism. 2013;62(11):1513–21.
2. Bluher M. Adipokines - removing road blocks to obesity and diabetes therapy. Mol Metab. 2014;3(3):230–40.
3. Steppan CM, Bailey ST, Bhat S, Brown EJ, Banerjee RR, Wright CM, Patel HR, Ahima RS, Lazar MA. The hormone resistin links obesity to diabetes. Nature. 2001;409(6818):307–12.
4. Filkova M, Haluzik M, Gay S, Senolt L. The role of resistin as a regulator of inflammation: Implications for various human pathologies. Clin Immunol. 2009;133(2):157–70.
5. Neumann E, Junker S, Schett G, Frommer K, Muller-Ladner U. Adipokines in bone disease. Nat Rev Rheumatol. 2016;12(5):296–302.
6. Tang CH, Chiu YC, Tan TW, Yang RS, Fu WM. Adiponectin enhances IL-6 production in human synovial fibroblast via an AdipoR1 receptor, AMPK, p38, and NF-kappa B pathway. J Immunol. 2007;179(8):5483–92.
7. Choi HM, Lee YA, Lee SH, Hong SJ, Hahm DH, Choi SY, Yang HI, Yoo MC, Kim KS. Adiponectin may contribute to synovitis and joint destruction in rheumatoid arthritis by stimulating vascular endothelial growth factor, matrix metalloproteinase-1, and matrix metalloproteinase-13 expression in fibroblast-like synoviocytes more than proinflammatory mediators. Arthritis Res Ther. 2009;11(6):R161.
8. Kitahara K, Kusunoki N, Kakiuchi T, Suguro T, Kawai S. Adiponectin stimulates IL-8 production by rheumatoid synovial fibroblasts. Biochem Biophys Res Commun. 2009;378(2):218–23.
9. Huang Q, Tao SS, Zhang YJ, Zhang C, Li LJ, Zhao W, Zhao MQ, Li P, Pan HF, Mao C, et al. Serum resistin levels in patients with rheumatoid arthritis and systemic lupus erythematosus: a meta-analysis. Clin Rheumatol. 2015;34(10):1713–20.
10. Yoshino T, Kusunoki N, Tanaka N, Kaneko K, Kusunoki Y, Endo H, Hasunuma T, Kawai S. Elevated serum levels of resistin, leptin, and adiponectin are associated with C-reactive protein and also other clinical conditions in rheumatoid arthritis. Intern Med. 2011;50(4):269–75.
11. Senolt L, Housa D, Vernerova Z, Jirasek T, Svobodova R, Veigl D, Anderlova K, Muller-Ladner U, Pavelka K, Haluzik M. Resistin in rheumatoid arthritis synovial tissue, synovial fluid and serum. Ann Rheum Dis. 2007;66(4):458–63.
12. Kusunoki N, Yamazaki R, Kawai S. Induction of apoptosis in rheumatoid synovial fibroblasts by celecoxib, but not by other selective cyclooxygenase 2 inhibitors. Arthritis Rheum. 2002;46(12):3159–67.
13. Shindo E, Nanki T, Kusunoki N, Shikano K, Kawazoe M, Sato H, Kaneko K, Muraoka S, Kaburaki M, Akasaka Y, et al. The growth factor midkine may play a pathophysiological role in rheumatoid arthritis. Mod Rheumatol. 2017;27(1):54–9.
14. Lee S, Lee HC, Kwon YW, Lee SE, Cho Y, Kim J, Lee S, Kim JY, Lee J, Yang HM, et al. Adenylyl cyclase-associated protein 1 is a receptor for human resistin and mediates inflammatory actions of human monocytes. Cell Metab. 2014;19(3):484–97.
15. Xie SS, Hu F, Tan M, Duan YX, Song XL, Wang CH. Relationship between expression of matrix metalloproteinase-9 and adenylyl cyclase-associated protein 1 in chronic obstructive pulmonary disease. J Int Med Res. 2014; 42(6):1272–84.
16. Tarkowski A, Bjersing J, Shestakov A, Bokarewa MI. Resistin competes with lipopolysaccharide for binding to toll-like receptor 4. J Cell Mol Med. 2010; 14(6b):1419–31.
17. Daquinag AC, Zhang Y, Amaya-Manzanares F, Simmons PJ, Kolonin MG. An isoform of decorin is a resistin receptor on the surface of adipose progenitor cells. Cell Stem Cell. 2011;9(1):74–86.

18. Sanchez-Solana B, Laborda J, Baladron V. Mouse resistin modulates adipogenesis and glucose uptake in 3T3-L1 preadipocytes through the ROR1 receptor. Mol Endocrinol. 2012;26(1):110–27.

19. Strieter RM, Polverini PJ, Kunkel SL, Arenberg DA, Burdick MD, Kasper J, Dzuiba J, Van Damme J, Walz A, Marriott D, et al. The functional role of the ELR motif in CXC chemokine-mediated angiogenesis. J Biol Chem. 1995; 270(45):27348–57.

20. Strieter RM, Burdick MD, Gomperts BN, Belperio JA, Keane MP. CXC chemokines in angiogenesis. Cytokine Growth Factor Rev. 2005;16(6):593–609.

21. Rubbert A, Combadiere C, Ostrowski M, Arthos J, Dybul M, Machado E, Cohn MA, Hoxie JA, Murphy PM, Fauci AS, et al. Dendritic cells express multiple chemokine receptors used as coreceptors for HIV entry. J Immunol. 1998;160(8):3933–41.

22. Ritchlin C. Fibroblast biology. Effector signals released by the synovial fibroblast in arthritis. Arthritis Res. 2000;2(5):356–60.

23. Krishnamurthy A, Joshua V, Haj Hensvold A, Jin T, Sun M, Vivar N, Ytterberg AJ, Engstrom M, Fernandes-Cerqueira C, Amara K, et al. Identification of a novel chemokine-dependent molecular mechanism underlying rheumatoid arthritis-associated autoantibody-mediated bone loss. Ann Rheum Dis. 2016; 75(4):721–9.

24. Kraan MC, Patel DD, Haringman JJ, Smith MD, Weedon H, Ahern MJ, Breedveld FC, Tak PP. The development of clinical signs of rheumatoid synovial inflammation is associated with increased synthesis of the chemokine CXCL8 (interleukin-8). Arthritis Res. 2001;3(1):65–71.

25. Haringman JJ, Smeets TJ, Reinders-Blankert P, Tak PP. Chemokine and chemokine receptor expression in paired peripheral blood mononuclear cells and synovial tissue of patients with rheumatoid arthritis, osteoarthritis, and reactive arthritis. Ann Rheum Dis. 2006;65(3):294–300.

26. Koch AE, Kunkel SL, Harlow LA, Johnson B, Evanoff HL, Haines GK, Burdick MD, Pope RM, Strieter RM. Enhanced production of monocyte chemoattractant protein-1 in rheumatoid arthritis. J Clin Invest. 1992;90(3):772–9.

27. Deshmane SL, Kremlev S, Amini S, Sawaya BE. Monocyte chemoattractant protein-1 (MCP-1): an overview. J Interferon Cytokine Res. 2009;29(6):313–26.

28. Nanki T, Nagasaka K, Hayashida K, Saita Y, Miyasaka N. Chemokines regulate IL-6 and IL-8 production by fibroblast-like synoviocytes from patients with rheumatoid arthritis. J Immunol. 2001;167(9):5381–5.

29. Koch AE, Kunkel SL, Shah MR, Hosaka S, Halloran MM, Haines GK, Burdick MD, Pope RM, Strieter RM. Growth-related gene product alpha. A chemotactic cytokine for neutrophils in rheumatoid arthritis. J Immunol. 1995;155(7):3660–6.

30. Hosaka S, Akahoshi T, Wada C, Kondo H. Expression of the chemokine superfamily in rheumatoid arthritis. Clin Exp Immunol. 1994;97(3):451–7.

31. Hogan M, Sherry B, Ritchlin C, Fabre M, Winchester R, Cerami A, Bucala R. Differential expression of the small inducible cytokines GRO alpha and GRO beta by synovial fibroblasts in chronic arthritis: possible role in growth regulation. Cytokine. 1994;6(1):61–9.

32. Koch AE, Kunkel SL, Harlow LA, Mazarakis DD, Haines GK, Burdick MD, Pope RM, Walz A, Strieter RM. Epithelial neutrophil activating peptide-78: a novel chemotactic cytokine for neutrophils in arthritis. J Clin Invest. 1994;94(3):1012–8.

8

Rheumatoid arthritis bone marrow environment supports Th17 response

Ewa Kuca-Warnawin[1*], Weronika Kurowska[1], Monika Prochorec-Sobieszek[2,3], Anna Radzikowska[1], Tomasz Burakowski[1], Urszula Skalska[1], Magdalena Massalska[1], Magdalena Plebańczyk[1], Barbara Małdyk-Nowakowska[4], Iwona Słowińska[4], Robert Gasik[4] and Włodzimierz Maśliński[1]

Abstract

Background: Rheumatoid arthritis (RA) is a systemic, autoimmune disease leading to joint destruction and ultimately disability. Bone marrow (BM) is an important compartment in RA, where pathological processes from "outside the joint" can occur. IL-17 is a cytokine that exerts proinflammatory effects and participates in the process of bone destruction. It is believed that IL-17 is involved in pathogenesis of RA. However, little is known about the biology of this cytokine in BM. In the present study we investigated Th17-related cytokines in RA BM.

Methods: BM samples were obtained from RA and osteoarthritis (OA) patients during total hip replacement surgery. Levels of IL-17AF, IL-17AA, IL-17FF, IL-1β, IL-6, IL-23, TGF-β and CCL20 in BM plasma were determined by specific enzyme-linked immunosorbent assay tests. Percentage of IL-17-producing cells in BM was evaluated by flow cytometry. The effect of IL-15 stimulation on IL-17 production by BM mononuclear cells was examined in vitro.

Results: Increased levels of IL-17AF were observed in BM plasma of RA patients in comparison to OA patients. Increased concentrations of IL-1β, IL-6 and CCL20 were observed in RA compared to OA BM plasma. Concordant with these findings, significantly increased percentages of $CD3^+CD4^+IL-17^+$ and $CD3^+CD4^+IL-17^+IFN-\gamma^+$ cells were present in RA BM in comparison to OA BM samples. Finally, abundant in RA BM, IL-15 increased IL-17 production by cultured BM mononuclear cells.

Conclusions: In the course of RA, the BM microenvironment can promote the development of Th17 cell responses and overproduction of IL-17AF that may lead to increased inflammation and tissue destruction in RA BM.

Keywords: Bone marrow, IL-17, IL-15, CCL20, Rheumatoid arthritis

Background

Rheumatoid arthritis (RA) is a systemic, autoimmune disease leading to joint destruction and ultimately disability [1]. Data obtained in the last decade indicate that bone marrow (BM) is an important compartment in RA, where pathological processes from "outside the joint" can occur. The cellular infiltrates found in RA BM consist of immunological cells that may form aggregates resembling germinal centres in secondary lymphoid organs [2]. Our previous flow cytometry analyses showed an increased number of mononuclear cells and accumulation of activated T cells and B cells in the BM of RA patients in comparison to osteoarthritis (OA) patients [2, 3]. Increased levels of proinflammatory cytokines and chemokines in RA BM were also observed, indicating an ongoing inflammatory process in this compartment. One of these cytokines is IL-15, which can be involved in T-cell activation [2, 4–6].

Interleukin-17 is predominantly expressed by a specific subset of human T-helper cells—Th17 cells. In addition, recent evidence indicates that IL-17 could also be produced by several innate immune cells and activated or inflammatory T cells [7]. It is assumed that this cytokine overproduction plays a crucial role in inflammation and the development of several autoimmune diseases, including RA. However, little is known about biology of this cytokine in BM. There are six known isoforms of

---

* Correspondence: ewa.kuca-warnawin@spartanska.pl
[1]Department of Pathophysiology and Immunology, National Institute of Geriatrics, Rheumatology and Rehabilitation (NIGRR), Spartanska 1, 02-637 Warsaw, Poland
Full list of author information is available at the end of the article

IL-17 (IL-17A–IL-17 F). Th17 cells are able to produce only proinflammatory IL-17A and IL-17 F, where IL-17A is considered more potent than IL-17 F. These two isoforms create dimers: in body fluids, homodimers IL-17AA and IL-17FF and also heterodimer IL-17AF could be detected [8]. Differentiation of human naïve T cells into Th17 cells requires the presence of TGF-β and at least one of the following proinflammatory cytokines: IL-1β, IL-6, IL-21 and IL-23 [9, 10]. In turn, Th1-related cytokine IFN-γ and Th2-related IL-4 suppress differentiation of Th17 cells [11, 12]. The proinflammatory cytokine IL-15 may also be involved in IL-17 production. Concentrations of IL-17 were demonstrated previously to correlate with concentrations of IL-15 in both serum and synovial fluid of RA patients [13]. Macrophage inflammatory protein-3α (MIP-3α/CCL20) has been reported to preferentially attract Th17 cells (via CCR6 binding) to the inflamed rheumatoid joints and the small intestine [14, 15].

In the present study we hypothesized that the RA BM microenvironment supports the development of Th17 cells and Th17 cell response. To verify this hypothesis, we examined the frequency of Th1, Th2 and Th17 cell populations as well as the concentrations of cytokines involved in Th17 cell differentiation and migration in BM from RA and OA patients. We analysed the concentrations of IL-17AA, IL-17AF and IL-17FF in the BM plasma and peripheral blood plasma of RA and OA patients. Moreover, because of the potential stimulatory effect of IL-15, the impact of this cytokine on IL-17 production has also been evaluated in vitro.

Methods

Patients

BM and peripheral blood were obtained from patients with RA and from patients with OA diagnosed according to American College of Rheumatology revised criteria for RA or for OA [16, 17]. Peripheral blood and BM samples were obtained from patients undergoing total hip replacement surgery. Patients' demographic and clinical characteristics are summarized in Table 1.

Immunohistochemistry

Bone marrow samples obtained from six OA patients and six RA patients were examined histopathologically. BM samples were fixed in Oxford fixative (formaldehyde 40%, glacial acetic acid 2%, sodium chloride 8.7%, distilled water), routinely processed and embedded in paraffin wax. Sections 3 μm thick were cut and stained with haematoxylin and eosin. The following antibodies were then used for further staining: anti-CD8 (polyclonal Ab, dilution 1:50; Dako, Glostrup, Denmark), anti-CD4 (clone 4B12, dilution 1:10; Novocastra, now part of Leica Microsystems, Wetzlar, Germany) and anti-IL-17A

Table 1 Patients' demographic and clinical characteristics

	RA ($n = 67$)	OA ($n = 43$)
Age, median (minimum–maximum)	58 (31–69)	59 (30–69)
Sex, female/male	54/15	42/21
ESR (mm/h), median (minimum–maximum)	37 (5–91)	11 (2–38)
CRP (mg/l), median (minimum–maximum)	21 (0–74)	3 (0–28)
Methotrexate	40	0
Steroids	54	0
Biologics	0	0

CRP C-reactive protein, *ESR* erythrocyte sedimentation rate, *OA* osteoarthritis, *RA* rheumatoid arthritis

(dilution 1:50; Santa Cruz). Staining was performed according to the manufacturer's instructions. The EnVision Detection System (Dako Denmark A/S, Glostrup, Denmark) was used for detection. Positive controls were performed on human tonsils. Negative (isotype) controls were performed using ready-to-use FLEX Negative Control Mouse (cocktail of murine IgG1, IgG2a, IgG2b, IgG3 and IgM, code number IR750; Dako Denmark A/ S). Samples were reviewed for expression of these proteins by a qualified histopathologist who was blinded to outcome. Appropriate cellular localization for immunostaining was membrane for CD8 and CD4 and cytoplasmatic for IL-17A. All photographs were taken using Olympus microscope cameras: DP72 Olympus BX63 and DP12 Olympus BX (Olympus, Tokyo, Japan).

BM plasma concentration of cytokines

Bone marrow plasma samples were obtained as we described previously [2, 4]. Concentrations of tested cytokines IL-17AA, IL-17AF, IL-17FF, IL-17A, TGF-β, IL-23, IL-1β, TNF-α, IL-4, IFN-γ, IL-6, CCL20 and IL-15 were detected using specific enzyme-linked immunosorbent assays (ELISAs). All measurements were performed in duplicate.

Concentrations of homodimer IL-17AA, homodimer IL-17FF and heterodimer IL-17AF were analysed by respective ELISA Ready-SET-Go kits (eBioscience, San Diego, CA, USA) according to the manufacturer's instructions. The detection limits were 4 pg/ml for IL-17AA, 16 pg/ml for IL-17FF and 30 pg/ml for IL-17AF.

Concentrations of TGF-β, IL-15, IL-1β and CCL20 were measured by respective ELISA Duo Set test (R&D Systems, Minneapolis, MN, USA) according to the manufacturer's instructions. The detection limits were 31 pg/ml for TGB-β, 3.9 pg/ml for IL-1β and 15.6 pg/ml for CCL20 and IL-15.

The concentration of IL-23 was assessed using polyclonal rat IgG anti-IL-23p19 as a coating Ab and biotinylated mouse IgG anti-IL-23 p40/70 as a detecting Ab (both Abs from Nautec, eBiosciences, San Diego, CA, USA). After staining with detecting antibody, samples were incubated with streptavidin conjugated with horseradish peroxidase (Sigma). Recombinant human IL-23 (R&D Systems) was used as a standard. The peroxidase reaction was developed using *o*-phenylenediamine dihydrochloride (Sigma). The optical density was measured at 492 nm with an automatic ELISA reader. The detection limit was 15 pg/ml.

Concentrations of IL-6 were analysed as described previously [18].

Isolation, culture and IL-15 stimulation of BM mononuclear cells

Bone marrow mononuclear cells (BMMC) were isolated by density gradient centrifugation using Ficoll-Paque (GE Healthcare Bio-Sciences, Uppsala, Sweden). Cells $(2 \times 10^6/\text{ml})$ were cultured in 24-well plates (Nunc, Roskilde, Denmark) in RPMI 1640 medium (Invitrogen, Paisley, UK) supplemented with 2 mM L-glutamine (Invitrogen), 10% heat-inactivated fetal calf serum (FCS) (Biochrom AG, Berlin, Germany), 100 U/ml penicillin, 100 µg/ml streptomycin (both antibiotics from Polfa Tarchomin, Warsaw, Poland), 30 µg/ml kanamycin (Sigma, St Louis, MO, USA) and 1 mM HEPES (Invitrogen) for 24 hours. For IL-15 stimulation, BMMC were cultured for an additional 72 hours in the presence of IL-15 (25 ng/ml) (R&D Systems).

Flow cytometry evaluation of IL-15 receptor complex expression on CD3$^+$CD4$^+$ cells

To estimate the surface expression of IL-15R receptor complex (CD122, CD132, CD215), BMMC were washed first in PBS (without Mg^{2+}/Ca^{2+}) buffer containing 1% BSA and 0.06% NaN_3, and then with glycine buffer (0.1 M, pH 3.0). In the next step BMMC were stained with antibodies anti-CD3-APC-Cy7, anti-CD4-PeCy7 (Becton Dickinson, San Diego, CA, USA), anti-CD122-FITC, anti-CD132-APC and anti-CD215-PE (R&D Systems). After the washing step, cells were incubated with 7-AAD to stain and exclude dead cells. Cells were acquired and analysed using FACSAria and Diva software (BD).

Measurement of secretory and intracellular IL-17 production upon IL-15 stimulation

Supernatants from BMMC cultured with or without IL-15 were collected for secretory IL-17A concentration measurement using Quantikine ELISA (R&D Systems) according to the manufacturer's instructions. Supernatants from unstimulated cell cultures served as control. In experiments designed for intracellular staining, BMMC were treated with PMA, ionomycin and Golgi-Stop 6 hours before the end of the culture. After staining of respective membrane antigens using anti-CD3 APC,

anti-CD4 FITC and anti-CD8 APC-Cy7 Abs, cells were fixed and permeabilized. The cells were then stained for intracellular expression of IL-17A using anti-IL-17A Ab conjugated with PE. Washed cells were acquired and analysed using FACSAria and Diva software (BD).

Flow cytometry evaluation of Th1/Th2/Th17 cell subsets in BM

Freshly isolated BMMC from patients' BM samples were treated for 6 hours with PMA (50 ng/ml) and ionomycin (1 µg/ml) in the presence of GolgiStop protein transport inhibitor. The cells were then harvested and stained for respective membrane antigens using anti-CD3 PerCp-Cy5.5, anti-CD4 Pe-Cy7 and anti-CD8 APC-Cy7 murine Abs. In the next step, cells were fixed and permeabilized using BD Cytofix/Cytoperm kit. Subsequently, intracellular staining using anti-IL-17A-PE, anti-IFN-γ-FITC and IL-4-APC Abs were performed. After the washing step, cells were acquired and analysed using a FACSAria cell sorter/cytometer and Diva software. All used reagents were purchased from Becton Dickinson (San Jose, CA, USA).

Statistical analysis

Data were analysed using GraphPad Prism 6 software. As obtained data were not normally distributed, according to the D'Agostino–Pearson omnibus normality test and the Shapiro–Wilk normality test, non-parametric tests were used for estimation of statistical significance of results. Comparisons between RA and OA were analysed by two-tailed Mann–Whitney U test. Correlations between the concentrations of cytokines were assessed using the Spearman test. The differences in IL-17 production after IL-15 stimulation were tested for statistical significance using the Wilcoxon test. $p < 0.05$ was considered statistically significant. Data are shown in the text as the median. Data are shown in the figures as the median with interquartile range or dots representing individual results.

Results

IL-17-positive cells are present in BM of RA patients

Immunohistopathological examination showed the presence of IL-17A-positive cells in BM samples obtained both from RA and OA patients (Fig. 1a–f). In immunohistochemical experiments we used an antibody against IL-17A monomer. We consider that positive staining with this antibody reflects the presence of both IL-17AA and IL-17AF dimers. Importantly, using ELISA, we found statistically significantly higher concentration of IL-17AF heterodimer in BM plasma of patients with RA (126.6 pg/ml, $n = 28$) compared to OA (92.96 pg/ml, $n = 32$) (Fig. 1g), indicating enhanced secretion of IL-17AF in RA BM. It is noteworthy that in both groups of patients the

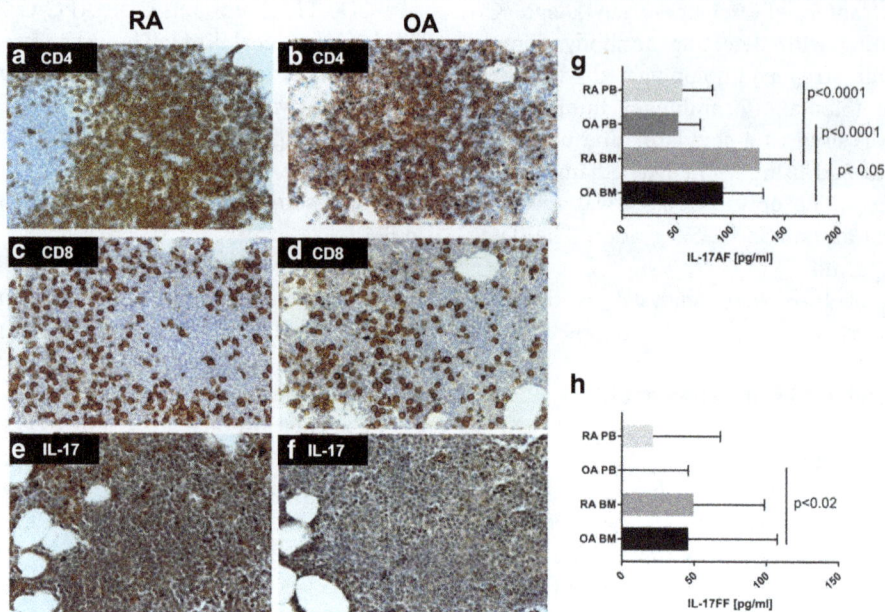

Fig. 1 a–f Immunohistochemical staining of BM samples obtained from patients with RA (*n* = 6) and OA (*n* = 6); EnVision stain, ×200. **a, b** CD4+ T cells in lymphoid follicle. **c, d** CD8+ T cells in lymphoid follicle. **e, f** IL-17A expression in lymphocytes in lymphoid follicle. **g** Concentration of IL-17AF in OA and RA BM plasma (OA *n* = 32; RA *n* = 28) and in OA and RA blood plasma (OA *n* = 21; RA *n* = 15). **h** Concentration of IL-17FF in OA and RA BM plasma (OA *n* = 34; RA *n* = 28) and in OA and RA blood plasma (OA *n* = 23; RA *n* = 15). Differences between groups were calculated using Mann–Whitney *U* test. BM bone marrow, IL interleukin, OA osteoarthritis, PB peripheral blood, RA rheumatoid arthritis

concentration of IL-17AF heterodimer was higher in BM plasma than in peripheral blood plasma. Surprisingly, there were no differences in IL-17FF homodimer concentration between OA BM (45.98 pg/ml) and RA BM (49.59 pg/ml) (Fig. 1h). The IL-17AA homodimer was detected only in 3 of 32 OA samples and 2 of 28 RA samples (data not shown). These results support other authors' observations that IL-17A exists mainly as an IL-17AF heterodimer [19]. Since on the basis of our experiments IL-17AA is hardly detectable in RA and OA BM plasma and IL-17FF levels are similar in both groups of patients, in the next flow cytometry experiments only intracellular expression of IL-17A was studied and positively stained cells were considered as the cells producing IL-17AF heterodimer.

Frequency of IL-17-positive cells is increased in RA BM

The percentage of CD3+CD4+IL-17+ cells was significantly higher in BM of RA patients in comparison to OA patients (1.0% vs 0.6%, *p* < 0.001) (Fig. 2b). Similarly, the percentage of CD3+CD4+IL-17+IFN-γ+ cells was higher in BM of RA patients in comparison to BM of OA patients (0.2% vs 0.1%, *p* < 0.03) (Fig. 2c). Both differences were statistically significant. We did not observe significant differences in BM percentage of CD3+CD4 +IL-4+ (4.0% vs 3.1%) and CD3+CD4+IFN-γ+ (12.9% vs 7.65%) between RA and OA patients (Fig. 2d, e).

Increased frequency of CD3+CD4+IL-17+ cells in RA BM suggests the recruitment of Th17 cells from the periphery or Th17 cell differentiation/stimulation in situ. Our next experiments were performed in order to test these two possibilities.

Proinflammatory milieu of RA BM microenvironment

In the next step the concentrations of cytokines involved in human Th17 cell differentiation were investigated in BM patient samples. We found an increased concentration of IL-6 (1105 pg/ml vs 198 pg/ml, *p* < 0.05) and IL-1β (2589 pg/ml vs 354 pg/ml, *p* < 0.01) in RA BM plasma in comparison to OA BM plasma (Fig. 3a, b). However, the differences in IL-23 (981 pg/ml vs 2034 pg/ml) and TGF-β (18.9 pg/ml vs 24.3 pg/ml) concentrations in both groups of patients were not statistically significant (Fig. 3c, d). Concentrations of Th1-related cytokine IFN-γ (46 pg/ml vs 68 pg/ml) and Th2-related IL-4 (2.6 pg/ml vs 3.2 pg/ml) were similar in both groups of patients (Fig. 3e, f). In addition, we found an increased concentration of TNF-α, an important player in the proinflammatory cytokine network, in RA BM plasma in comparison to OA BM plasma (966.7 pg/ml vs 435.5 pg/ml, *p* < 0.05) (Fig. 3g). An important chemokine that attracts Th17 cells by binding to receptor CCR6 is CCL20. CCR6 is also a known marker of Th17 cells [20]. Interestingly, we found increased concentration of CCL20 chemokine in RA BM (median value 46.7 pg/ml) in

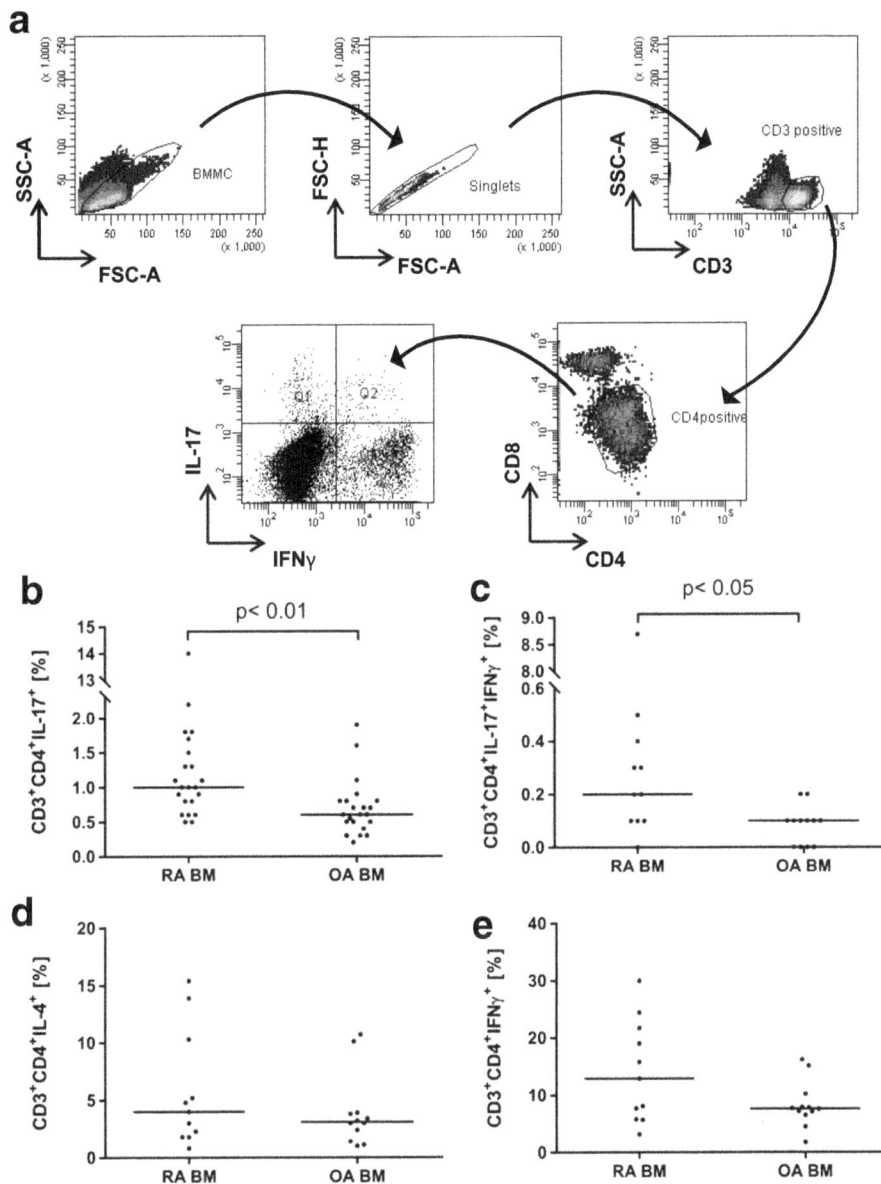

Fig. 2 Flow cytometry analysis of Th1, Th2 and Th17 lymphocyte subpopulations in OA and RA BM. **a** Representative gating strategy for FACS of RA BMMC, showing CD3$^+$CD4$^+$ lymphocytes with intracellular staining for IL-17 and IFN-γ after PMA/ionomycin stimulation. **b** Percentage of CD3$^+$CD4$^+$IL-17A$^+$ cells (OA $n = 22$; RA $n = 22$) **c** Percentage of CD3$^+$CD4$^+$IL-17A$^+$IFN-γ$^+$ cells (OA $n = 12$; RA $n = 11$). **d** Percentage of CD3$^+$CD4$^+$IL-4$^+$ cells (OA $n = 12$; RA $n = 11$). **e** Percentage of CD3$^+$CD4$^+$IFN-γ$^+$ cells (OA $n = 12$; RA $n = 11$). Differences between groups were calculated using Mann-Whitney U test. BM bone marrow, BMMC bone marrow mononuclear cells, FSC forward scatter, IFN interferon, IL interleukin, OA osteoarthritis, RA rheumatoid arthritis, SSC side scatter

comparison to OA BM (median value 0 pg/ml) (Fig. 3h), which could be responsible for the increased number of Th17 cells in RA BM.

IL-15 increases IL-17 secretion by RA BMMC

Our previous data indicate that IL-15 concentration is elevated in RA BM [2]. It was also shown that IL-15 levels correlate with IL-17 levels in sera of RA patients [13]. Our present data show that IL-15

concentration correlated with IL-17AF concentration in RA BM but did not correlate with IL-17FF concentration (Table 2).

In the next step we investigated the impact of IL-15 stimulation on IL-17 production by BMMC. Although in both groups of patients we observed a statistically significant increase in IL-17A secretion after stimulation with IL-15 (Fig. 4a), such an effect was more profound in BMMC derived from the RA patient group.

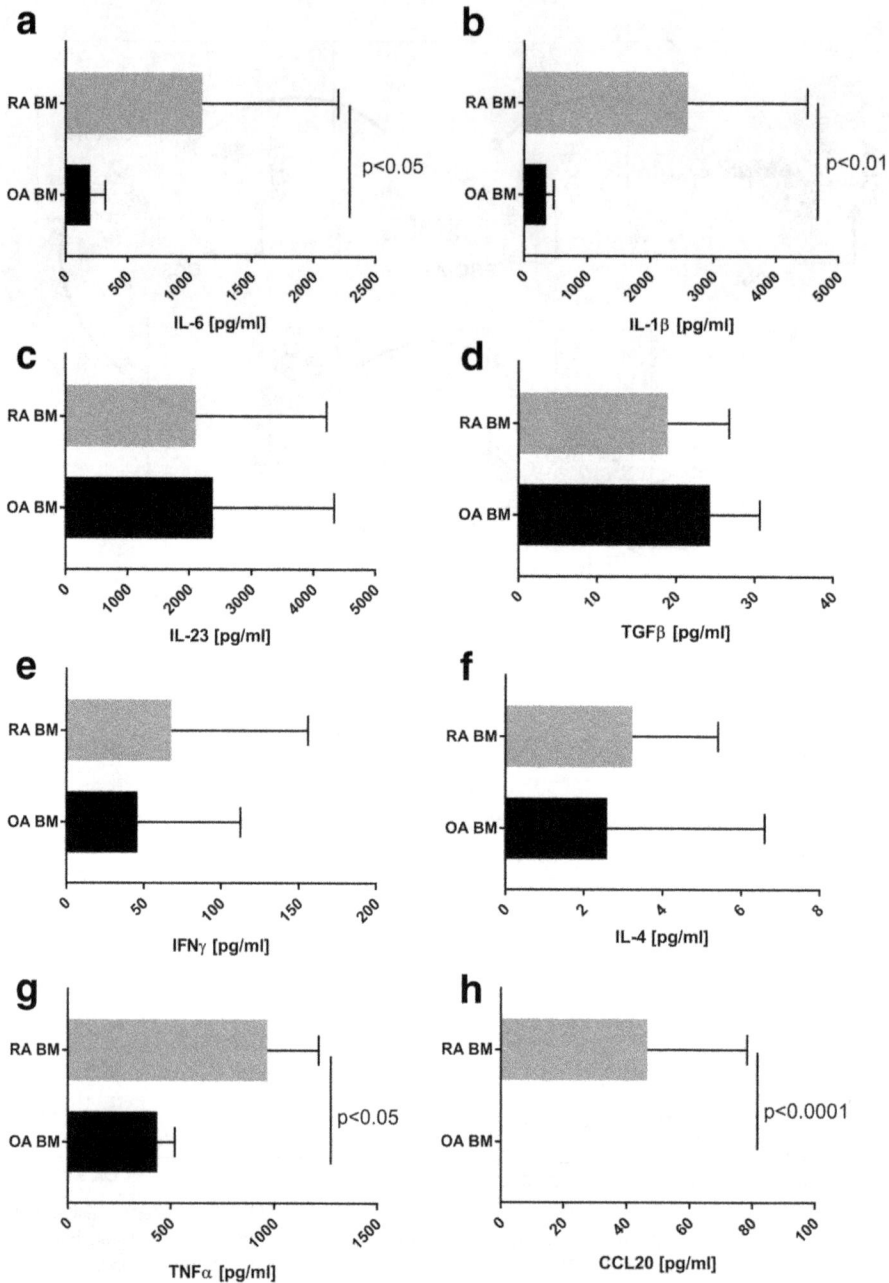

Fig. 3 Concentrations of selected cytokines associated with Th17 cell differentiation and activity in BM plasma of RA and OA patients. All cytokine concentrations detected using specific ELISAs. **a–d** Concentration of IL-6, IL-1β, IL-23 and TGF-β (OA $n = 13$–15; RA $n = 10$–14). **e, f** Concentrations of IFN-γ and IL-4 (OA $n = 28$–29; RA $n = 27$). **g** Concentration of TNF-α (OA $n = 14$; RA $n = 12$). **h** Concentration of CCL20 (OA $n = 35$; RA $n = 28$). Differences between groups were calculated using Mann–Whitney U test. BM bone marrow, IFN interferon, IL interleukin, OA osteoarthritis, RA rheumatoid arthritis, TGF transforming growth factor, TNF tumour necrosis factor

Table 2 Correlation coefficients (r) and significance values (p) between levels of IL-17AF, IL-17FF and IL-15 in BM plasma of RA patients ($n = 28$)

		r	p
RA BM IL-17AF	RA BM IL-15	0.38	<0.05
RA BM IL-17FF	RA BM IL-15	0.034	ns

BM bone marrow, IL interleukin, ns not significant, RA rheumatoid arthritis

IL-15 does not influence Th17 differentiation

The next experiments were designed to clarify whether IL-15 stimulation influences Th17 cell differentiation. BMMC derived from RA and OA were stimulated for 72 hours with IL-15 and at the end of culture the percentage of IL-17A-positive cells was measured by flow cytometry. In RA patients as well as in OA patients,

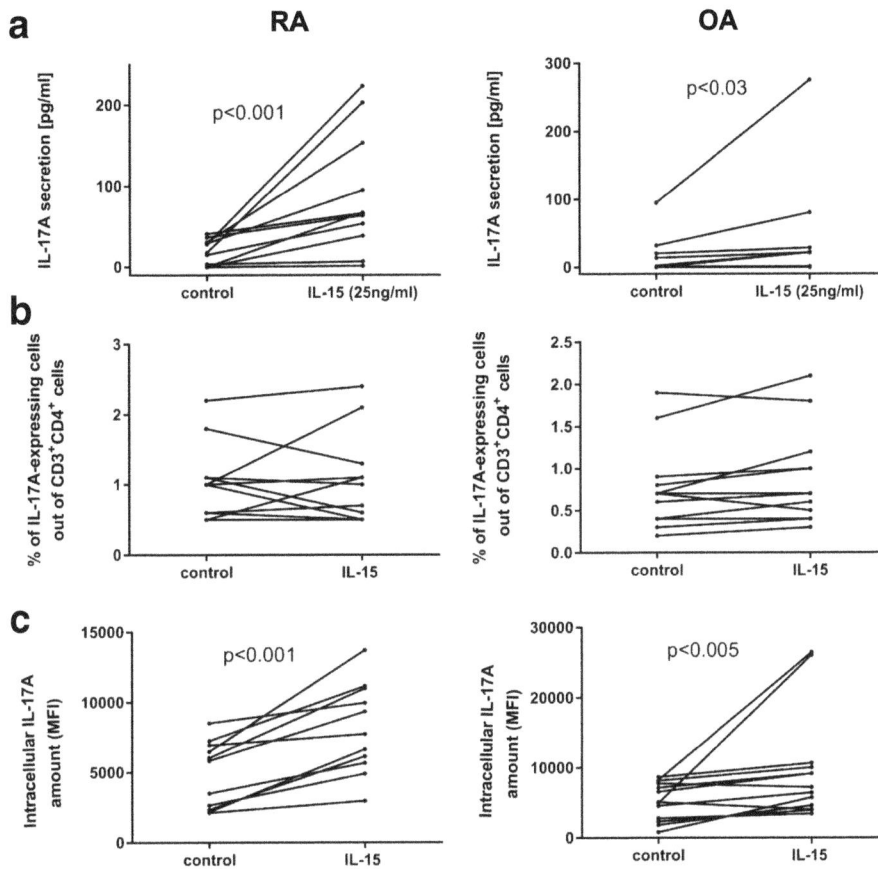

Fig. 4 Impact of IL-15 stimulation on IL-17 production and on Th17 differentiation. BMMC from OA (right panel) and RA (left panel) patients cultured for 72 hours without (control) or with addition of IL-15 (25 ng/ml). At the end of cell culture, supernatants were collected for ELISA (**a**) and cells were designated for FACS analysis (**b, c**). **a** Concentration of secreted IL-17A in cell culture supernatants (RA $n = 11$; OA $n = 11$). **b** Percentage of IL-17A-expressing CD3$^+$CD4$^+$ cells out of total CD3$^+$CD4$^+$ cells (RA $n = 11$; OA $n = 13$). **c** Intracellular amount of IL-17A (reflected by MFI) in CD3$^+$CD4$^+$ cells (RA $n = 11$; OA $n = 13$). IL interleukin, MFI mean fluorescence intensity, OA osteoarthritis, RA rheumatoid arthritis

stimulation with IL-15 did not increase the percentage of IL-17A-producing cells in the culture, suggesting the lack of IL-15 impact on Th17 differentiation (Fig. 4b). However, in both groups of patients an increased intracellular production of IL-17A (mean fluorescence intensity value (MFI)) in CD3$^+$CD4$^+$ cells was noted upon IL-15 stimulation (Fig. 4c). These results suggest that IL-15 stimulation enhances IL-17A production in existing/already differentiated Th17 cells.

IL-15 receptor complex is present on CD3$^+$CD4$^+$ cells isolated from bone marrow

The heterotrimeric IL-15 receptor complex consists of a unique IL-15Rα subunit (CD215), IL-2/IL-15Rβ (CD122) and the common gamma-chain/IL-15Rγ subunit (CD132). IL-15 binds with high affinity to IL-15Rα (Kd = 10–11 M). IL-15/IL-15Rα then associates with a complex composed of the IL-2/IL-15Rβ and common gamma-chain/IL-15Rγ subunits, expressed either on the same cell (cis presentation) or on a different cell (trans

presentation). In some experimental models, IL-15 bound to the IL-15Rα acts much more efficiently than soluble IL-15. We found that the percentage of CD3$^+$CD4$^+$CD215$^+$ cells was similar in BM of RA patients in comparison to OA patients (1.6% vs 1.9%, ns) (Fig. 5a). Also, the percentage of CD3$^+$CD4$^+$CD122$^+$ cells was similar in BM of RA and OA patients (6.5% vs 5.2%, ns) (Fig. 5b). In addition, we did not observe any differences in MFI value of CD215 and CD122 on CD3$^+$CD4$^+$ cells in both studied patients groups (Fig. 5d, e). However, we noted a significantly higher percentage of CD3$^+$CD4$^+$CD132$^+$ cells in RA BM in comparison to OA BM (18.7% vs 8.9%, $p < 0.005$) (Fig. 5c). Furthermore, MFI value of CD132 on CD3$^+$CD4$^+$CD132$^+$ cells obtained from RA BM was found to be higher in comparison to the same type of cells obtained from OA BM (625 vs 458, $p < 0.05$) (Fig. 5f). Therefore, increased expression of CD132 my be responsible for stronger response of RA BM CD3$^+$CD4$^+$ cells for IL-15 stimulation.

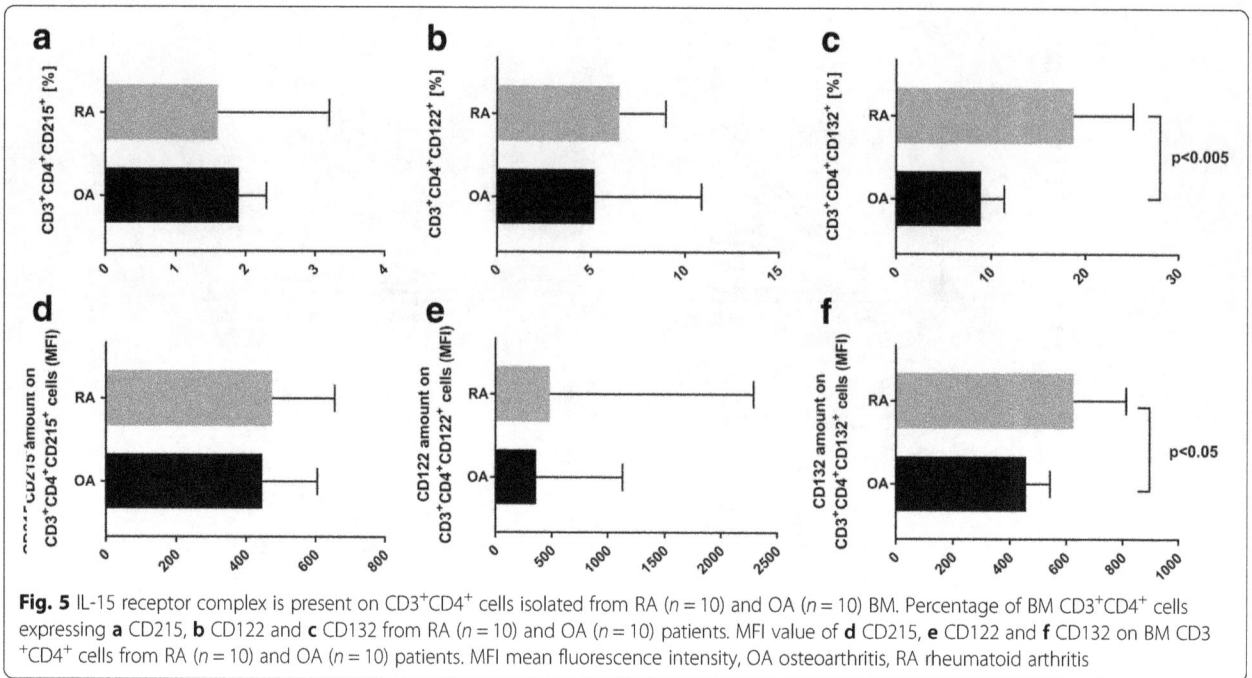

Fig. 5 IL-15 receptor complex is present on CD3$^+$CD4$^+$ cells isolated from RA ($n = 10$) and OA ($n = 10$) BM. Percentage of BM CD3$^+$CD4$^+$ cells expressing **a** CD215, **b** CD122 and **c** CD132 from RA ($n = 10$) and OA ($n = 10$) patients. MFI value of **d** CD215, **e** CD122 and **f** CD132 on BM CD3$^+$CD4$^+$ cells from RA ($n = 10$) and OA ($n = 10$) patients. MFI mean fluorescence intensity, OA osteoarthritis, RA rheumatoid arthritis

Discussion

In the recent years, there has been growing evidence supporting implication of the BM compartment in initiation and perpetuation of the inflammatory processes in RA. Elegant studies confirmed that BM oedema, which is often present in RA patients, reflects true BM inflammation [21]. Moreover, numerous studies have reported that BM oedema represents an independent predictor of RA development and radiographic progression in patients with undifferentiated arthritis [22–26]. Such ongoing inflammatory processes in BM are also reflected by the activation of B cells and T cells. As we reported previously, ligation of Toll-like receptors (TLR) triggered BM-derived B-cell activation [3], and the number of recently activated T cells was significantly elevated in RA BM [2].

Overproduction of several proinflammatory cytokines, including TNF-α, IL-1β, IL-6, IL-15 and relatively recently added IL-17, contribute to pathological processes in RA [6, 27]. Tissue-specific IL-17 exacerbates tissue damage and disease chronicity. It was shown that expression of IL-17 mRNA and protein are higher in RA joints compared to healthy controls [28]. However, there are no data regarding BM production of IL-17 in the course of RA. In the present study we investigated the Th17 compartment in RA BM. In the first sets of experiments the concentrations of IL-17 dimers in BM were measured. We found a significantly higher concentration of IL-17AF in BM of patients with RA than those with OA (Fig. 1). Moreover, in both patient groups, IL-17AF levels in BM plasma were higher than in peripheral blood plasma. There were no differences in BM IL-17FF levels in the OA and RA patient groups. Nonetheless, the IL-17FF concentration in BM plasma was also increased when compared to blood plasma (in both groups of patients). Thus, our results show that BM represents an important source of both IL-17AF and IL-17FF and that overproduction of IL-17AF seems to be characteristic for RA BM.

IL-17 is an important player in the proinflammatory cytokine network. This cytokine may induce production of various proteins in tissues, but when acting alone its effects are not highly pronounced. In contrast, its interaction with other cytokines such as TNF-α, IL-1β, IFN-γ or IL-22 leads to synergistically increased production of IL-6 and IL-8 [29–31]. IL-17 also contributes to increased osteoclastogenesis: it can directly induce differentiation of osteoclasts from monocytes and is able to up-regulate RANKL synthesis by RA fibroblast-like synoviocytes [32]. As we have reported before [33], the RANKL concentration was elevated in RA BM plasma in comparison to OA BM plasma. Thus, the increased production of IL-17A in RA BM may be associated with bone and cartilage destruction observed in the course of RA.

The optimal conditions for Th17 differentiation are still a highly debated issue. There is general agreement that IL-6 and IL-23 participate in the differentiation and survival of murine Th17 [34]. However, even in the murine model, the role of TGF-β remains controversial. For example, there is a study showing that murine, highly pathogenic Th17 lymphocytes differentiate in the absence of TGF-β [35].

Several cytokines, including IL-1β, IL-6, IL-23 and TGF-β, were demonstrated to participate in the differentiation and survival of human Th17 cells. However, it has also been shown that only IL-6 and IL-1β, but not TGF-β, are essential for Th17 differentiation [36]. On the other hand, in some studies the presence of TGF-β is necessary for RORc expression in human CD4 cells [37].

We compared concentrations of IL-1β, IL-6, IL-23 and TGF-β in BM samples obtained from patients with RA and OA in order to investigate whether RA BM creates suitable conditions for Th17 lymphocyte differentiation/survival. We found significantly increased levels of IL-1β and IL-6 in RA BM (Fig. 3a, b). IL-23 and TGF-β were also present in RA and OA BM, although at the comparable levels in both patient groups (Fig. 3c, d). In addition, we observed an increased percentage of Th17 cells in the BM of RA patients compared to the BM of OA patients (Fig. 2), indicating that all necessary cytokines described in the literature required for human Th17 cell differentiation are present in BM in sufficient concentrations to trigger differentiation of Th17 cells. It is likely that levels of TGF-β and IL-23, although not different between RA and OA, are sufficient for supporting Th17 cell differentiation while highly elevated levels of IL-1β and IL-6 may be responsible for the higher number of Th17 cells in RA BM. There are observations that Th1-related and Th2-related cytokines (IFN-γ, IL-4) suppress differentiation of Th17 cells [11, 12]. However, in our experiments we did not observe increased levels of these cytokines in RA BM in comparison to OA BM (Fig. 3e, f).

The role of IL-15 in Th17 cell differentiation is not clearly defined. The IL-15 concentration is known to correlate with the concentration of IL-17 in synovial fluid from RA patients [13]. In addition, the contribution of IL-15 to the increased level of IL-17 in the course of collagen-induced arthritis has been also reported [38]. Our research demonstrated increased production of IL-17 in RA BMMC after IL-15 stimulation (Fig. 4a). Interestingly, flow cytometry experiments showed that although IL-15 did not affect the percentage of BM cells producing IL-17 in vitro, it increased the amount of intracellular IL-17 (referred as MFI, Fig. 4). Additionally, we found correlation between concentrations of IL-17AF and IL-15 in RA BM plasma. These results suggest that IL-15 may contribute to the phenotype stabilization and survival of Th17 cells as well as the increased production of IL-17. It is noteworthy that such an effect is not characteristic only for RA, but also for OA. However, BMMC obtained from RA patients reacted to IL-15 slightly better, indicating the increased sensitivity of T cells from RA BM to IL-15. Our analysis showed the presence of IL-15 receptor complex on CD3$^+$CD4$^+$ cells isolated from BM. Interestingly, the higher percentage of CD3$^+$CD4$^+$ cells bearing CD132 present in RA BM than in OA BM may explain why CD3$^+$CD4$^+$ cells from RA patients react stronger to IL-15 stimulation. It should, however, be noted that the stimulatory effect of IL-15 on IL-17 production in BMMC culture may result from direct stimulation of Th17 cells or other cells capable of producing cytokines involved in Th17 cell differentiation [39].

Another explanation for increased IL-17AF concentration in BM of RA patients could be the increased migration of Th17 cells into the BM. We reported previously the increased levels of some chemokines in BM of patients with RA that indicate the possibility of impaired cell migration in the course of the disease [4]. However, previously we did not evaluate the concentration of CCL20, the key chemokine regulating Th17 migration. CCL20 recruits Th17 cells and dendritic cells to the inflammatory site [20]. CCL20 is typically expressed at a low basal level, but can be strongly induced by proinflammatory cytokine TNF-α [40]. In the present study we found elevated concentrations of CCL20 as well as TNF-α in RA BM plasma. Highly elevated CCL20 in BM of RA patients may participate in the observed increased percentage of Th17 cells as well as the formation of germinal centres in this tissue as we reported before [2].

Conclusions

Our results indicate that in the course of RA the BM microenvironment can promote the development of Th17 responses and overproduction of IL-17AF. Our observations support the notion that BM actively participates in pathogenesis of RA.

Abbreviations
7-AAD: 7-Aminoactinomycin D; Ab: Antibody; APC: Allophycocyanin; APC-Cy7: Allophycocyanin tandem conjugate with cyanine; BM: Bone marrow; BMMC: Bone marrow mononuclear cells; ELISA: Enzyme-linked immunosorbent assay; FITC: Fluorescein isothiocyanate; IFN-γ: interferon gamma; IL: Interleukin; MFI: Mean fluorescence intensity; NaN$_3$: Sodium azide; OA: Osteoarthritis; PE: Phycoerythrin; PE-Cy7: Phycoerythrin tandem conjugate with cyanine; PerCp-Cy5.5: Peridinin-chlorophyll proteins tandem conjugate with cyanine; PMA: Phorbol 12-myristate 13-acetate; RA: Rheumatoid arthritis; TGF-β: Transforming growth factor beta; Th: T-helper; TNF-α: Tumour necrosis factor alpha

Funding
This work was partially funded by grant number UMO-2011/03/B/NZ6/05035 from National Science Centre, Poland and a core grant to National Institute of Geriatrics, Rheumatology and Rehabilitation from Polish Ministry of Science and Higher Education.

Authors' contributions
EK-W conceived and designed the study, performed flow cytometry experiments, data analysis and data interpretation, and wrote the manuscript. WK participated in manuscript writing and performed ELISA tests. MP-S performed immunohistochemical analysis. TB was responsible for cell isolation and culture. BM-N, IS and RG helped with recruited patients and acquired and analysed clinical data. MP, AR and MM performed ELISA tests. US participated in manuscript writing. WM participated in study design.

All authors drafted the manuscript, and all authors read and approved the final manuscript. All authors meet authorship requirements according to the International Committee of Medical Journal Editors.

Competing interests

The authors declare that they have no conflicts of interest.

Author details

[1]Department of Pathophysiology and Immunology, National Institute of Geriatrics, Rheumatology and Rehabilitation (NIGRR), Spartanska 1, 02-637 Warsaw, Poland. [2]Department of Pathology, National Institute of Geriatrics, Rheumatology, and Rehabilitation (NIGRR), Warsaw, Poland. [3]Department of Diagnostic Hematology, Institute of Hematology and Transfusion Medicine, Warsaw, Poland. [4]Department of Rheumoorthopaedic Surgery, National Institute of Geriatrics, Rheumatology and Rehabilitation (NIGRR), Warsaw, Poland.

References

1. Scott DL, Wolfe F, Huizinga TWJ. Rheumatoid arthritis. Lancet. 2010; 376(9746):1094–108.
2. Kuca-Warnawin E, Burakowski T, Kurowska W, Prochorec-Sobieszek M, Radzikowska A, Chorazy-Massalska M, Maldyk P, Kontny E, Maslinski W. Elevated number of recently activated T cells in bone marrow of patients with rheumatoid arthritis: a role for interleukin 15? Ann Rheum Dis. 2011; 70(1):227–33.
3. Rudnicka W, Burakowski T, Warnawin E, Jastrzebska M, Bik M, Kontny E, Chorazy-Massalska M, Radzikowska A, Buler M, Maldyk P, et al. Functional TLR9 modulates bone marrow B cells from rheumatoid arthritis patients. Eur J Immunol. 2009;39(5):1211–20.
4. Kuca-Warnawin EH, Kurowska WJ, Radzikowska A, Massalska MA, Burakowski T, Kontny E, Slowinska I, Gasik R, Maslinski W. Different expression of chemokines in rheumatoid arthritis and osteoarthritis bone marrow. Reumatologia. 2016;54(2):51–3.
5. JongenLavrencic M, Peeters HRM, Wognum A, Vreugdenhil G, Breedveld FC, Swaak AJG. Elevated levels of inflammatory cytokines in bone marrow of patients with rheumatoid arthritis and anemia of chronic disease. J Rheumatol. 1997;24(8):1504–9.
6. Papadaki HA, Kritikos HD, Gemetzi C, Koutala H, Marsh JC, Boumpas DT, Eliopoulos GD. Bone marrow progenitor cell reserve and function and stromal cell function are defective in rheumatoid arthritis: evidence for a tumor necrosis factor alpha-mediated effect. Blood. 2002;99(5):1610–9.
7. Beringer A, Noack M, Miossec P. IL-17 in chronic inflammation: from discovery to targeting. Trends Mol Med. 2016;22(3):230–41.
8. Wright JF, Guo YJ, Quazi A, Luxenberg DP, Bennett F, Ross JF, Qiu YC, Whitters MJ, Tomkinson KN, Dunussi-Joannopoulos K, et al. Identification of an interleukin 17F/17A heterodimer in activated human CD4+ T cells. J Biol Chem. 2007;282(18):13447–55.
9. Veldhoen M, Hocking RJ, Atkins CJ, Locksley RM, Stockinger B. TGFβ in the context of an inflammatory cytokine milieu supports de novo differentiation of IL-17-producing T cells. Immunity. 2006;24(2):179–89.
10. Volpe E, Servant N, Zollinger R, Bogiatzi SI, Hupe P, Barillot E, Soumelis V. A critical function for transforming growth factor-beta, interleukin 23 and proinflammatory cytokines in driving and modulating human T(H)-17 responses. Nat Immunol. 2008;9(6):650–7.
11. Park H, Li Z, Yang XO, Chang SH, Nurieva R, Wang YH, Wang Y, Hood L, Zhu Z, Tian Q, et al. A distinct lineage of CD4 T cells regulates tissue inflammation by producing interleukin 17. Nat Immunol. 2005;6(11):1133–41.
12. van Hamburg JP, Mus AM, de Bruijn MJ, de Vogel L, Boon L, Cornelissen F, Asmawidjaja P, Hendriks RW, Lubberts E. GATA-3 protects against severe joint inflammation and bone erosion and reduces differentiation of Th17 cells during experimental arthritis. Arthritis Rheum. 2009;60(3):750–9.
13. Ziolkowska M, Koc A, Luszczykiewicz G, Ksiezopolska-Pietrzak K, Klimczak E, Chwalinska-Sadowska H, Maslinski W. High levels of IL-17 in rheumatoid arthritis patients: IL-15 triggers in vitro IL-17 production via cyclosporin A-sensitive mechanism. J Immunol. 2000;164(5):2832–8.
14. Hirota K, Yoshitomi H, Hashimoto M, Maeda S, Teradaira S, Sugimoto N, Yamaguchi T, Nomura T, Ito H, Nakamura T, et al. Preferential recruitment of CCR6-expressing Th17 cells to inflamed joints via CCL20 in rheumatoid arthritis and its animal model. J Exp Med. 2007;204(12):2803–12.
15. Esplugues E, Huber S, Gagliani N, Hauser AE, Town T, Wan YY, O'Connor Jr W, Rongvaux A, Van Rooijen N, Haberman AM, et al. Control of TH17 cells occurs in the small intestine. Nature. 2011;475(7357):514–8.
16. Altman R, Alarcon G, Appelrouth D, Bloch D, Borenstein D, Brandt K, Brown C, Cooke TD, Daniel W, Feldman D, et al. The American College of Rheumatology criteria for the classification and reporting of osteoarthritis of the hip. Arthritis Rheum. 1991;34:505–14.
17. Arnett FC, Edworthy SM, Bloch DA, McShane DJ, Fries JF, Cooper NS, Healey LA, Kaplan SR, Liang MH, Luthra HS, et al. The American Rheumatism Association 1987 revised criteria for the classification of rheumatoid arthritis. Arthritis Rheum. 1988;31(3):315–24.
18. Kontny E, Grabowska A, Kowalczewski J, Kurowska M, Janicka I, Marcinkiewicz J, Maslinski W. Taurine chloramine inhibition of cell proliferation and cytokine production by rheumatoid arthritis fibroblast-like synoviocytes. Arthritis Rheum. 1999;42(12):2552–60.
19. Wright JF, Guo Y, Quazi A, Luxenberg DP, Bennett F, Ross JF, Qiu Y, Whitters MJ, Tomkinson KN, Dunussi-Joannopoulos K, et al. Identification of an interleukin 17F/17A heterodimer in activated human CD4+ T cells. J Biol Chem. 2007;282(18):13447–55.
20. Chabaud M, Page G, Miossec P. Enhancing effect of IL-1, IL-17, and TNF-alpha on macrophage inflammatory protein-3alpha production in rheumatoid arthritis: regulation by soluble receptors and Th2 cytokines. J Immunol. 2001;167(10):6015–20.
21. Jimenez-Boj E, Nobauer-Huhmann I, Hanslik-Schnabel B, Dorotka R, Wanivenhaus AH, Kainberger F, Trattnig S, Axmann R, Tsuji W, Hermann S, et al. Bone erosions and bone marrow edema as defined by magnetic resonance imaging reflect true bone marrow inflammation in rheumatoid arthritis. Arthritis Rheum. 2007;56(4):1118–24.
22. Boyesen P, Haavardsholm EA, Ostergaard M, van der Heijde D, Sesseng S, Kvien TK. MRI in early rheumatoid arthritis: synovitis and bone marrow oedema are independent predictors of subsequent radiographic progression. Ann Rheum Dis. 2011;70(3):428–33.
23. Haavardsholm EA, Boyesen P, Ostergaard M, Schildvold A, Kvien TK. Magnetic resonance imaging findings in 84 patients with early rheumatoid arthritis: bone marrow oedema predicts erosive progression. Ann Rheum Dis. 2008;67(6):794–800.
24. Solau-Gervais E, Legrand JL, Cortet B, Duquesnoy B, Flipo RM. Magnetic resonance imaging of the hand for the diagnosis of rheumatoid arthritis in the absence of anti-cyclic citrullinated peptide antibodies: a prospective study. J Rheumatol. 2006;33(9):1760–5.
25. Boutry N, Do Carmo CC, Flipo RM, Cotten A. Early rheumatoid arthritis and its differentiation from other joint abnormalities. Eur J Radiol. 2009; 71(2):217–24.
26. Duer-Jensen A, Horslev-Petersen K, Hetland ML, Bak L, Ejbjerg BJ, Hansen MS, Johansen JS, Lindegaard HM, Vinterberg H, Moller JM, et al. Bone edema on magnetic resonance imaging is an independent predictor of rheumatoid arthritis development in patients with early undifferentiated arthritis. Arthritis Rheum. 2011;63(8):2192–202.
27. Jongen-Lavrencic M, Peeters HR, Wognum A, Vreugdenhil G, Breedveld FC, Swaak AJ. Elevated levels of inflammatory cytokines in bone marrow of patients with rheumatoid arthritis and anemia of chronic disease. J Rheumatol. 1997;24(8):1504–9.
28. Shahrara S, Huang Q, Mandelin AM, Pope RM. TH-17 cells in rheumatoid arthritis Arthritis Research & Ther. 2008;10(4):R93.
29. Onishi RM, Gaffen SL. Interleukin-17 and its target genes: mechanisms of interleukin-17 function in disease. Immunology. 2010;129(3):311–21.
30. Chabaud M, Fossiez F, Taupin JL, Miossec P. Enhancing effect of IL-17 on IL-1-induced IL-6 and leukemia inhibitory factor production by rheumatoid arthritis synoviocytes and its regulation by Th2 cytokines. J Immunol. 1998; 161(1):409–14.
31. Zrioual S, Ecochard R, Tournadre A, Lenief V, Cazalis MA, Miossec P. Genome-wide comparison between IL-17A- and IL-17F-induced effects in human rheumatoid arthritis synoviocytes. J Immunol. 2009;182(5):3112–20.
32. Kim KW, Kim HR, Kim BM, Cho ML, Lee SH. Th17 cytokines regulate osteoclastogenesis in rheumatoid arthritis. Am J Pathol. 2015;185(11):3011–24.

33. Radzikowska ABT, Maldyk P, Michalak C, Jung L, Maslinski W. Soluble and cell-surfac expressed RANKL and osteoprotegerin in bone marrow from rheumatoid aerhritis patients. Ann Rheum Dis. 2007;66:267.

34. Kimura A, Kishimoto T. IL-6: regulator of Treg/Th17 balance. Eur J Immunol. 2010;40(7):1830–5.

35. Ghoreschi K, Laurence A, Yang XP, Tato CM, McGeachy MJ, Konkel JE, Ramos HL, Wei L, Davidson TS, Bouladoux N, et al. Generation of pathogenic T(H)17 cells in the absence of TGF-beta signalling. Nature. 2010; 467(7318):967–71.

36. Acosta-Rodriguez EV, Napolitani G, Lanzavecchia A, Sallusto F. Interleukins 1beta and 6 but not transforming growth factor-beta are essential for the differentiation of interleukin 17-producing human T helper cells. Nat Immunol. 2007;8(9):942–9.

37. Burgler S, Ouaked N, Bassin C, Basinski TM, Mantel PY, Siegmund K, Meyer N, Akdis CA, Schmidt-Weber CB. Differentiation and functional analysis of human T(H)17 cells. J Allergy Clin Immunol. 2009;123(3):588–95. 595 e581–7.

38. Yoshihara K, Yamada H, Hori A, Yajima T, Kubo C, Yoshikai Y. IL-15 exacerbates collagen-induced arthritis with an enhanced CD4+ T cell response to produce IL-17. Eur J Immunol. 2007;37(10):2744–52.

39. Harris K, Fasano A, Mann D. Monocytes differentiated with IL-15 support Th17 and Th1 responses to wheat gliadin: implications for celiac disease. Clin Immunol. 2010;135(3):430–9.

40. Schutyser E, Struyf S, Van Damme J. The CC chemokine CCL20 and its receptor CCR6. Cytokine Growth Factor Rev. 2003;14(5):409–26.

9

Effectiveness and safety of tofacitinib in rheumatoid arthritis

Marina Amaral de Ávila Machado[1], Cristiano Soares de Moura[1], Steve Ferreira Guerra[1], Jeffrey R. Curtis[2], Michal Abrahamowicz[1,3] and Sasha Bernatsky[1,3]*

Abstract

Background: Tofacitinib is the first oral Janus kinase inhibitor approved for the treatment of rheumatoid arthritis (RA). We compared the effectiveness and safety of tofacitinib, disease-modifying antirheumatic drugs (DMARDs), tumor necrosis factor inhibitors (TNFi), and non-TNF biologics in patients with RA previously treated with methotrexate.

Methods: We used MarketScan® databases (2011–2014) to study methotrexate-exposed patients with RA who were newly prescribed tofacitinib, DMARDs other than methotrexate, and biologics. The date of first prescription was defined as the cohort entry. The therapy was considered effective if all of the following criteria from a claims-based algorithm were achieved at the first year of follow-up: high adherence, no biologic or tofacitinib switch or addition, no DMARD switch or addition, no increase in dose or frequency of index drug, no more than one glucocorticoid joint injection, and no new/increased oral glucocorticoid dose. The safety outcome was serious infections requiring hospitalization. Non-TNF biologics comprised the reference group.

Results: We included 21,832 patients with RA, including 0.8% treated with tofacitinib, 24.7% treated with other DMARDs, 61.2% who had started therapy with TNFi, and 13.3% treated with non-TNF biologics. The rates of therapy effectiveness were 15.4% for tofacitinib, 11.1% for DMARDs, 18.6% for TNFi, and 19.8% for non-TNF biologics. In adjusted analyses, tofacitinib and non-TNF biologics appeared to have similar effectiveness rates, whereas DMARD initiators were less effective than non-TNF biologics. We could not clearly establish if tofacitinib was associated with a higher rate of serious infections.

Conclusions: In patients with RA previously treated with methotrexate, our comparisons of tofacitinib with non-TNF biologics, though not definitive, did not demonstrate differences with respect to hospitalized infections or effectiveness.

Keywords: Rheumatoid arthritis, Tofacitinib, Disease-modifying antirheumatic drug, Biologic therapy, Comparative effectiveness research

Background

New strategies have been developed to treat rheumatoid arthritis (RA) by inhibiting Janus kinase (JAK) pathways. The first JAK inhibitor approved for the treatment of RA in the United States (November 2012) was tofacitinib. This drug is an oral small molecule and recommended by both the American College of Rheumatology (ACR) and the European League Against Rheumatism (EULAR) as an alternative to biologic drugs when a patient remains with moderate or high disease activity after a first-line disease-modifying antirheumatic drug (DMARD), usually methotrexate, in patients with established RA [1, 2].

Indirect comparisons have suggested that patients with RA in whom DMARD treatment fails experience similar efficacy in response to tumor necrosis factor inhibitors (TNFi), abatacept, tocilizumab, or tofacitinib (monotherapy or in combination with methotrexate). However, caution must be taken when interpreting that result because indirect comparisons are potentially biased [3]. Researchers studying a cohort derived from U.S. administrative

* Correspondence: sasha.bernatsky@mcgill.ca
[1]Division of Clinical Epidemiology, Research Institute of McGill University Health Centre, 5252 de Maisonneuve West, Montreal, QC, Canada
[3]Department of Epidemiology, Biostatistics and Occupational Health, Research Institute of McGill University Health Centre, 5252 de Maisonneuve West, Montreal, QC, Canada
Full list of author information is available at the end of the article

databases (2012–2014) reported that patients using tofacitinib, etanercept, adalimumab, and abatacept had similar persistence and adherence at the end of the first year of therapy [4]. In terms of drug safety, it is well known that RA therapies can exacerbate the risk for herpes virus, and evidence from phase III and long-term extension of randomized controlled trials (RCTs) suggests that patients treated with tofacitinib have a higher incidence of herpes virus infection than those treated with placebo or adalimumab [5]. Another systematic review demonstrated that RCTs might not be sensitive enough to compare the risk of adverse events with tofacitinib [6], whereas researchers in one cohort study reported a higher risk for herpes virus infection with tofacitinib than with abatacept, TNFi, and other RA biologics [7]. Thus, the long-term safety of tofacitinib remains mostly uncertain.

More real-world evidence generated during routine clinical practice and obtained outside the context of RCTs is needed [8]. RCTs are typically planned to assess efficacy outcomes and are underpowered for detecting adverse events. Also, follow-up duration in RCTs is short, and long-term extension studies are potentially affected by healthy user bias. Evidence on new drug therapies is required throughout the entire product life cycle, therefore there has been increased interest in comparative effectiveness research on interventions to inform regulatory bodies for health care decision-making and to support optimization of practitioners' strategies for the management of RA [9].

To provide direct comparative evidence for tofacitinib's effectiveness and to expand the safety literature as well, we performed a study using real-world population data of tofacitinib, DMARDs, TNFi, and non-TNF biologics for patients with RA. ACR and EULAR recommend tofacitinib after a trial of methotrexate [1, 2]; thus, we studied patients with RA who had been or were exposed to methotrexate.

Methods

In this retrospective cohort study, we used data from the MarketScan® Commercial Claims and Encounters database and the MarketScan Medicare Supplemental and Coordination of Benefits database (Truven Health Analytics, Ann Arbor, MI, USA) for the period between January 1, 2010, and December 31, 2014. These databases contain claims data for millions of privately insured individuals and their dependents, with many different health plans from large employers, indemnity plans, and health maintenance organizations as well as Medicare-covered patients. These databases include inpatient and outpatient visits, emergency room visits, and outpatient prescription drug information and have been widely used for diverse studies, including RA [10, 11].

We studied adult individuals with RA (at least 18 years old) who were previously treated with methotrexate (oral or subcutaneous) and newly dispensed other DMARDs, biologics, and tofacitinib between January 1, 2011, and December 30, 2014 (see below for complete list of drugs). Patients could be currently using methotrexate. The date of the first medication claim, either an outpatient prescription or a procedure claim (in-office drug administration), was defined as the cohort entry. We selected individuals with no use of these medications any time before cohort entry (minimum 12 months), although previous use of DMARDs was allowed for individuals in the biologic and tofacitinib groups. Patients with RA were identified as individuals with at least one inpatient or two outpatient claims (30 to 365 days apart) with an International Classification of Diseases, Ninth Revision, Clinical Modification (ICD-9-CM), code for RA (714.0x or 714.3x). Patients were excluded if they had another diagnosis before cohort entry for which relevant biologics are also approved: ankylosing spondylitis (ICD-9-CM code 720.0x), chronic lymphocytic leukemia (204.1 x), Crohn's disease (555.xx), juvenile idiopathic arthritis (714.3x), non-Hodgkin's lymphoma (200.xx, 202.xx), plaque psoriasis (696.1x), psoriatic arthritis (696.0x), or ulcerative colitis (556.xx) [12–14]. We also restricted our analysis to individuals with 12 continuous months of medical and pharmacy coverage prior to cohort entry and for the duration of follow-up.

Effectiveness analysis

Patients were classified in mutually exclusive groups according to the medication classes dispensed/administered at the cohort entry: (1) DMARDs (sulfasalazine, leflunomide, hydroxychloroquine, and chloroquine), (2) TNFi (adalimumab, etanercept, infliximab, certolizumab, and golimumab) with or without DMARDs, (3) non-TNF biologics (abatacept, rituximab, and tocilizumab) with or without DMARDs, and (4) tofacitinib with or without DMARDs. For this analysis, each patient contributed one therapy episode in one group.

A given therapy was considered effective if the six criteria of a validated claims-based algorithm [14, 15] were achieved throughout 1 year after cohort entry. This algorithm was validated with a gold standard (Disease Activity Score in 28 joints) and presented high sensitivity (72%), specificity (91%), positive predictive value (76%), and negative predictive value (90%) [15]. For this analysis, we considered only patients with at least 1 year of follow-up. The algorithm criteria relate to changes in the initial therapy: (1) high adherence, (2) no biologic or tofacitinib switch or addition, (3) no DMARD switch or addition, (4) no increase in dose or frequency of index drug, (5) no more than one glucocorticoid joint injection, and (6) no new/increased oral glucocorticoid dose. The details of all criteria are presented in Table 1. Adherence

Table 1 Claims-based algorithm for accessing effectiveness after one year of follow-up in patients with rheumatoid arthritis

Criteria	Description of criteria

Criterion 1
High adherence
	Adherence to therapy was defined as follows:
	• For medications with pharmacy claims only: MPR ≥ 80%[a]
	• For medications with procedure claims only:
	  Etanercept: ≥ 48 procedures
	  Adalimumab: ≥ 22 procedures
	  Certolizumab: ≥ 22 procedures
	  Golimumab: ≥ 11 procedures
	  Infliximab: ≥ 8 procedures
	  Rituximab: ≥ 4 procedures
	  Abatacept: ≥ 11 procedures
	  Tocilizumab: ≥ 11 procedures

Criterion 2 No prescription or procedure of a new biologic or tofacitinib during follow-up	No prescription or procedure of a new biologic or tofacitinib during follow-up
Criterion 3 No DMARD switch or addition	No prescription of a new DMARD between months 4 and 12 of follow-up

Criterion 4
No increase in dose or frequency of index drug
	No increase in dose or frequency of index drug
	• For medications with pharmacy claims only: ≥ 10% of the daily dose at any time during follow-up compared with the daily dose at cohort entry
	• For medications with procedure claims only:
	  Adalimumab: > 25 procedures
	  Certolizumab: > 25 procedures
	  Golimumab: > 12 procedures
	  Infliximab: > 9 procedures
	  Rituximab: > 5 procedures
	  Abatacept: > 13 procedures
	  Tocilizumab: > 12 procedures
	  Etanercept: > 55 procedures

Criterion 5 No more than one procedure for glucocorticoid joint injection between months 4 and 12 of follow-up	No more than one procedure for glucocorticoid joint injection between months 4 and 12 of follow-up
Criterion 6 No new/increased oral glucocorticoid dose	No increase in dose of oral glucocorticoid • For patients who received no prescriptions for oral glucocorticoids 6 months prior to cohort entry: > 30 days of cumulative oral glucocorticoid between months 4 and 12 of follow-up • For patients who received prescriptions for oral glucocorticoids 6 months prior to cohort entry: cumulative dose between months 7 and 12 of follow-up ≥ 120% cumulative dose 6 months prior to cohort entry

MPR Medication possession ratio, DMARD Disease-modifying antirheumatic drug
Adapted from Curtis et al., 2011 [15]
[a]A patient was considered highly adherent if the total days' supply of drug divided by the total days of follow-up was ≥ 80%

to prescribed medication was evaluated using the medication possession ratio (MPR), calculated as the total days' supply of drug divided by the total follow-up days. Patients with MPRs ≥ 80% were considered highly adherent (i.e., meeting criterion 1).

For procedure claims, we used the recommended treatment interval in the U.S. prescribing information to calculate adherence (criterion 1) and increase in biologic dose or frequency (criterion 4) [16–23]. To take into account the differences between prescription and procedure claims regarding the measures of both criteria 1 and 4 (as described above), we excluded patients with a mix of pharmacy and procedure claims for the same index biologic during the follow-up.

In each exposure group, we estimated the separate proportion and the 95% CIs of patients who met individual criteria, as well as the overall proportion of patients for whom the therapy was effective (according to the claims-based algorithm). We estimated adjusted risk ratios with 95% CIs using Poisson regression with robust variance to quantify the relationships between the initiation of treatment with drugs in each exposure group and the effectiveness of the therapy, with non-TNF biologics with or without DMARDs as the reference category, given our particular interest in assessing second-line and subsequent therapies in RA. The models were adjusted for sex, age at entry, and year of cohort entry, as well as for potential confounders measured during 1 year prior to cohort entry: Charlson comorbidity index; hospitalized infection; binary indicators of use of selective cyclooxygenase-2 inhibitors and nonsteroidal anti-inflammatory drugs; oral glucocorticoid use categorized as no use, use of ≤ 7.5 mg/day of prednisone equivalent dose, or ever use of > 7.5 mg/day of prednisone equivalent dose (assessed for each filled prescription); and four indicators of health service use, assessed by the number of (1) emergency department visits, (2) physician visits, (3) rheumatology visits, and (4) hospitalizations.

We performed two sensitivity analyses in which we tested the modified claims-based algorithm for assessing therapy effectiveness while eliminating one of the criteria. First, we excluded criterion 1 (high adherence) to avoid bias estimating adherence of drugs with different administration routes using health claims. Second, we excluded criterion 4 (no increase in dose or frequency of index drug), because patients starting therapy with tofacitinib and some biologics usually do not change the initial dose and/or the frequency.

Safety analysis

For the safety analysis, current drug exposure was modeled as a time-dependent variable. Accordingly, each subject's follow-up time was divided into consecutive time intervals with a new interval starting whenever the patient changed, interrupted, and/or started treatment with one of the drug groups of interest. Switching to another drug within the same exposure group was not considered a change of drug exposure. Patients were considered exposed during the days supplied for the pre-scribed medication or, in the case of an outpatient pro-cedure, the number of days in the recommended treatment interval. We applied a maximum grace period of 90 days, implying that subjects were assumed to re-main exposed for the most recently presented drug until 90 days after the end of the prescription or the start of a new drug, whichever came earlier. Within each interval, a patient was classified into one of the same exposure categories as above, plus a no-use category, based on his/her current medication exposure: (1) DMARDs, (2) TNFi with or without DMARDs, (3) non-TNF biologics with or without DMARDs, (4) tofacitinib with or with-out DMARDs, or (5) nonuse (if not currently in use of any of the drugs in these categories). The outcome was defined as the occurrence of serious infection requiring hospitalization identified from the primary diagnosis recorded in the hospitalization discharge records (ICD-9-CM codes 001-139 or 480–486).

We estimated the rate of serious infections per 100 patient-years for each exposure group. We also estimated the adjusted HRs with 95% CIs, using multivariable time-dependent Cox proportional hazards regression to assess the risk of serious infections associated with the current use of drugs in different categories, represented by time-dependent binary indicators (dummy variables). The non-TNF biologics with or without DMARDs group was the reference category. Adjustments were made for the same covariates described for the effectiveness analysis and additionally for four time-dependent variables indicating current use of methotrexate, current use of glucocorticoid (no use, ≤ 7.5 mg/day, and > 7.5 mg/day), previous use of biologics, and previous use of other DMARDs.

Patients were followed from cohort entry until the earliest date of either (1) the event (i.e., the first occur-rence of a serious infection) or (2) censoring at the time of loss of medical or pharmacy coverage, inpatient death, or the end of the study (December 31, 2014). Thus, we considered only one event per patient. In the primary analyses, we allowed patients to continue in the analyses after a drug change placed them in a different exposure category, but in a sensitivity analysis we censored them after they stopped/switched their initial therapy.

We restricted this analysis to only patients covered by Medicare in a sensitivity analysis. The rationale was that patients from commercial health plans enter and leave the cohort according to their drug insurance plan, which can change over time as their employment changes,

whereas the Medicare coverage was expected to be more stable. Thus, for commercially insured people, the data we held is only a sampling of their entire health history, and missing information for the remaining periods could have affected the accuracy of the analyses. The Medicare patients, on the other hand, remained in the cohort for the entire follow-up period.

In an additional sensitivity analysis of safety, we repeated our work in a new cohort of patients with RA requiring them to be exposed to biologics and then to have initiated a new biologic agent or tofacitinib. All analyses were conducted using SAS version 9.4 software (SAS Institute, Cary, NC, USA).

Results

A total of 21,832 patients with RA previously exposed to methotrexate met the inclusion criteria. The therapy at cohort entry included TNFi with or without DMARDs (61.2%), DMARDs alone (24.7%), non-TNF biologics with or without DMARDs (13.3%), and tofacitinib with or without DMARDs (0.8%). Baseline characteristics were similar across groups (Table 2).

Effectiveness

Overall, therapy effectiveness was rather low, below 20% for each exposure group (first row of Table 3), with the low-est rates being in the DMARDs-alone group (11%). Patients using either TNFi or non-TNF biologics reached better effectiveness rates, followed by tofacitinib. Among the six criteria, high adherence had the lowest rates in all groups and was especially low for DMARDs alone and tofacitinib. For criterion 2 (no biologic or tofacitinib switch or addition), the highest rate observed was among tofacitinib users. For criterion 3 (no DMARD switch or addition), DMARDs had the lowest rate. All patients using tofacitinib met criterion 4 (no dose escalation). Joint injections (criter-ion 5) occurred less often among patients using DMARDs, and oral glucocorticoid dose increases (criterion 6) were least likely to happen in the TNFi group (Table 3).

In the multivariable analyses, DMARDs were sig-nificantly less likely than non-TNF biologics to be classified as effective (Table 4). For TNFi and the tofacitinib groups, the 95% CIs around the point es-timates were fairly wide and precluded definitive conclusions.

The algorithm without criterion 1 (high adherence) showed that tofacitinib was more likely than non-TNF biologics to reach effectiveness (Additional file 1). When we excluded criterion 4 (no increase in dose or frequency of index drug), most of the multivariate re-sults were similar to the primary analysis, but in addition TNFi were less effective than non-TNF bio-logics (Additional file 1).

Table 2 Baseline characteristics of patients with rheumatoid arthritis included in the study

Variable	All patients (n = 21,832)	DMARDs (n = 5399)	TNFi ± DMARDs (n = 13,367)	Non-TNF biologics ± DMARDs (n = 2902)	Tofacitinib ± DMARDs (n = 164)
Female sex, %	77.0	76.8	76.1	81.4	78.7
Age, years, median (IQR)	56 (48–63)	57 (49–63)	56 (48–63)	58 (50–65)	58 (50–64)
Year of cohort entry, %					
2011	48.5	25.9	52.3	70.5	0
2012	21.6	27.2	20.5	14.1	0.6
2013	14.7	21.9	13.1	8.7	43.9
2014	15.2	25.0	14.1	6.7	55.5
Urban residency, %	82.6	81.1	83.2	82.8	89.4
Oral glucocorticoid use, %					
No use	32.3	29.2	33.4	33.0	31.0
≤ 7.5 mg/day of prednisone equivalent dose	63.0	65.1	62.2	62.2	64.9
> 7.5 mg/day of prednisone equivalent dose	4.7	5.7	4.4	4.8	4.0
Nonsteroidal anti-inflammatory drug use, %	60.7	60.3	62.1	54.9	51.8
Selective COX-2 inhibitor use, %	12.8	10.9	12.9	16.0	13.4
Charlson comorbidity index, mean (SD)	0.61 (0.93)	0.73 (1.04)	0.54 (0.84)	0.73 (1.02)	0.86 (1.14)
Infection-related hospitalization, %	1.6	1.9	1.3	2.6	1.8
Number of emergency department visits, mean (SD)	0.44 (1.20)	0.48 (1.39)	0.42 (1.14)	0.44 (1.05)	0.43 (0.83)
Number of physician visits, mean (SD)	17.99 (13.26)	17.32 (14.07)	17.37 (12.24)	22.21 (15.24)	16.70 (14.24)
Number of rheumatology visits, mean (SD)	4.51 (4.92)	3.39 (3.85)	4.54 (4.71)	6.47 (6.75)	3.88 (3.26)
Number of hospitalizations, mean (SD)	0.16 (0.50)	0.16 (0.54)	0.14 (0.45)	0.23 (0.62)	0.17 (0.62)

Abbreviations: DMARD Disease-modifying antirheumatic drug, *TNFi* Tumor necrosis factor inhibitor, *COX-2* Cyclooxygenase-2
Baseline variables were collected at cohort entry (sex, age, year of cohort entry, and place of residence) or 1 year prior to cohort entry (use of drugs, Charlson comorbidity index, hospitalized infection, and indicators of health service use)

Safety

Current use of tofacitinib was associated with a rate of serious infections of 3.67 per 100 patient-years, and the 95% CI for this estimate (2.21; 5.75) overlapped with the rate of serious infections for the other drug groups (Table 5). In the multivariate analyses, the hazards of serious infection for DMARDs, TNFi, and tofacitinib were not significant different compared with non-TNF biologic. Current use of methotrexate, previous use of biologics, use of oral glucocorticoid in the year before cohort entry, and current use

Table 3 Proportion of patients who achieved therapy effectiveness and individual criteria at 1 year of follow-up (n = 16,305)

Effectiveness criteria	DMARDs		TNFi ± DMARDs		Non-TNF biologics ± DMARDs		Tofacitinib ± DMARDs	
	Percent	95% CI	Percent	95% CI	Percent	95% CI	Percent	95% CI
Effective therapy (satisfied all six criteria)	11.1	10.1–12.1	18.6	17.9–19.4	19.8	18.2–21.4	15.4	6.6–24.2
Criterion 1 High adherence	26.6	25.1–28.0	44.0	43.0–44.9	53.3	51.3–55.3	27.7	16.8–38.6
Criterion 2 No biologic or tofacitinib switch or addition	72.7	71.2–74.1	64.3	63.4–65.2	82.1	80.5–83.6	84.6	75.8–93.4
Criterion 3 No DMARD switch or addition	85.3	84.2–86.5	96.1	95.8–96.5	95.5	94.6–96.3	98.5	95.5–100
Criterion 4 No increase in dose or frequency of index drug	92.0	91.1–92.9	94.0	93.5–94.4	88.9	87.6–90.1	100.0[a]	–
Criterion 5 No more than one glucocorticoid joint injection	91.3	90.3–92.2	88.8	88.2–89.4	72.8	71.0–74.6	87.7	79.7–95.7
Criterion 6 No new/increased oral glucocorticoid dose	81.4	80.2–82.7	83.3	82.6–84.1	78.0	76.3–79.7	76.9	66.7–87.2

DMARD Disease-modifying antirheumatic drug, *TNFi* Tumor necrosis factor inhibitors
[a]Standard tofacitinib dose is usually not increased

Table 4 Adjusted risk ratio and 95% CI for medication effectiveness (algorithm result) (n = 16,305)

Parameter	Adjusted risk ratio	95% CI
Drug therapy		
Non-TNF biologics ± DMARDs	Reference	–
DMARDs	0.58	0.51–0.66
TNFi ± DMARDs	0.94	0.86–1.03
Tofacitinib ± DMARDs	0.75	0.42–1.34
Sex (female)	0.94	0.87–1.02
Age	1.01	1.00–1.01
Year of cohort entry		
2011	Reference	–
2012	0.87	0.8–0.95
2013	1.00	0.91–1.1
Oral glucocorticoid use 1 year prior to cohort entry		
No use	Reference	–
Use of ≤ 7.5 mg/day of prednisone equivalent dose	0.94	0.88–1.02
Use of > 7.5 mg/day of prednisone equivalent dose	1.07	0.90–1.26
Nonsteroidal anti-inflammatory drug use 1 year prior to cohort entry	0.94	0.88–1.01
Selective COX-2 inhibitors use 1 year prior to cohort entry	0.98	0.88–1.08
Charlson comorbidity index 1 year prior to cohort entry	0.91	0.86–0.95
Infection-related hospitalization 1 year prior to cohort entry	0.84	0.60–1.19
Number of emergency department visits 1 year prior to cohort entry	0.96	0.90–1.01
Number of physician visits 1 year prior to cohort entry	1.00	0.99–1.00
Number of rheumatology visits 1 year prior to cohort entry	1.00	1.00–1.01
Number of hospitalizations 1 year prior to cohort entry	0.97	0.89–1.06

Abbreviations: DMARD Disease-modifying antirheumatic drug, *TNFi* Tumor necrosis factor inhibitors, *COX-2* Cyclooxygenase-2

Table 5 Crude incidence and 95% CIs of serious infection (n = 21,832)

Drug therapy	Events	Total person-years	Crude rate (per 100 patient-year)	95% CI
DMARDs	104	5196.02	2.01	1.65–2.42
TNFi ± DMARDs	490	22,736.79	2.16	1.98–2.36
Non-TNF biologic ± DMARDs	173	6936.41	2.49	2.14–2.88
Tofacitinib ± DMARDs	17	474.48	3.67	2.21–5.75

DMARDs Disease-modifying antirheumatic drugs, *TNFi* Tumor necrosis factor inhibitors

of oral glucocorticoid were associated with significant increases in the current hazard of infections (Table 6).

Our findings were similar in the sensitivity analysis, where we censored patients after they discontinued or switched their initial therapy (Additional file 2). The analysis limited to Medicare data reduced the sample to 5200 patients. The incidence of serious infection was higher in the Medicare patients than in the primary analyses, across all exposure groups, but the HRs were generally similar to the primary analysis, despite the wide CIs (Additional file 3). Finally, in an additional sensitivity analysis in a new cohort of patients with RA previously exposed to a biologic agent, the results also indicated that tofacitinib was not significantly different from non-TNF biologics (Additional file 4).

Discussion

In this retrospective cohort study of patients previously treated with methotrexate, we evaluated the effectiveness and risk of serious infection of tofacitinib compared with DMARDs, TNFi, and non-TNF biologics. Effectiveness at 1 year of follow-up, estimated by a claims-based algorithm, was noted in 15% of tofacitinib users, 11% of DMARD users, and around 19% of TNFi and non-TNF biologic users. The adjusted analysis showed that patients using tofacitinib were as likely as non-TNF biologic users to show effectiveness. The algorithm measures effectiveness on the basis of changes of the initial therapy that can capture both lack of or low effectiveness as well as drug intolerance and side effects. Therefore, it may be expected that our results show lower "success" rates than RCTs. In addition of course, our "real-world" data reflect a different population from the relatively narrow and homogeneous range of subjects enrolled in RCTs, which also will result in different "success" rates as compared with RCTs.

Adherence was an important component in our effectiveness algorithms: less than half of patients in the TNFi and non-TNF biologic groups and only one-third in the tofacitinib and DMARD groups continued their initial therapy. This criterion does not distinguish between actual noncompliance with the treatment and intolerance or adverse events. Switching/addition was another important factor contributing to overall algorithm failure, particularly in the TNFi group. Note that patients using tofacitinib did not increase their initial dose, given that there is only one Food and Drug Administration-approved dose. The adjusted comparisons of the final algorithm result suggested greater effectiveness for TNFi or non-TNF biologics than for DMARDs, and we were unable to establish differences for tofacitinib and DMARDs. In effect, tofacitinib appeared as effective as biologics on the basis of most criteria. Researchers in another cohort study using pharmacy claims reported a

Table 6 Adjusted HRs and 95% CIs for time to serious infection (n = 21,832)

Parameter	Adjusted HR	95% CI
Drug therapy		
Non-TNF biologic ± DMARDs	Reference	–
DMARDs	0.80	0.62–1.03
TNFi ± DMARDs	1.14	0.95–1.37
Tofacitinib ± DMARDs	1.54	0.93–2.56
Current use of methotrexate[a]	1.19	1.04–1.37
Previous use of biologics[a]	1.32	1.12–1.57
Previous use of other DMARDs[a]	1.04	0.86–1.27
Sex (female)	1.02	0.87–1.18
Age	1.04	1.03–1.04
Year of cohort entry		
2011	Reference	–
2012	1.10	0.92–1.31
2013	0.85	0.66–1.08
2014	0.97	0.70–1.35
Oral glucocorticoid use one year prior to cohort entry		
No use	Reference	–
Use of ≤ 7.5 mg/day of prednisone equivalent dose	1.23	1.05–1.44
Use of > 7.5 mg/day of prednisone equivalent dose	1.36	1.00–1.84
Current use of oral glucocorticoid[a]		
No use	Reference	–
Use of ≤ 7.5 mg/day of prednisone equivalent dose	1.90	1.64–2.20
Use of > 7.5 mg/day of prednisone equivalent dose	2.83	1.37–5.83
Nonsteroidal anti-inflammatory drugs use 1 year prior to cohort entry	0.93	0.81–1.06
Selective COX-2 inhibitors use 1 year prior to cohort entry	1.13	0.95–1.35
Charlson comorbidity index 1 year prior to cohort entry	1.72	1.49–1.99
Infection related hospitalization 1 year prior to cohort entry	2.19	1.68–2.86
Number of emergency department visits 1 year prior to cohort entry	1.04	1.01–1.06
Number of physician visits 1 year prior to cohort entry	1.01	1.00–1.01
Number of rheumatology visits 1 year prior to cohort entry	1.00	0.99–1.02
Number of hospitalizations 1 year prior to cohort entry	1.33	1.24–1.43

DMARDs Disease-modifying antirheumatic drug, *TNFi* Tumor necrosis factor inhibitors
[a]Time-varying covariates

similar proportion of persistence and adherence (measured by proportion of days covered) at the first year of therapy among patients using tofacitinib, etanercept, adalimumab, and abatacept. A greater proportion of patients using etanercept and adalimumab switched to tofacitinib or another biologic. Finally, dose increase happened in 5% of patients using tofacitinib [4].

Our study shows that the unadjusted incidence of hospitalizations for infection was 3.6 per 100 patient-years for tofacitinib, compared with 2.2 and 2.5 per 100 patient-years in individuals using TNFi and non-TNF biologics, respectively. Higher rates were observed in each of these groups in the cohort containing only patients covered by Medicare (aged > 65 years). Recent cohort studies showed different point estimates for DMARDs and biologic agents [24–26], which may be explained by the difference in the definition of serious infections, by differences in patients' profiles regarding other risk factors for infections, or perhaps by chance alone. Our adjusted comparisons did not demonstrate that tofacitinib users had an increased risk of serious (hospitalized) infections compared with those treated with non-TNF biologics. One recent study using Medicare and Market-Scan databases showed that patients using tofacitinib had a higher risk for herpes virus infection than those using biologic drugs [7]. Although the aim of our study was not to directly compare infection risk of tofacitinib patients with that of those treated with anti-TNF drugs only, we performed this comparison and did not find a significant difference. Factors that were associated with higher risk of infection in our study were current use of methotrexate, use of oral glucocorticoid before cohort entry, and previous use of biologics.

In our sample, after a first treatment with methotrexate, tofacitinib was not commonly prescribed. Although the ACR and EULAR guidelines recommend the use of tofacitinib after failure of therapy with DMARDs in patients with established RA, others argue that the JAK inhibitors (owing to the uncertainty about long-term safety and cost-effectiveness) should be used only after insufficient response to initial biologic treatment [27]. The dearth of evidence from observational studies to date was in part the motivation for our work in this analysis to inform the comparative effectiveness and safety of tofacitinib. Our additional analysis of tofacitinib after failure of a first biologic therapy for patients with RA showed similar safety in terms of serious (hospitalized) infection.

Our study has potential limitations. First, we obtained a small sample of tofacitinib users, which was expected for a novel therapy. The patients were not clinically confirmed, but we did use a validated RA definition; our patients were all previously exposed to the cornerstone RA therapy (methotrexate); and we excluded patients with other indications for various RA drug exposures (e.g., cancer, other rheumatic diseases). Still, although MarketScan databases collect data on a large population, it lacks data on important clinical variables and reasons for changing the initial therapy. As a result, we indirectly measured therapy effectiveness using an algorithm based on registers of drug prescriptions or drug administration. This algorithm is composed of criteria related to actionable interventions used by physicians. Although the algorithm has previously been validated for anti-TNF and DMARD therapy in RA, it seemed reasonable to apply the same set of criteria to measure the response to non-TNF biologics and tofacitinib as we did in our study. In addition, herpes zoster (which usually does not require hospitalization) is potentially an important infectious outcome but not one we focused on in this analysis.

All observational studies are at risk of "channeling"; that is, persons are not allocated drugs randomly, and the characteristics of certain people who tend to receive certain drugs may become confounders (e.g., RA disease duration and prior biologic use, which have been shown to be confounders of infection risk [28]) if those are also associated with the outcome of interest. So, for example, it may be that people assigned to tofacitinib were more or less likely (because of their past response to drugs in terms of effectiveness or infection) to have the outcome of interest. We aimed to overcome this potential issue by studying only those patients with RA with previous methotrexate exposure, and we also controlled for proxies of disease severity (e.g., past drugs and rheumatology visits).

We note that in the dataset that we used, patients' follow-up could have happened because of a loss or change in their health insurance. Medicare completely captures patients' claims, and the analysis restricted to those patients showed similar risk for infections, despite the lower precision.

As a final point that should be taken into account when interpreting and comparing our results, in our analyses, patients using biologics or tofacitinib could also be taking one or more DMARDs, including MTX. However, most of these combinations would be with drugs such as hydroxychloroquine, which itself tends not to increase infection risk.

Conclusions

In summary, in this report of a large population-based cohort study, we present novel data on real-world use of tofacitinib in patients with RA previously treated with methotrexate. Our study estimated similar (relatively low) effectiveness rates at 1 year of follow-up for patients starting tofacitinib after therapy with methotrexate, as opposed to initiators of non-TNF biologics. Our comparisons of tofacitinib versus non-TNF biologics,

though not definitive, did not clearly demonstrate differences with respect to hospitalized infections.

Additional files

Additional file 1: Proportion and adjusted risk ratio of patients who achieved therapy effectiveness based on the modified algorithm ($n = 16,305$).

Additional file 2: Adjusted HR for time to serious infection in patients censored after they stopped/switched their initial therapy ($n = 21,832$).

Additional file 3: Adjusted HR for time to serious infection in patients covered by Medicare ($n = 5200$).

Additional file 4: Crude incidence of serious infection in patients with RA previously exposed to a biologic agent ($n = 14,875$). Adjusted HR for time to serious infection in patients with RA previously exposed to a biologic agent ($n = 14,875$).

Abbreviations
ACR: American College of Rheumatology; COX-2: Cyclooxygenase-2; DMARD: Disease-modifying antirheumatic drug; EULAR: European League Against Rheumatism; ICD-9-CM: International Classification of Diseases, Ninth Revision, Clinical Modification; JAK: Janus kinase; MPR: Medication possession ratio; RA: Rheumatoid arthritis; RCT: Randomized controlled trial; TNFi: Tumor necrosis factor inhibitor(s)

Acknowledgements
Hassan Behlouli provided analytical support.

Funding
This work was funded by the Canadian Institutes of Health Research.

Authors' contributions
MAAM contributed to the design, data analyses, data interpretation, and manuscript preparation. CSM contributed to the design, data analyses, data interpretation, and manuscript preparation. SFG contributed to data analyses and manuscript preparation. JRC contributed to the design, data interpretation, and manuscript preparation. MA contributed to acquisition of data, data analyses, data interpretation, and manuscript preparation. SB contributed to acquisition of data, study concept and design, data interpretation, and manuscript preparation. All authors read and approved the final manuscript.

Competing interests
The authors declare that they have no competing interests.

Author details
[1]Division of Clinical Epidemiology, Research Institute of McGill University Health Centre, 5252 de Maisonneuve West, Montreal, QC, Canada. [2]Division of Clinical Immunology and Rheumatology, University of Alabama at Birmingham, 619 19th Street South, Birmingham, AL SRC 076, USA. [3]Department of Epidemiology, Biostatistics and Occupational Health, Research Institute of McGill University Health Centre, 5252 de Maisonneuve West, Montreal, QC, Canada.

References
1. Singh JA, Saag KG, Bridges SL Jr, Akl EA, Bannuru RR, Sullivan MC, et al. 2015 American College of Rheumatology Guideline for the Treatment of Rheumatoid Arthritis. Arthritis Rheumatol. 2016;68(1):1–26.
2. Smolen JS, Landewé R, Bijlsma J, Burmester G, Chatzidionysiou K, Dougados M, et al. EULAR recommendations for the management of rheumatoid

arthritis with synthetic and biological disease-modifying antirheumatic drugs: 2016 update. Ann Rheum Dis. 2017;76(6):960–77.

3. Buckley F, Finckh A, Huizinga TW, Dejonckheere F, Jansen JP. Comparative efficacy of novel DMARDs as monotherapy and in combination with methotrexate in rheumatoid arthritis patients with inadequate response to conventional DMARDs: a network meta-analysis. J Manag Care Spec Pharm. 2015;21(5):409–23.

4. Harnett J, Gerber R, Gruben D, Koenig AS, Chen C. Evaluation of real-world experience with tofacitinib compared with adalimumab, etanercept, and abatacept in RA patients with 1 previous biologic DMARD: data from a U.S. administrative claims database. J Manag Care Spec Pharm. 2016;22(12): 1457–71.

5. Winthrop KL, Yamanaka H, Valdez H, Mortensen E, Chew R, Krishnaswami S, et al. Herpes zoster and tofacitinib therapy in patients with rheumatoid arthritis. Arthritis Rheumatol. 2014;66(10):2675–84.

6. Souto A, Maneiro JR, Salgado E, Carmona L, Gomez-Reino JJ. Risk of tuberculosis in patients with chronic immune-mediated inflammatory diseases treated with biologics and tofacitinib: a systematic review and meta-analysis of randomized controlled trials and long-term extension studies. Rheumatology (Oxford). 2014;53(10):1872–85.

7. Curtis JR, Xie F, Yun H, Bernatsky S, Winthrop KL. Real-world comparative risks of herpes virus infections in tofacitinib and biologic-treated patients with rheumatoid arthritis. Ann Rheum Dis. 2016;75(10):1843–7.

8. Berger ML, Sox H, Willke RJ, Brixner DL, Eichler HG, Goettsch W, et al. Good practices for real-world data studies of treatment and/or comparative effectiveness: recommendations from the joint ISPOR-ISPE Special Task Force on real-world evidence in health care decision making. Pharmacoepidemiol Drug Saf. 2017;26(9):1033–9.

9. Berger ML, Dreyer N, Anderson F, Towse A, Sedrakyan A, Normand SL. Prospective observational studies to assess comparative effectiveness: the ISPOR good research practices task force report. Value Health. 2012;15(2):217–30.

10. Gu NY, Huang XY, Fox KM, Patel VD, Baumgartner SW, Chiou CF. Claims data analysis of dosing and cost of TNF antagonists. Am J Pharm Benefits. 2010;2:351–9.

11. Petri H, Maldonato D, Robinson NJ. Data-driven identification of co-morbidities associated with rheumatoid arthritis in a large US health plan claims database. BMC Musculoskelet Disord. 2010;11:247.

12. Curtis JR, Schabert VF, Harrison DJ, Yeaw J, Korn JR, Quach C, et al. Estimating effectiveness and cost of biologics for rheumatoid arthritis: application of a validated algorithm to commercial insurance claims. Clin Ther. 2014;36(7):996–1004.

13. Sauer BC, Teng CC, He T, Leng J, Lu CC, Curtis JR, Cannon GW. Effectiveness and costs of biologics in veterans with rheumatoid arthritis. Am J Pharm Benefits. 2015;7(6):280–9.

14. Bonafede M, Johnson BH, Princic N, Shah N, Harrison DJ. Cost per patient-year in response using a claims-based algorithm for the 2 years following biologic initiation in patients with rheumatoid arthritis. J Med Econ. 2015; 18(5):376–89.

15. Curtis JR, Baddley JW, Yang S, Patkar N, Chen L, Delzell E, et al. Derivation and preliminary validation of an administrative claims-based algorithm for the effectiveness of medications for rheumatoid arthritis. Arthritis Res Ther. 2011;13(5):R155.

16. Genentech I. Actemra (tocilizumab) prescribing information. South San Francisco, CA: Genentech, Inc.; 2017.

17. UCB, Inc. Cimzia (certolizumab pegol) prescribing information. Smyrna, GA: UCB, Inc.; 2013.

18. Corporation I. Enbrel (etanercept) prescribing information. Thousand Oaks, CA: Immunex Corporation; 2013.

19. Laboratories A. Humira (adalimumab) prescribing information. North Chicago, IL: Abbott Laboratories; 2014.

20. Bristol-Myers Squibb Company. Orencia (abatacept) prescribing information. Princeton, NJ: Bristol-Myers Squibb Company; 2014.

21. Centocor Ortho Biotech, Inc. Remicade (infliximab) prescribing information. Malvern, PA: Centocor Ortho Biotech, Inc.; 2013.

22. Biogen/Genentech USA, Inc. Rituxan (rituximab) prescribing information. South San Francisco, CA: Biogen/Genentech USA, Inc.; 2016.

23. Biotech J. Inc. Simponi (golimumab) prescribing information. Horsham, PA: Janssen Biotech, Inc.; 2014.

24. Dixon WG, Symmons DP, Lunt M, Watson KD, Hyrich KL, British Society for Rheumatology Biologics Register Control Centre Consortium, et al. Serious infection following anti-tumor necrosis factor alpha therapy in patients with rheumatoid arthritis: lessons from interpreting data from observational studies. Arthritis Rheum. 2007;56(9):2896–904.

25. Curtis JR, Yang S, Patkar NM, Chen L, Singh JA, Cannon GW, et al. Risk of hospitalized bacterial infections associated with biologic treatment among US veterans with rheumatoid arthritis. Arthritis Care Res (Hoboken). 2014; 66(7):990–7.

26. Kawashima H, Kagami SI, Kashiwakuma D, Takahashi K, Yokota M, Furuta S, et al. Long-term use of biologic agents does not increase the risk of serious infections in elderly patients with rheumatoid arthritis. Rheumatol Int. 2017; 37(3):369–76.

27. Kissin EY. The "dirty little secret" exposed in the 2013 EULAR recommendations for rheumatoid arthritis therapy. Clin Ther. 2014;36(7): 1114–6.

28. Curtis JR, Xie F, Chen L, Baddley JW, Beukelman T, Saag KG, et al. The comparative risk of serious infections among rheumatoid arthritis patients starting or switching biological agents. Ann Rheum Dis. 2011;70(8):1401–6.

10

Smoking, body mass index, disease activity, and the risk of rapid radiographic progression in patients with early rheumatoid arthritis

Emil Rydell[1,2]* , Kristina Forslind[3,4], Jan-Åke Nilsson[1,2], Lennart T. H. Jacobsson[1,5] and Carl Turesson[1,2]

Abstract

Background: Identification of risk factors for rapid joint destruction in early rheumatoid arthritis (RA) can be helpful for optimizing treatment, and improving our understanding of destructive arthritis and its mechanisms. The objective of this study was to investigate the relationship between early RA patient characteristics and subsequent rapid radiographic progression (RRP).

Methods: An inception cohort of patients with early RA (symptom duration < 12 months), recruited during 1995–2005 from a defined area (Malmö, Sweden), was investigated. Radiographs of the hands and feet were scored in chronological order according to the modified Sharp–van der Heijde score (SHS), by a trained reader. RRP was defined as an increase of ≥ 5 points in SHS per year.

Results: Two hundred and thirty-three patients were included. Radiographs were available from 216 patients at baseline, 206 patients at 1 year, and 171 patients at 5 years. Thirty-six patients (22%) had RRP up to 5 years. In logistic regression models, rheumatoid factor (RF) and anti-cyclic citrullinated peptides (anti-CCP), and increased erythrocyte sedimentation rate (ESR) or C-reactive protein (CRP) at baseline, predicted RRP over 5 years. Patients identified as overweight or obese had a significantly reduced risk of RRP up to 5 years (odds ratio (OR) 0.26; 95% confidence interval (CI) 0.11–0.63; adjusted for RF, baseline erosions, and ESR). Similar point estimates were obtained when stratifying for antibody status, and in models adjusted for smoking. A history of ever smoking was associated with a significantly increased risk of RRP up to 5 years, independent of body mass index (BMI) (OR 3.17; 95% CI 1.22–8.28; adjusted for BMI). At the 1-year follow-up, erosive changes, Disease Activity Score of 28 joints, Health Assessment Questionnaire, swollen joint count, and patient's global assessment of disease activity and pain were also significantly associated with RRP up to 5 years.

Conclusions: A history of smoking, presence of RF and/or anti-CCP and early erosions, high initial disease activity and active disease at 1 year, all increase the risk of RRP. Patients with a high BMI may have a reduced risk of severe joint damage. This pattern was not explained by differences in disease activity or antibody status. The results of this study suggest independent effects of smoking and BMI on the risk of RRP.

Keywords: Rheumatoid arthritis, Radiographic progression, Joint damage, Smoking, Body mass index, Disease activity

* Correspondence: emil.rydell@med.lu.se
[1]Rheumatology, Department of Clinical Sciences, Malmö, Lund University, Jan Waldenströms gata 35, SE-202 13 Malmö, Sweden
[2]Department of Rheumatology, Skåne University Hospital, Inga Marie Nilssons gata 32, SE-214 28 Malmö, Sweden
Full list of author information is available at the end of the article

Background

In order to optimize treatment in patients with early rheumatoid arthritis (RA), with the intention to stop progression of joint destruction, it is important at an early stage to identify patients at high risk of rapid radiographic progression (RRP). Finding early risk factors is therefore of key importance. Previous research shows that patients with rheumatoid factor (RF) and anti-citrullinated protein antibodies (ACPA) have more severe disease with more extensive radiographic progression [1, 2]. Early joint erosions as well as high levels of markers of inflammation have also been associated with worse radiographic outcomes [3–6]. Environmental factors, such as smoking, may also affect the course of RA. Smoking is a risk factor for developing RA [7, 8], as well as for extra-articular manifestations in patients with established disease [9]. In addition, it has been suggested that smoking increases the risk for radiographic progression [10]. However, results from previous studies on smoking and radiographic damage are mixed [10–14]. Intricate relationships between smoking, antibodies, body composition, treatment response, and disease activity as well as differences in the design of previous studies make it difficult to assess the independent effect of smoking on the risk of radiographic progression.

Furthermore, although a high level of inflammation in the early stages of disease is a known risk factor for radiographic progression, the utility of the commonly used composite measure Disease Activity Score of 28 joints (DAS28) for identifying patients at risk and the importance of persistent disease activity are less clear [12, 15–17]. Previous research has indicated better outcomes for patients receiving disease-modifying antirheumatic drugs (DMARDs) at an early stage [18, 19]. However, such effects may vary across populations and depend on current treatment strategies.

Patients with high body mass index (BMI) have been shown in large studies to have higher disease activity [20, 21], to be less likely to respond to treatment [22], and to have more extensive disability [23]. Despite this, high BMI has been associated with reduced radiographic progression in a limited number of studies [24–28].

The purpose of this study was to investigate how patient characteristics, smoking status, disease activity measures over time, BMI, and time to initiation of DMARD treatment relate to subsequent RRP in patients with early RA.

Methods

Patients

An inception cohort of 233 consecutive patients with early RA was investigated. The catchment area was the city of Malmö, Sweden (population 259,579 in 2000). Patients were recruited from the rheumatology outpatient clinic of Malmö University Hospital, the only hospital serving the city, or from the four rheumatologists in private practice in the area, between 1995 and 2005.

The patients were diagnosed with RA by a specialist in rheumatology, fulfilled the 1987 American College of Rheumatology classification criteria for RA [29], and had a duration of symptoms ≤ 12 months at the time of inclusion. There were no additional exclusion criteria. All patients gave their written consent for participation in the study, including data collection and inclusion in the database. The study was approved by the Regional Ethical Review Board for southern Sweden (Lund, Sweden), and complied with the Declaration of Helsinki.

Results on clinical parameters and grip strength in a subset of the included patients have been reported previously [30].

Clinical assessment

Patients were followed according to a structured program with evaluations at inclusion, 12 months, and 60 months. The same rheumatologist performed all of the clinical examinations. Patient characteristics and disease activity parameters were recorded, and radiographs of the hands and feet were obtained. The presence of erosions (present vs absent) was determined by a radiologist as part of standard clinical practice. Disability was assessed using the Swedish version of the Stanford Health Assessment Questionnaire (HAQ) [31]. Visual analogue scales (VASs) were used to evaluate the patients' global assessment of disease activity and the patient's assessment of pain. All patients were managed according to usual care with no prespecified protocol for antirheumatic treatment. The patients were included before the current practice of treat to target [32] was implemented, and before early treatment with biologic DMARDs came into widespread use. Information on height, weight, and smoking history (current/previous/never) was collected at inclusion through a self-administered questionnaire. For confirmation, information on smoking was also gathered through case-record reviews, with previous smoking being defined as a history of daily smoking for more than 6 months at anytime earlier in the patient's life. The time from symptom onset to first start of DMARD treatment was assessed based on a review of medical records.

Data on treatment with biologic DMARDs at any time during the study period were obtained through linkage to a regional biologics register [33].

Changes in disease activity (DAS28) from baseline to the 1-year follow-up were categorized according to the European League Against Rheumatism (EULAR) response criteria [34].

Laboratory investigations

RF and antibodies to cyclic citrullinated peptides (anti-CCP) were analyzed using standard ELISA methods at the immunology laboratories of the University Hospitals in Malmö and Lund. IgM RF was analyzed using ELISA, which was calibrated against the World Health Organization (WHO) RF reference preparation. Anti-CCP antibodies were analyzed using the Quanta Lite CCP IgG ELISA (INOVA Diagnostics, USA). The erythrocyte sedimentation rate (ESR) and C-reactive protein (CRP) were assessed according to standard methods at the Department of Clinical Chemistry, Malmö University Hospital.

Radiographic assessment

Radiographs of the hands and feet were scored in chronological order according to the modified Sharp–van der Heijde score (SHS), by a trained reader (KF, coauthor) who was blinded to the clinical data. The intraclass correlation coefficient (ICC) from two readings with 2-week intervals for a subset of the cohort ($n = 30$) was 0.97. Based on the excellent ICC, a single reading was performed. The primary outcome, RRP, was defined as an increase of ≥ 5 points in SHS per year [35]. We also assessed SHS progression above the median as an outcome.

Statistical analysis

Potential associations between each individual baseline variable with RRP over the first 5 years, as well as with above median progression of SHS during the same time period, were assessed using logistic regression analyses. Furthermore, the relation between 1-year variables and RRP between the follow-ups at 1 and 5 years was evaluated.

The covariates for the multivariate models were chosen based on the literature and the unadjusted analyses. Due to colinearity, we did not include both RF and anti-CCP. RF was chosen over anti-CCP due to the smaller number of patients with missing data for RF. The final multivariate analyses were adjusted for RF and for the presence of erosions according to standard radiologist assessment (independent of SHS scoring).

During part of the study period, high-sensitivity CRP analysis was not available and CRP values between 0 and 9 mg/l were reported by the laboratory as < 9 mg/l. In logistic regression models, CRP was therefore included as a dichotomized variable; that is, above versus below the median (9 mg/l) at inclusion and above versus below the 75th percentile (10 mg/l) at 1 year (since the median at 1 year was < 9 mg/l). Current smoking, previous smoking, and ever smoking were each compared to the reference category, never smoking.

BMI was included as a continuous variable. Furthermore, the risk of RRP in individuals fulfilling the WHO criteria for overweight or obesity (≥ 25 kg/m^2), overweight ($25–29.99$ kg/m^2), or obesity (≥ 30 kg/m^2) was compared to that in individuals with normal BMI ($18.5–24.99$ kg/m^2).

Predictors of SHS progression above the median were assessed in the same manner.

Statistical analysis was performed using IBM SPSS Statistics version 22.0 (IBM Corp. Armonk, NY, USA).

Results

Patient characteristics

A total of 233 patients with early RA (median symptom duration 7 months; interquartile range (IQR) 5–10) were included in this study. Characteristics at baseline and at the 1-year follow-up in patients with available radiographic data are presented in Table 1. A majority of the patients was treated with methotrexate (MTX) (Table 1), and 17% of all patients in the cohort ($n = 40$) were treated with a biologic DMARD at some time during the first 5 years. Among those with radiographic data, the most frequently used type of non-MTX DMARD was antimalarials (29% at inclusion, 20% at 1 year). Combination treatment (≥ 2 DMARDs) was used in three patients at baseline (2%) and in 13 patients (8%) at 1 year.

Radiographic progression

Radiographs were available for 216 patients at baseline, 206 patients at 1 year, and 171 patients at 5 years. Mean progression of SHS from baseline to 1 year, from baseline to 5 years, and from 1 year to 5 years was 4.0 ($n = 194$, standard deviation (SD) = 6.3), 17.4 ($n = 162$, SD = 20.0), and 13.8 ($n = 161$, SD = 19.0), respectively. Compared to baseline SHS values, 60 patients (31%) had RRP at 1 year (21 men, 39 women) and 36 patients (22%) up to 5 years (11 men, 25 women). Thirty-six patients (22%) had RRP from the 1-year follow-up to the 5-year follow-up (9 men, 27 women). The median SHS progression from baseline to 5 years was 12.

Baseline predictors of RRP

Results of analyses of associations between baseline variables and RRP up to 5 years as well as above median progression in SHS up to 5 years are presented in Tables 2 and 3, respectively. Crude estimates and estimates adjusted for RF and baseline presence of erosions are presented. Age and sex were not significant predictors of RRP at 5 years in crude or adjusted analysis (Table 2).

Disease severity

Positive RF was a significant predictor of RRP over 5 years (odds ratio (OR) 5.23; 95% confidence interval (CI) 1.73–15.86; adjusted for baseline erosions). Significant associations for baseline variables with RRP up to 5 years were seen in adjusted models for anti-CCP positivity, ESR, and CRP (Table 2). No significant

Table 1 Characteristics of patients with radiographic data

	Data available at inclusion and 5 years ($n = 162$)	Data available at 1 year and 5 years ($n = 161$)
	Characteristics at inclusion	Characteristics at 1 year
Demographics and history		
Female sex, n (%)	114 (70)	116 (72)
Age at inclusion (years)	62 (52–70)	62 (52–70)
Symptom duration at inclusion (months)	7 (5–10)	7 (5–10)
Time to first DMARD (months)[a]	5 (3–7)	5 (3–7)
Current treatment		
DMARD (any), n (%)	138 (85)	135 (84)
MTX, n (%)	85 (52)	97 (60)
MTX dose (mg/week)	10.0 (7.5–10.0)	10.0 (7.5–15.0)
Other DMARDs, n (%)	56 (35)	51 (32)
Concurrent prednisolone, n (%)	60 (37)	45 (28)
Prednisolone dose (mg/day)	7.5 (5.0–15.0)	5.0 (3.75–7.5)
Anthropometrics		
BMI (kg/m^2)	25 (23–28)	NR
Obese[b], n (%)	19 (12)	NR
Overweight[b], n (%)	69 (45)	NR
Normal BMI[b], n (%)	66 (43)	NR
Cigarette smoking status		
Current smokers, n (%)	49 (32)	NR
Previous smokers, n (%)	51 (33)	NR
Never smokers, n (%)	55 (36)	NR
Disease parameters		
RF-positive at inclusion, n (%)	105 (65)	104 (65)
Anti-CCP antibody-positive at inclusion, n (%)	83 (59)	80 (58)
Modified Sharp–van der Heijde score	2 (0–8)	6 (1–16)
Joint space narrowing score	0 (0–6)	4 (0–11)
Erosion score	0 (0–2)	2 (0–4)
Erosions present[c], n (%)	28 (17)	47 (30)
DAS28	4.7 (3.6–5.7)	3.6 (2.7–4.4)
Remission[d], n (%)	12 (8)	36 (23)
Low disease activity[d], n (%)	27 (17)	56 (36)
Moderate disease activity[d], n (%)	75 (47)	80 (51)
High disease activity[d], n (%)	59 (37)	21 (13)
HAQ	0.75 (0.38–1.25)	0.50 (0.13–0.88)
Swollen joint count (out of 28)	7 (5–11)	4 (2–6)
Tender joint count (out of 28)	4 (2–9)	2 (0–5)
ESR (mm/h)	22 (11–43)	16 (8–30)

Table 1 Characteristics of patients with radiographic data *(Continued)*

	Data available at inclusion and 5 years (*n* = 162)	Data available at 1 year and 5 years (*n* = 161)
	Characteristics at inclusion	Characteristics at 1 year
CRP (mg/l)[e]	9 (< 9–28)	< 9 (< 9–11)
Patient's global assessment (VAS 0–100)	46 (21–65)	24 (11–48)
Pain (VAS 0–100)	40 (19–61)	24 (11–44)

Median (interquartile range) presented unless otherwise stated
For characteristics in patients with radiographic data available and included in the analysis for inclusion/1 year, missing numbers were as follows: symptom duration = 1/NA, time to DMARD = 15/NA, BMI = 5/NR, cigarette smoking status = 7/NR, RF = 1/1, anti-CCP = 22/22, erosion present = 1/2, DAS28 = 1/4, HAQ = 1/0, swollen joint count = 1/1, tender joint count = 1/1, ESR = 1/3, CRP = 1/2, patient's global assessment = 1/2, pain = 1/2
DMARD disease-modifying antirheumatic drug, *MTX* methotrexate, *BMI* body mass index, *NR* not reported, *RF* rheumatoid factor, *anti-CCP* antibodies to cyclic citrullinated peptides, *DAS28* Disease Activity Score of 28 joints, *HAQ* Health Assessment Questionnaire, *ESR* erythrocyte sedimentation rate, *CRP* C-reactive protein, *VAS* visual analogue scale, *NA* not applicable
[a]Duration from rheumatoid arthritis symptom onset to start of first DMARD
[b]Definitions based on BMI: obese ≥ 30 kg/m^2; overweight 25–29.99 kg/m^2; normal 18.5–24.99 kg/m^2. Three patients with BMI ≤ 18.5 kg/m^2 were excluded from this analysis
[c]By standard radiographic evaluation, independent of modified Sharp–van der Heijde scoring
[d]Definitions based on DAS28: remission ≤ 2.6; low ≤ 3.2; moderate > 3.2 to ≤ 5.1; high > 5.1
[e]Analysis sensitivity differs, with some data ranging from 0 to 9 (mg/l) only reported as < 9 (mg/l)

associations were observed for DAS28, HAQ, swollen and tender joint counts, VAS for patients' global assessment of disease activity or pain, or time from symptom onset to DMARD initiation, when analyzed as continuous variables, for RRP up to 5 years (Table 2). Separate analysis of the baseline category of disease activity revealed a significantly increased risk of RRP up to 5 years for patients with high baseline DAS28 (> 5.1) compared to those with low to moderate disease activity (Table 2).

Baseline presence of erosions tended to predict RRP up to 5 years in unadjusted analysis (OR 2.29; 95% CI 0.95–5.53) (Table 2).

Results of analyses of predictors of SHS progression above the median (Table 3) were largely similar to the main results.

Smoking and BMI
Significant associations with RRP from baseline up to 5 years were observed for current and ever smoking in crude and adjusted models (Table 2). Similar point estimates for the impact of ever smoking on the risk of RRP were obtained in analyses additionally adjusted for ESR (OR 2.69; 95% CI 0.98–7.44) or for DAS28 (OR 2.51; 95% CI 0.93–6.76). The pattern was similar for current smoking.

Obese or overweight patients had a reduced risk of RRP up to 5 years compared to those with normal BMI, with a numerically stronger effect for those who fulfilled the criteria for obesity (Table 2). The estimated impact of overweight/obesity (BMI > 25 kg/m^2) on RRP up to 5 years was similar in RF-positive (OR 0.27; 95% CI 0.11–0.65) and RF-negative (OR 0.27; 95% CI 0.03–2.80) patients, and also in analyses stratified for anti-CCP status (positive OR 0.25 (95% CI 0.09–0.68); negative OR 0.26 (95% CI 0.03–2.70)). The presence of overweight/obesity was associated with a significantly reduced risk

of RRP up to 5 years in analyses adjusted for RF and presence of erosions at baseline (Table 2), and also when additionally adjusting for ESR (OR 0.26; 95% CI 0.11–0.63). There were no major differences in baseline CRP, ESR, or DAS28 across categories of BMI (data not shown). In analyses stratified by sex, the negative association for overweight/obesity reached statistical significance in men (OR 0.17; 95% CI 0.04–0.74), with a similar trend in women (OR 0.43; 95% CI 0.17–1.07).

In multivariate analyses, adjusted for BMI, current smoking (OR 3.54; 95% CI 1.24–10.13) and ever smoking (OR 3.17; 95% CI 1.22–8.28) were both predictive of RRP over 5 years. Overweight/obesity was negatively associated with 5-year RRP, adjusted for ever smoking (OR 0.29; 95% CI 0.13–0.67), with a similar trend in analysis adjusted for current smoking (OR 0.44; 95% CI 0.16–1.23).

There were no significant associations between smoking or overweight/obesity and SHS progression above the median (Table 3).

One-year variables as predictors of RRP
Disease activity parameters at 1 year had a significant impact on subsequent RRP up to 5 years (Table 4). Not only high ESR and CRP, but also DAS28, HAQ, swollen joint count, VAS global, and VAS pain analyzed as continuous variables, as well as the presence of erosions at the 1-year radiographic evaluation, were significantly associated with RRP up to 5 years in crude and adjusted models (Table 4). Additional analyses of erosive changes during the first year revealed that progression of SHS, total change in SHS, as well as RRP up to 1 year also significantly predicted RRP up to 5 years, in unadjusted models (Table 4). Numerically, presence of erosions, RRP during first year, CRP > 10 mg/l, and high/moderate disease activity at 1 year were the strongest predictors. Correspondingly, decreasing disease activity at 1 year,

Table 2 Baseline predictors of rapid radiographic progression up to 5 years

	Crude		Adjusted[a]	
	OR	95% CI	OR	95% CI
Demographics and anthropometrics				
Male sex	1.06	(0.47–2.37)	0.81	(0.34–1.89)
Age (per SD)[b]	1.20	(0.81–1.77)	1.34	(0.86–2.10)
Time to first DMARD (per SD)[b]	0.57	(0.25–1.30)	0.57	(0.23–1.42)
BMI (per SD)[b]	0.76	(0.51–1.15)	0.67	(0.44–1.03)
Normal BMI[c] (reference)	1.00		1.00	
Obese[c]	0.10	(0.01–0.83)	0.07	(0.01–0.58)
Obese or overweight[c]	0.32	(0.15–0.71)	0.27	(0.12–0.63)
Overweight[c]	0.39	(0.18–0.88)	0.36	(0.15–0.84)
Smoking habits				
Never smoker (reference)	1.00		1.00	
Current smoker	3.60	(1.27–10.22)	2.92	(1.00–8.56)
Ever smoker	3.18	(1.22–8.24)	2.69	(1.01–7.18)
Previous smoker	2.79	(0.97–8.03)	2.50	(0.83–7.55)
Baseline disease parameters				
RF positivity	5.70	(1.90–17.10)	NA	NA
Anti-CCP positivity	6.04	(1.98–18.47)	3.69	(1.12–12.17)
Erosions present[d]	2.29	(0.95–5.53)	NA	NA
DAS28 (per SD)[b]	1.47	(0.99–2.18)	1.41	(0.94–2.11)
Disease activity[c]				
Low/moderate (reference)	1.00		1.00	
High	2.76	(1.29–5.89)	2.70	(1.21–6.03)
HAQ (per SD)[b]	1.37	(0.96–1.96)	1.55	(1.05–2.28)
ESR (per SD)[b]	1.89	(1.33–2.69)	1.70	(1.17–2.46)
CRP below median (reference)	1.00		1.00	
CRP above median (> 9 mg/l)	2.89	(1.31–6.39)	2.36	(1.04–5.38)
Swollen joint count (per SD)[b]	1.26	(0.87–1.84)	1.26	(0.86–1.86)
Tender joint count (per SD)[b]	0.85	(0.55–1.32)	0.94	(0.60–1.48)
Patient's global assessment (VAS; per SD)[b]	1.36	(0.92–2.00)	1.29	(0.85–1.94)
Pain (VAS; per SD)[b]	1.16	(0.79–1.69)	1.18	(0.79–1.77)

OR odds ratio, *CI* confidence interval, *SD* standard deviation, *DMARD* disease-modifying antirheumatic drug, *BMI* body mass index, *NA* not applicable, *RF* rheumatoid factor, *anti-CCP* antibodies to cyclic citrullinated peptides, *DAS28* Disease Activity Score of 28 joints, *HAQ* Health Assessment Questionnaire, *ESR* erythrocyte sedimentation rate, *CRP* C-reactive protein, *VAS* visual analogue scale

[a]Adjusted for RF and presence of erosions

[b]SD: age 15 years; time to first DMARD 5.8 months; BMI 4.0 kg/m^2; DAS28 1.4; HAQ 0.64; ESR 26 mm/h; swollen joint count 4.9; tender joint count 5.8; patient's global assessment 26; pain 26

[c]For definitions see Table 1

[d]By standard radiographic evaluation, independent of modified Sharp–van der Heijde scoring

demonstrated by a greater change in DAS28 from baseline to 1 year or defined according to the EULAR response criteria as a good response at 1 year, drastically decreased the risk of RRP between the 1-year and 5-year follow-ups (Table 5).

Discussion

In this inception cohort study, over 20% of patients with early RA had a substantial radiographic progression over the first 5 years of follow-up. There was a reduced risk of RRP in overweight and obese patients, and smoking was predictive of RRP, independent of BMI. These exposures appeared to affect the risk of rapid progression, rather than minor joint damage, as they were not significantly associated with SHS progression above the median (12 units over 5 years) in this study. Our results on the predictive value of seropositivity, erosions and high inflammatory markers at baseline are in agreement with the literature [36].

Table 3 Baseline predictors of radiographic progression with change in SHS above the median (i.e. > 12) up to 5 years

	Crude		Adjusted[a]	
	OR	95% CI	OR	95% CI
Demographics and anthropometrics				
Male sex	1.25	(0.64–2.46)	0.96	(0.46–1.98)
Age (per SD)[b]	1.18	(0.86–1.62)	1.23	(0.88–1.74)
Time to first DMARD (per SD)[b]	1.08	(0.80–1.45)	1.06	(0.74–1.53)
BMI (per SD)[b]	0.93	(0.67–1.29)	0.84	(0.59–1.19)
Normal BMI[c] (reference)	1.00		1.00	
Obese[c]	0.98	(0.35–2.74)	0.79	(0.26–2.37)
Obese or overweight[c]	0.71	(0.37–1.34)	0.67	(0.33–1.34)
Overweight[c]	0.64	(0.33–1.27)	0.64	(0.31–1.33)
Smoking habits				
Never smoker (reference)	1.00		1.00	
Current smoker	2.16	(0.99–4.73)	1.82	(0.80–4.16)
Ever smoker	1.83	(0.93–3.57)	1.55	(0.76–3.16)
Previous smoker	1.56	(0.72–3.37)	1.39	(0.61–3.17)
Baseline disease parameters				
RF positivity	3.18	(1.60–6.34)	NA	NA
Anti-CCP positivity	2.47	(1.24–4.94)	1.41	(0.64–3.13)
Erosions present[d]	4.00	(1.59–10.06)	NA	NA
DAS28 (per SD)[b]	1.07	(0.78–1.47)	1.06	(0.75–1.49)
Disease activity[c]				
Low/moderate (reference)	1.00		1.00	
High	1.44	(0.76–2.75)	1.44	(0.72–2.86)
HAQ (per SD)[b]	0.99	(0.73–1.34)	1.08	(0.78–1.49)
ESR (per SD)[b]	1.73	(1.23–2.44)	1.57	(1.10–2.24)
CRP below median (reference)	1.00		1.00	
CRP above median (> 9 mg/l)	2.07	(1.11–3.88)	1.64	(0.84–3.19)
Swollen joint count (per SD)[b]	0.94	(0.68–1.30)	0.93	(0.66–1.32)
Tender joint count (per SD)[b]	0.61	(0.42–0.89)	0.66	(0.45–0.98)
Patient's global assessment (VAS; per SD)[b]	1.16	(0.84–1.60)	1.13	(0.80–1.60)
Pain (VAS; per SD)[b]	0.99	(0.72–1.36)	1.03	(0.73–1.44)

OR odds ratio, *CI* confidence interval, *SD* standard deviation, *DMARD* disease-modifying antirheumatic drug, *BMI* body mass index, *NA* not applicable, *RF* rheumatoid factor, *anti-CCP* antibodies to cyclic citrullinated peptides, *DAS28* Disease Activity Score of 28 joints, *HAQ* Health Assessment Questionnaire, *ESR* erythrocyte sedimentation rate, *CRP* C-reactive protein, *VAS* visual analogue scale

[a]Adjusted for RF and presence of erosions

[b]SD: age 15 years; time to first DMARD 5.8 months; BMI 4.0 kg/m²; DAS28 1.4; HAQ 0.64; ESR 26 mm/h; swollen joint count 4.9; tender joint count 5.8; patient's global assessment 26; pain 26

[c]For definitions see Table 1

[d]By standard radiographic evaluation, independent of modified Sharp–van der Heijde scoring

Previous research on the influence of smoking on radiographic progression has been somewhat inconclusive. Several studies have indicated an association between smoking and worse radiographic outcomes [10–12, 37–40], while some have shown no such association [13, 14, 41, 42]. Differences in adjustments for other possible contributors to joint damage, such as RF, ACPA, and disease activity, when examining the effects of smoking on radiographic progression limit

comparability between studies. Another concern is the effect of smoking on body composition and BMI, which could be of importance in this context. However, our study suggests that smoking and BMI have independent effects on radiographic outcomes in RA.

The finding that patients with high BMI at inclusion were less likely to have rapidly progressive joint damage is consistent with previous research in the field [24–28]. In the Swedish SWEFOT study, a similar negative

Table 4 One-year predictors of rapid radiographic progression up to 5 years

	Crude		Adjusted[a]	
	OR	95% CI	OR	95% CI
1-year disease parameters				
Erosions present[b]	6.16	(2.77–13.73)	NA	NA
First-year progression (≥ 1 unit increase in SHS)	5.25	(1.90–14.47)	NA	NA
First-year change in SHS (per SD)[c]	2.31	(1.51–3.54)	NA	NA
RRP during first year	6.87	(2.98–15.82)	NA	NA
DAS28 (per SD)[c]	2.89	(1.81–4.61)	2.54	(1.54–4.19)
Disease activity[d]				
Low (reference)	1.00		1.00	
Moderate	7.13	(2.02–25.13)	6.14	(1.68–22.40)
High	13.25	(3.11–56.44)	9.05	(1.91–42.84)
HAQ (per SD)[c]	1.62	(1.12–2.33)	1.75	(1.18–2.61)
ESR (per SD)[c]	2.82	(1.77–4.50)	2.10	(1.30–3.37)
CRP below 75th percentile (reference)	1.00		1.00	
CRP above 75th percentile (> 10 mg/l)	10.32	(4.44–24.00)	6.98	(2.85–17.14)
Swollen joint count (per SD)[c]	1.97	(1.35–2.87)	1.79	(1.18–2.70)
Tender joint count (per SD)[c]	1.49	(1.01–2.19)	1.46	(0.94–2.29)
Patient's global assessment (VAS; per SD)[c]	1.59	(1.08–2.34)	1.71	(1.10–2.66)
Pain (VAS; per SD)[c]	1.71	(1.16–2.52)	1.86	(1.19–2.91)

OR odds ratio, CI confidence interval, NA not applicable, SHS Sharp–van der Heijde score, SD standard deviation, RRP rapid radiographic progression, DAS28 Disease Activity Score of 28 joints, HAQ Health Assessment Questionnaire, ESR erythrocyte sedimentation rate, CRP C-reactive protein, VAS visual analogue scale
[a]Adjusted for rheumatoid factor and presence of erosions
[b]By standard radiographic evaluation, independent of modified SHS
[c]SD: first year change in SHS 6.3; DAS28 1.3; HAQ 0.58; ESR 19 mm/h; swollen joint count 4.0, tender joint count 4.1; patient's global assessment 23; pain 23
[d]For definitions see Table 1

association between obesity and SHS progression over 2 years was observed, although it did not reach significance in the fully adjusted model, which included current smoking [43]. Apart from the SWEFOT study, only one other previously published study on this subject included adjustment for smoking [25], whereas others did not [24, 26–28]. In previous studies, the

Table 5 DAS28 response at 1 year and risk of rapid radiographic progression up to 5 years

	Crude		Adjusted[a]	
	OR	95% CI	OR	95% CI
Change in DAS28 (per SD)[b]	0.52	(0.34–0.81)	0.53	(0.33–0.86)
EULAR response[c]				
No response (reference)	1.00		1.00	
Moderate response	0.54	(0.24–1.21)	0.58	(0.24–1.41)
Good response	0.06	(0.01–0.49)	0.08	(0.01–0.64)
Moderate response (reference)	1.00		1.00	
Good response	0.12	(0.01–0.93)	0.14	(0.02–1.14)

DAS28 Disease Activity Score of 28 joints, OR odds ratio, CI confidence interval, SD standard deviation, EULAR European League Against Rheumatism
[a]Adjusted for rheumatoid factor and presence of erosions at 1 year
[b]Standard deviation: 1.6
[c]Moderate response n = 61 (39%); good response n = 33 (21%)

association with high BMI and less radiographic progression was found only to be significant among seropositive patients [25, 26]. Although the statistical power was limited for subanalyses of the RF or ACPA-negative patients in the present study, crude estimates on the impact of overweight/obesity in these subsets were similar to seropositive patients.

A recent study demonstrated a negative association between BMI and MRI-detected synovitis and bone marrow edema in patients with RA, while the reverse was observed for other types of arthritis [44]. This suggests that high BMI is specifically associated with downregulation of destructive arthritis in RA. The underlying pathways could be related to differences in adipokine production [45, 46], or other metabolic or hormonal factors, and should be furthered studied. The worse clinical symptoms observed in obese RA patients [47] may be due to other mechanisms including nonspecific pain, comorbidities, and immobility.

The associations for high baseline disease activity and failure to reduce DAS28 within 1 year with RRP are in accordance with some [12, 15, 17, 48], but not all [16, 49], previous studies. Differences in follow-up and in baseline disease activity and rates of radiographic progression may explain these discrepancies. Taken together, the ability to identify patients at higher risk of radiographic progression may improve when analyzing DAS28 over time, as both patients with high initial disease activity and those with active disease 1 year after diagnosis appear to be more prone to developing severe radiographic damage. Finally, early development of joint damage was a strong predictor of RRP.

In our study, time to initiation of DMARD treatment was not associated with RRP. Previous studies have shown that early treatment may alter the long-term course of disease and is of great importance in order to reduce radiographic progression over time [50]. Generally, short disease duration and small individual differences in time to initiation of treatment in our cohort are possible explanations for our results.

Limitations in this study include the relatively small sample size, which affects statistical power for the multivariate analyses. As data on smoking and BMI were only available at baseline, longitudinal evaluation of the impact of these factors was not possible. Since high-sensitivity CRP was not available during part of the follow-up, we could only estimate the impact of CRP by treating it as a dichotomous variable (see Statistical analysis section for further details).

Strengths of our study include the structured longitudinal follow-up of an inception cohort from a defined catchment area. Therefore, selection bias is not a major issue in this study, and the results could be generalized to patients with RA seen in clinical practice.

Conclusion

A history of smoking, presence of RF and/or anti-CCP and early erosions, high initial disease activity and active disease at 1 year, all increase the risk of RRP. Patients with a high BMI may have a reduced risk of severe joint damage. This pattern was not explained by differences in disease activity or antibody status. The results of this study suggest independent effects of smoking and BMI on the risk of RRP.

Abbreviations
ACPA: Anti-citrullinated protein antibodies; Anti-CCP: Antibodies to cyclic citrullinated peptides; BMI: Body mass index; CI: Confidence interval; CRP: C-reactive protein; DAS28: Disease Activity Score of 28 joints; DMARD: Disease-modifying antirheumatic drug; ESR: Erythrocyte sedimentation rate; EULAR: European League Against Rheumatism; HAQ: Health Assessment Questionnaire; IQR: Interquartile range; MTX: Methotrexate; OR: Odds ratio; RA: Rheumatoid arthritis; RF: Rheumatoid factor; RRP: Rapid radiographic progression; SD: Standard deviation; SHS: Sharp–van der Heijde score; VAS: Visual analogue scale; WHO: World Health Organization

Acknowledgements
Christina Book, MD, PhD, initiated this project and performed a major part of the data collection. She passed away before preparation of this manuscript.

Funding
This work was supported by Lund University (ALFSKANE-446501 to CT), the Swedish Rheumatism Association (R-481821 to CT), the Swedish Research Council (2015–02228 to CT), and the Foundation for Assistance to Disabled People in Skåne (to KF).

Authors' contributions
ER participated in the study design, performed the statistical analysis, participated in the interpretation of the results, and drafted the manuscript. KF reviewed and scored the radiographs, and participated in the interpretation of the results. J-ÅN gave expert advice on the statistical analysis, and participated in the interpretation of the results. LTHJ participated in the study design and in the interpretation of the results. CT participated in the study design and the interpretation of the results, and helped draft the manuscript. All authors participated in the critical revision of the manuscript, and read and approved the final manuscript.

Competing interests
The authors declare that they have no competing interests.

Author details
[1]Rheumatology, Department of Clinical Sciences, Malmö, Lund University, Jan Waldenströms gata 35, SE-202 13 Malmö, Sweden. [2]Department of Rheumatology, Skåne University Hospital, Inga Marie Nilssons gata 32, SE-214 28 Malmö, Sweden. [3]Department of Research and Education, Helsingborg Hospital, Charlotte Yhlens gata 10, SE-251 87 Helsingborg, Sweden. [4]Rheumatology, Department of Clinical Sciences, Helsingborg, Lund University, Svartbrödragränden 3–5, SE-251 87 Helsingborg, Sweden. [5]Department of Rheumatology and Inflammation Research, Sahlgrenska Academy at Gothenburg University, Guldhedsgatan 10 A, SE-405 30 Göteborg, Sweden.

References
1. van Steenbergen HW, Ajeganova S, Forslind K, Svensson B, van der Helm-van Mil AH. The effects of rheumatoid factor and anticitrullinated peptide antibodies on bone erosions in rheumatoid arthritis. Ann Rheum Dis. 2015;74:e3.
2. Forslind K, Ahlmen M, Eberhardt K, Hafstrom I, Svensson B, BARFOT Study Group. Prediction of radiological outcome in early rheumatoid arthritis in clinical practice: role of antibodies to citrullinated peptides (anti-CCP). Ann Rheum Dis. 2004;63:1090–5.
3. Combe B, Dougados M, Goupille P, Cantagrel A, Eliaou JF, Sibilia J, et al. Prognostic factors for radiographic damage in early rheumatoid arthritis: a multiparameter prospective study. Arthritis Rheum. 2001;44:1736–43.
4. Visser K, Goekoop-Ruiterman YP, de Vries-Bouwstra JK, Ronday HK, Seys PE, Kerstens PJ, et al. A matrix risk model for the prediction of rapid radiographic progression in patients with rheumatoid arthritis receiving different dynamic treatment strategies: post hoc analyses from the BeSt study. Ann Rheum Dis. 2010;69:1333–7.
5. Tobon G, Saraux A, Lukas C, Gandjbakhch F, Gottenberg JE, Mariette X, et al. First-year radiographic progression as a predictor of further progression in early arthritis: results of a large national French cohort. Arthritis Care Res (Hoboken). 2013;65:1907–15.
6. Lindqvist E, Eberhardt K, Bendtzen K, Heinegard D, Saxne T. Prognostic laboratory markers of joint damage in rheumatoid arthritis. Ann Rheum Dis. 2005;64:196–201.
7. Silman AJ, Newman J, MacGregor AJ. Cigarette smoking increases the risk of rheumatoid arthritis. Results from a nationwide study of disease-discordant twins. Arthritis Rheum. 1996;39:732–5.
8. Bergstrom U, Jacobsson LT, Nilsson JA, Berglund G, Turesson C. Pulmonary dysfunction, smoking, socioeconomic status and the risk of developing rheumatoid arthritis. Rheumatology (Oxford). 2011;50:2005–13.

9. Nyhall-Wåhlin BM, Petersson IF, Nilsson JA, Jacobsson LT, Turesson C, BARFOT study group. High disease activity disability burden and smoking predict severe extra-articular manifestations in early rheumatoid arthritis. Rheumatology (Oxford). 2009;48:416–20.
10. Ruiz-Esquide V, Gomez-Puerta JA, Canete JD, Graell E, Vazquez I, Ercilla MG, et al. Effects of smoking on disease activity and radiographic progression in early rheumatoid arthritis. J Rheumatol. 2011;38:2536–9.
11. de Rooy DP, van Nies JA, Kapetanovic MC, Kristjansdottir H, Andersson ML, Forslind K, et al. Smoking as a risk factor for the radiological severity of rheumatoid arthritis: a study on six cohorts. Ann Rheum Dis. 2014;73:1384–7.
12. Saevarsdottir S, Rezaei H, Geborek P, Petersson I, Ernestam S, Albertsson K, et al. Current smoking status is a strong predictor of radiographic progression in early rheumatoid arthritis: results from the SWEFOT trial. Ann Rheum Dis. 2015;74:1509–14.
13. Westhoff G, Rau R, Zink A. Rheumatoid arthritis patients who smoke have a higher need for DMARDs and feel worse, but they do not have more joint damage than non-smokers of the same serological group. Rheumatology (Oxford). 2008;47:849–54.
14. Vesperini V, Lukas C, Fautrel B, Le Loet X, Rincheval N, Combe B. Association of tobacco exposure and reduction of radiographic progression in early rheumatoid arthritis: results from a French multicenter cohort. Arthritis Care Res (Hoboken). 2013;65:1899–906.
15. Svensson B, Andersson M, Forslind K, Ajeganova S, Hafstrom I, BARFOT study group. Persistently active disease is common in patients with rheumatoid arthritis, particularly in women: a long-term inception cohort study. Scand J Rheumatol. 2016;45:448–55.
16. Fautrel B, Granger B, Combe B, Saraux A, Guillemin F, Le Loet X. Matrix to predict rapid radiographic progression of early rheumatoid arthritis patients from the community treated with methotrexate or leflunomide: results from the ESPOIR cohort. Arthritis Res Ther. 2012;14:R249.
17. Welsing PM, Landewe RB, van Riel PL, Boers M, van Gestel AM, van der Linden S, et al. The relationship between disease activity and radiologic progression in patients with rheumatoid arthritis: a longitudinal analysis. Arthritis Rheum. 2004;50:2082–93.
18. Kyburz D, Gabay C, Michel BA, Finckh A, physicians of SCQM-RA. The long-term impact of early treatment of rheumatoid arthritis on radiographic progression: a population-based cohort study. Rheumatology (Oxford). 2011; 50:1106–10.
19. Mottonen T, Hannonen P, Korpela M, Nissila M, Kautiainen H, Ilonen J, et al. Delay to institution of therapy and induction of remission using single-drug or combination-disease-modifying antirheumatic drug therapy in early rheumatoid arthritis. Arthritis Rheum. 2002;46:894–8.
20. Jawaheer D, Olsen J, Lahiff M, Forsberg S, Lahteenmaki J, da Silveira IG, et al. Gender, body mass index and rheumatoid arthritis disease activity: results from the QUEST-RA Study. Clin Exp Rheumatol. 2010;28:454–61.
21. Ajeganova S, Andersson ML, Hafström I, BARFOT Study Group. Association of obesity with worse disease severity in rheumatoid arthritis as well as with comorbidities: a long-term followup from disease onset. Arthritis Care Res (Hoboken). 2013;65:78–87.
22. Heimans L, van den Broek M, le Cessie S, Siegerink B, Riyazi N, Han KH, et al. Association of high body mass index with decreased treatment response to combination therapy in recent-onset rheumatoid arthritis patients. Arthritis Care Res (Hoboken). 2013;65:1235–42.
23. Giles JT, Bartlett SJ, Andersen RE, Fontaine KR, Bathon JM. Association of body composition with disability in rheumatoid arthritis: impact of appendicular fat and lean tissue mass. Arthritis Rheum. 2008;59:1407–15.
24. Kaufmann J, Kielstein V. Relation between body mass index and radiological progression in patients with rheumatoid arthritis. J Rheumatol. 2003;30:2350–5.
25. Westhoff G, Rau R, Zink A. Radiographic joint damage in early rheumatoid arthritis is highly dependent on body mass index. Arthritis Rheum. 2007;56:3575–82.
26. van der Helm-van Mil AH, van der Kooij SM, Allaart CF, Toes RE, Huizinga TW. A high body mass index has a protective effect on the amount of joint destruction in small joints in early rheumatoid arthritis. Ann Rheum Dis. 2008;67:769–74.
27. de Rooy DP, van der Linden MP, Knevel R, Huizinga TW, van der Helm-van Mil AH. Predicting arthritis outcomes—what can be learned from the Leiden Early Arthritis Clinic? Rheumatology (Oxford). 2011;50:93–100.
28. Baker JF, Ostergaard M, George M, Shults J, Emery P, Baker DG, et al. Greater body mass independently predicts less radiographic progression on X-ray and MRI over 1-2 years. Ann Rheum Dis. 2014;73:1923–8.
29. Arnett FC, Edworthy SM, Bloch DA, McShane DJ, Fries JF, Cooper NS, et al. The American Rheumatism Association 1987 revised criteria for the classification of rheumatoid arthritis. Arthritis Rheum. 1988;31:315–24.
30. Rydholm M, Book C, Wikström I, Jacobsson L, Turesson C. Despite early improvement, patients with rheumatoid arthritis still have impaired grip force 5 years after diagnosis. Arthritis Care Res (Hoboken). 2017;70:491–498. https://doi.org/10.1002/acr.23318.
31. Ekdahl C, Eberhardt K, Andersson SI, Svensson B. Assessing disability in patients with rheumatoid arthritis. Use of a Swedish version of the Stanford Health Assessment Questionnaire. Scand J Rheumatol. 1988;17:263–71.
32. Smolen JS, Aletaha D, Bijlsma JW, Breedveld FC, Boumpas D, Burmester G, et al. Treating rheumatoid arthritis to target: recommendations of an international task force. Ann Rheum Dis. 2010;69:631–7.
33. Geborek P, Nitelius E, Noltorp S, Petri H, Jacobsson L, Larsson L, et al. Population based studies of biological antirheumatic drug use in southern Sweden: comparison with pharmaceutical sales. Ann Rheum Dis. 2005;64:1805–7.
34. van Gestel AM, Prevoo ML, van 't Hof MA, van Rijswijk MH, van de Putte LB, van Riel PL. Development and validation of the European League Against Rheumatism response criteria for rheumatoid arthritis. Comparison with the preliminary American College of Rheumatology and the World Health Organization/International League Against Rheumatism Criteria. Arthritis Rheum. 1996;39:34–40.
35. Vastesaeger N, Xu S, Aletaha D, St Clair EW, Smolen JS. A pilot risk model for the prediction of rapid radiographic progression in rheumatoid arthritis. Rheumatology (Oxford). 2009;48:1114–21.
36. Carpenter L, Nikiphorou E, Sharpe R, Norton S, Rennie K, Bunn F, et al. Have radiographic progression rates in early rheumatoid arthritis changed? A systematic review and meta-analysis of long-term cohorts. Rheumatology (Oxford). 2016;55:1053–1065. https://doi.org/10.1093/rheumatology/kew004.
37. Mattey DL, Hutchinson D, Dawes PT, Nixon NB, Clarke S, Fisher J, et al. Smoking and disease severity in rheumatoid arthritis: association with polymorphism at the glutathione S-transferase M1 locus. Arthritis Rheum. 2002;46:640–6.
38. Haye Salinas MJ, Retamozo S, Alvarez AC, Maldonado Ficco H, Dal Pra F, Citera G, et al. Effects of cigarette smoking on early arthritis: a cross-sectional study-data from the Argentine Consortium for Early Arthritis (CONAART). Rheumatol Int. 2015;35:855–9.
39. Papadopoulos NG, Alamanos Y, Voulgari PV, Epagelis EK, Tsifetaki N, Drosos AA. Does cigarette smoking influence disease expression, activity and severity in early rheumatoid arthritis patients? Clin Exp Rheumatol. 2005;23:861–6.
40. Saag KG, Cerhan JR. Cigarette smoking and rheumatoid arthritis severity. Ann Rheum Dis. 1997;56:463–9.
41. Manfredsdottir VF, Vikingsdottir T, Jonsson T, Geirsson AJ, Kjartansson O, Heimisdottir M, et al. The effects of tobacco smoking and rheumatoid factor seropositivity on disease activity and joint damage in early rheumatoid arthritis. Rheumatology (Oxford). 2006;45:734–40.
42. Quintana-Duque MA, Rondon-Herrera F, Calvo-Paramo E, Yunis JJ, Varela-Narino A, Iglesias-Gamarra A. The impact of smoking on disease activity, disability, and radiographic damage in rheumatoid arthritis: is cigarette protective? Rheumatol Int. 2017;37:2065–70.
43. Levitsky A, Brismar K, Hafstrom I, Hambardzumyan K, Lourdudoss C, van Vollenhoven RF, et al. Obesity is a strong predictor of worse clinical outcomes and treatment responses in early rheumatoid arthritis: results from the SWEFOT trial. RMD Open. 2017;3:e000458.
44. Mangnus L, Nieuwenhuis WP, van Steenbergen HW, Huizinga TW, Reijnierse M, van der Helm-van Mil AH. Body mass index and extent of MRI-detected inflammation: opposite effects in rheumatoid arthritis versus other arthritides and asymptomatic persons. Arthritis Res Ther. 2016;18:245.
45. Giles JT, Allison M, Bingham CO 3rd, Scott WM Jr, Bathon JM. Adiponectin is a mediator of the inverse association of adiposity with radiographic damage in rheumatoid arthritis. Arthritis Rheum. 2009;61:1248–56.
46. Meyer M, Sellam J. Serum level of adiponectin is a surrogate independent biomarker of radiographic disease progression in early rheumatoid arthritis: results from the ESPOIR cohort. Arthritis Res Ther. 2013;15:R210.
47. Vidal C, Barnetche T, Morel J, Combe B, Daien C. Association of body mass index categories with disease activity and radiographic joint damage in rheumatoid arthritis: a systematic review and metaanalysis. J Rheumatol. 2015;42:2261–9.

11

Factors associated with physicians' prescriptions for rheumatoid arthritis drugs not filled by patients

Hong J. Kan[1*], Kirill Dyagilev[2], Peter Schulam[3], Suchi Saria[3], Hadi Kharrazi[1], David Bodycombe[1], Charles T. Molta[4] and Jeffrey R. Curtis[5]

Abstract

Background: This study estimated the extent and predictors of primary nonadherence (i.e., prescriptions made by physicians but not initiated by patients) to methotrexate and to biologics or tofacitinib in rheumatoid arthritis (RA) patients who were newly prescribed these medications.

Methods: Using administrative claims linked with electronic health records (EHRs) from multiple healthcare provider organizations in the USA, RA patients who received a new prescription for methotrexate or biologics/tofacitinib were identified from EHRs. Claims data were used to ascertain filling or administration status. A logistic regression model for predicting primary nonadherence was developed and tested in training and test samples. Predictors were selected based on clinical judgment and LASSO logistic regression.

Results: A total of 36.8% of patients newly prescribed methotrexate failed to initiate methotrexate within 2 months; 40.6% of patients newly prescribed biologics/tofacitinib failed to initiate within 3 months. Factors associated with methotrexate primary nonadherence included age, race, region, body mass index, count of active drug ingredients, and certain previously diagnosed and treated conditions at baseline. Factors associated with biologics/tofacitinib primary nonadherence included age, insurance, and certain previously treated conditions at baseline. The area under the receiver operating characteristic curve of the logistic regression model estimated in the training sample and applied to the independent test sample was 0.86 and 0.78 for predicting primary nonadherence to methotrexate and to biologics/tofacitinib, respectively.

Conclusions: This study confirmed that failure to initiate new prescriptions for methotrexate and biologics/tofacitinib was common in RA patients. It is feasible to predict patients at high risk of primary nonadherence to methotrexate and to biologics/tofacitinib and to target such patients for early interventions to promote adherence.

Keywords: Rheumatoid arthritis, Primary nonadherence, Disease-modifying anti-rheumatic drugs, Methotrexate, Biologics, Predictive modeling

Background

Rheumatoid arthritis (RA) is a chronic autoimmune disease characterized by persistent synovitis, joint destruction, systemic inflammation, and immunological abnormalities. Available drug treatments for RA include nonsteroidal anti-inflammatory drugs (NSAIDs), glucocorticoids, and conventional disease-modifying anti-rheumatic drugs (DMARDs) such as hydroxychloroquine, leflunomide, methotrexate, and sulfasalazine. In addition, the last two decades heralded the arrival of biologic DMARDs including anti-tumor necrosis factor (anti-TNF) biologics such as adalimumab, certolizumab, etanercept, golimumab, and infliximab; and nonanti-TNF biologics such as abatacept, anakinra, rituximab, and tocilizumab, as well as newer synthetic DMARDs such as tofacitinib. Even though rheumatologists have many choices of medications to use for RA patients, patient adherence to RA medications is suboptimal [1–5], which has been one of the causes of suboptimal control

* Correspondence: hkan1@jhu.edu
[1]Center for Population Health IT, Department of Health Policy and Management, Johns Hopkins Bloomberg School of Public Health, Hampton House HH502, 624 N. Broadway, Baltimore, MD 21205, USA
Full list of author information is available at the end of the article

of RA disease [6, 7]. It is useful to distinguish two major types of nonadherence. Primary nonadherence occurs when patients do not fill a new (first) prescription written by their physicians; secondary nonadherence occurs when patients fill a new prescription one or more times but subsequently discontinue the treatment.

Secondary nonadherence to RA treatments has been studied extensively in terms of rates and relevant factors [1–5]. For example, systematic literature reviews found that rates of methotrexate persistence ranged widely from 50 to 94% at 1 year and from 25 to 79% at 5 years [1], and that persistence to biologic DMARDs ranged from 32 to 91% at 1 year [3]. While many factors may impact adherence, a review of factors for immune-mediated inflammatory diseases including RA found consistent associations with adherence for psychosocial factors, with the strongest evidence for the impact of the healthcare professional–patient relationship, perceptions of treatment concerns and depression, lower treatment self-efficacy and necessity beliefs, and practical barriers to treatment [4]. Specifically, another systematic review found that adherence to methotrexate was mostly strongly related to beliefs in the necessity and efficacy of methotrexate, absence of low mood, mild disease, and monotherapy [5]. More generally, the importance of patient beliefs on adherence including necessity for and concerns about treatments were confirmed as important factors for adherence among many other factors across chronic diseases [8, 9]. Drug-specific characteristics and concerns may motivate adherence. For example, methotrexate may cause adverse events such as fatigue, gastrointestinal symptoms including nausea and diarrhea, malaise, oral ulcers, and alopecia [10]. A variety of other AEs specific to RA biologics may also lead to discontinuation including common and serious infections, laboratory abnormalities, and gastrointestinal perforation [11].

In contrast to many published studies on secondary nonadherence in RA where patients have experience with the medication, failure to fill a new prescription for RA medications has been understudied. In particular, factors that influence not filling a new RA prescription are not well understood. In order to conduct such research, one must link physicians' prescriptions as written or ordered to patients' filling of those prescriptions. Among the few studies available, Yelin et al. [12], using a longitudinal patient survey, studied sociodemographic, disease, health system, and contextual factors affecting failure to initiate biologics for RA, and found that age, Hispanic ethnicity, being married, and rural residence were associated with a higher probability of initiating biologics. Fewer rheumatology visits and living in an area with at least one federally qualified health center were associated with a lower probability of biologic initiation despite being prescribed the therapy. Harnett et al. [13], using electronic health records

(EHRs) linked with claims, found that more than 50% of patients with RA who were prescribed injectable biologic DMARDs did not fill or receive administration within 30 days of the index prescription and that more than 40% of patients did not initiate treatment within 180 days. However, their study was limited to biologic DMARDs, and did not attempt to identify important predictors associated with primary nonadherence.

This population-based study of RA patients from multiple healthcare provider organizations in the USA estimated the extent of primary nonadherence to methotrexate (MTX), the most commonly prescribed conventional DMARD, and to biologic DMARDs or tofacitinib (B/T). The analysis focused on patients who were newly prescribed these medications, harnessing the power of an integrated EHRs and claims database that juxtaposes what a clinician prescribed based on EHRs and what that patient actually filled or received based on administrative claims. In addition, the study aimed to identify important predictors associated with primary nonadherence and to develop simple, transparent prediction models in order to identify RA patients at risk of primary nonadherence at the time that the prescription is written and target them for appropriate clinical interventions.

Methods
Sample selection
This study was designed as a retrospective cohort study of RA patients identified from Optum's de-identified Integrated Claims-Clinical dataset, which combines adjudicated administrative claims with Humedica's EHRs. The longitudinal clinical repository from Humedica is derived from 50+ healthcare provider organizations in the USA that include over 600 hospitals and 6500 clinics and treat more than 63 million patients. The integrated dataset includes historical administrative claim data from pharmacy claims, physician claims, and facility claims, linked with EHRs including medications prescribed and administered, laboratory results, vital signs, body measurements, diagnoses, and procedures. Clinical information from EHRs was derived from both structured EHR data fields (e.g., biometric and clinical observations) and unstructured free text using natural language processing (NLP) (e.g., signs, diseases and symptoms). The data extracted from free text using NLP rather than free text itself were made available for this study. The integrated dataset was statistically de-identified under the Expert Determination method consistent with the Health Insurance Portability and Accountability Act.

The integrated dataset contains linked claims and EHRs for about 120,000 RA patients from 2007 to 2015, from which a MTX cohort and a B/T cohort were independently extracted. The MTX cohort consists of patients newly prescribed oral or injectable methotrexate. The B/T cohort consists of patients newly prescribed a biologic DMARD or tofacitinib. The biologics and tofacitinib in the B/T cohort were treated as a single group of drugs in this study to focus on whether a patient initiated treatment after receiving a biologic or tofacitinib prescription or infusion order.

For inclusion in this analysis, patients were first required to have ≥ 2 RA diagnoses (International Classification of Diseases, Ninth Revision, Clinical Modification (ICD-9-CM): 714.0, 714.2, or 714.81) made by a physician (excluding laboratory, X-ray, and other provisional diagnoses) at least 7 days apart and within 12 months from inpatient and outpatient claims data. Subsequently, from EHRs, the first written prescription of MTX or the first prescription or infusion order for B/T after the first RA diagnosis was identified and defined as the index prescription. We conducted the search for the first RA diagnosis from claims and the first drug prescription from EHRs after diagnosis starting from 2007 onward in order to find patients at the earliest stage of disease possible allowed by the data. In addition, the following inclusion and exclusion criteria were applied. Patients must have been ≥ 18 years old at the time of the first RA diagnosis. Patients must have ≥ 12 months of continuous pharmacy and medical insurance coverage before and ≥ 2 (for MTX) or ≥ 3 (for B/T) months of continuous coverage after index prescription. Patients in the MTX cohort who ever had previous evidence of use of MTX, biologics, or tofacitinib in claims data using all available data before the index date were excluded. Patients in the B/T cohort who ever had evidence of use of biologics or tofacitinib in claims data using all available data before the index date were excluded. Also excluded were patients with diagnoses of other autoimmune diseases in claims data before the index, including psoriasis or psoriatic arthritis, inflammatory bowel disease, and ankylosing spondylitis or cancer (excluding nonmelanoma skin cancer). Patients with RA-related inpatient claims within 2 (for MTX) or 3 (for B/T) months after the index were also excluded as they may have received treatment in the hospital setting. This cohort definition is supported by previous research demonstrating that the positive predictive value of identifying RA patients exceeds 85% [14]. The 12-month period before the index prescription was defined as the baseline period during which potential predictors associated with primary nonadherence were identified from claims or EHRs.

The primary nonadherence concept was predicated on linking a new written prescription or infusion order in the EHR data to its filling/administration status in pharmacy claims or medical claims (for infused RA therapies). This study defined a new prescription as the very first prescription or infusion order of MTX or B/T after RA diagnosis. To find out how successfully these sample selection criteria identified new prescriptions, we calculated the percentage of patients with the first RA diagnosis in claims occurring at or after the first ever recorded EHR activity. This

criterion guaranteed overlap of EHRs with claims data after RA diagnosis. Thus, the calculated percentage also indicates the percentage of index prescriptions being the first prescription ever recorded in the EHR data after RA diagnosis according to our definition of new prescriptions. This is a conservative measure (i.e., actual percentage of index prescriptions being the first prescription could be higher) as a patient could have been registered in an EHR system before the first recorded EHR activity occurred.

Measures and outcomes

Primary nonadherence was defined as a new prescription of MTX or a new prescription or infusion order of B/T written by a physician as recorded in EHRs but not filled or administered within 2 months for MTX or 3 months for B/T based on claims. Since a drug filled/administered in claims could not be directly linked to a specific prescription in EHRs as administrative claims and EHR prescriptions/orders belong to two unlinked data systems, we searched for any MTX and any B/T filled/administered in claims after the index prescription and attributed the first such claim to the index prescription. Thus, we gave "credit" for any filled or administered B/T therapy, despite the fact that formulary restrictions might preclude use of certain targeted therapies and might require a different therapy to be used first. We compared the individual index B/T prescription with the first filled/administered B/T after the index, expecting that they would agree in most cases. More time was allowed for B/T initiation than for MTX as patients often need more time to clear clinical screening and insurance hurdles (e.g., screening for latent tuberculosis, prior authorization) and may face practical barriers such as scheduling and travel arrangement for infusions [15]. The time window of 2 and 3 months in the definition of primary nonadherence to MTX and B/T was also confirmed empirically by examining the distribution of time elapsed between a new prescription and the first filled or administered MTX and B/T. Infused and some self-injected biologics were identified in medical claims through the Healthcare Common Procedure Coding System, and all oral drugs and the majority of self-injected biologics were identified in pharmacy claims through National Drug Codes (NDCs).

The following baseline potential predictors for primary nonadherence were identified from claims or EHRs either at the index date or during 12 months before the index date. Using clinical judgment and subject matter expertise of the rheumatologist authors, 398 and 416 potential predictors at baseline were identified for the MTX and B/T cohorts, respectively. Baseline patient characteristics (30 variables for both the MTX and B/T samples) included age, sex, average household income (imputed values at the level of zip codes), percentage with college education (imputed values at the level of zip codes), geographic divisions, integrated delivery system (vs multispecialty practice), commercial insurance (vs Medicare), insurance products (e.g., health maintenance organization, point of service, preferred provider organization, exclusive provider organization), administrative service only, and a consumer-driven health plan which is typically associated with high out-of-pocket expenses [16]. Clinical and drug-related characteristics at baseline (17 variables for MTX and 19 variables for B/T) included the count of all active drug ingredients (not just RA related), count of chronic conditions, count of inpatient hospitalizations, count of emergency visits (all of the counts were derived from claims), number of days from RA diagnosis (derived from claims) to index prescription (derived from EHRs), number of RA diagnoses recorded in claims, calendar year of index prescription (from EHRs), prescription of both MTX and B/T within 2 months prior to index (from EHRs), and route of administration of index B/T prescriptions (namely, infusion, subcutaneous injection, or oral).

From structured EHR data fields, clinical observations (16 variables for both MTX and B/T) such as body mass index (BMI), smoking status (namely, never smoked, current smoker, not smoking now, previously smoking), pain score on a 0–10 scale, pulse, and respiration rate were included. When multiple clinical observations were available, the one closest to the index was chosen. A separate indicator for missing data was added for each clinical observation. From the NLP data extracted from free text in EHRs, we generated binary indicators (nine variables for both MTX and B/T) for the presence or absence of signs, diseases, and symptoms (pain, RA, swelling, tenderness, anxiety, depression, fatigue, weakness, and arthritis) as their mentions in free clinical text may serve as a dichotomous indicator for severity. No other measures of RA disease activity or severity were found from the current version of NLP data. Note that the NLP data extracted from free text were generated by Optum for general research purposes rather than specifically for this study or for RA.

In addition, the Johns Hopkins Adjusted Clinical Groups® (ACG®) risk adjustment/case mix system version 11.0 [17] was applied to claims data to generate general comorbidity indicators based on ICD-9-CM diagnosis codes from inpatient and outpatient claims and NDCs from pharmacy claims. These included diagnosis-based conditions called Expanded Diagnosis Clusters (EDCs; 253 variables for MTX and 234 for B/T), pharmacy-based conditions called Rx-defined Morbidity Groups (RxMGs; 59 variables for MTX and 58 for B/T), and Aggregated Diagnosis Groups (ADGs; 32 variables for both MTX and B/T). EDCs and RxMGs cover a large aggregate set of comorbidities including depression, anxiety, and sleep disorder. RxMGs represent treated conditions and do not completely overlap with EDCs which are based solely on diagnosis codes. ADGs are

an even higher level aggregation of diagnosed conditions based on clinical criteria such as time limited or not, requiring primary or specialty care, or addressing physical health or psychosocial needs, as well as expected need for healthcare resources.

Statistical analysis

Patient characteristics at baseline were summarized using mean, median, standard deviation (SD), and percentage. A chi-square test was applied to test association between two categorical variables when appropriate.

Entering all of the 400 or so potential predictors selected based on clinical judgment into a predictive model for primary nonadherence may result in overfitting given the relatively small sample size as well as inclusion of potentially irrelevant variables. To address the high-dimensional input data, the potential predictors were tested for their importance in predicting primary nonadherence using L1-penalized LASSO (least absolute shrinkage and selection operator) logistic regression. LASSO logistic regression conducts variable selection and model estimation at the same time [18]. Specifically, each cohort was first randomly divided into training (75%) and test (25%) samples. In the training sample, a 10-fold crossvalidated misclassification error was evaluated across a wide range of the L1-penalty parameter to determine the largest such penalty that was within one standard error of the parameter that achieved the minimum error. The one standard error criterion tends to select a more parsimonious model without compromising much predictive power. This is especially important for this study as we aimed to develop an interpretable, transparent model as a simple tool for clinical application to identify patients at risk of primary nonadherence. To obtain unbiased estimates of the variables selected by the LASSO logistic regression, a regular multivariate logistic regression model was estimated using the entire training sample. Age, sex, and race were forced into the final regression models regardless of variable selection by LASSO regression.

To assess generalizability of model estimates, the logistic regression estimated with the training sample was applied to the test sample. The area under the curve (AUC) of the receiver operating characteristic and the Hosmer–Lemeshow goodness-of-fit test were estimated in the test sample. To visually show the calibration of the model in the test sample, mean observed probability was plotted against mean predicted probability in each of the 10 deciles of predicted probabilities. All programming was performed in R version 3.2.2 [19] with the two key packages dplyr version 0.4.3 [20] and glmnet version 2.0–5 [21].

Results

The MTX and B/T cohorts consisted of 763 and 434 patients (Table 1). Requiring ≥ 1 prescriptions in EHRs, continuous medical and pharmacy benefits, and no prior

Table 1 Patient selection for methotrexate (MTX) and biologics/tofacitinib (B/T) cohorts

Inclusion/exclusion criteria	Number of patients for MTX cohort	Number of patients for B/T cohort
Patients with two RA inpatient/outpatient diagnoses 7 days apart and within 12 months of each other in claims; age ≥ 18 years at first such RA diagnosis	49,606	49,606
Requiring ≥ 1 prescriptions of corresponding drugs from EHR at or after first RA diagnosis (first prescription defined as index prescription)	8025	5129
Requiring ≥ 12 months before index and ≥ 2 (for MTX) or ≥ 3 (for B/T) months after index of continuous medical and pharmacy benefits coverage (≤ 45 days of insurance gap allowed)	2401	1266
Excluding patients with filling or administration of corresponding drugs in claims during 12+ months before index	968	483
Excluding patients with RA-related hospitalizations in claims within 2 (MTX) or 3 (B/T) months after index prescription	955	476
Excluding patients with B/T fills or administration in pharmacy and medical claims during 12+ months before index (i.e., biologic naïve)	848	–
Excluding patients with ≥ 2 diagnoses of psoriasis or psoriatic arthritis, inflammatory bowel disease, ankylosing spondylitis, or cancer (excluding nonmelanoma skin cancer) in claims during 12+ months before index (final sample size)	763	434

RA rheumatoid arthritis, EHR electronic health record

evidence of MTX and B/T use resulted in the largest loss of patients. In almost all of the patients (753 out of the 763 MTX patients; 430 out of the 434 B/T patients), the first identified RA diagnosis occurred at or after the first recorded EHR activity, indicating that the index prescription was indeed the very first prescription of corresponding drugs after RA diagnosis in almost all cases.

Among the 763 patients with a new MTX prescription, 281 failed to initiate a MTX treatment within 2 months, resulting in a MTX primary nonadherence rate of 36.8% (95% confidence interval (CI) ± 3.4%). Similarly, 176 out of the 434 patients with a new B/T prescription failed to initiate a B/T treatment within 3 months, resulting in a B/T primary nonadherence rate of 40.6% (95% CI ± 4.6%).

Table 2 presents patient characteristics at the index date or during 12 months before the index date. These characteristics (except for age, sex, and race) were selected as important variables by the LASSO logistic regression. At the index date, the mean age of B/T and MTX patients was 57.7 and 62.5 years, respectively. About 75% of the patients were female and about 80% were white in both the cohorts. More B/T patients (61.5%) had commercial insurance than MTX patients (47.7%). Although neither of them was selected as important predictors, the median percentage of patients with college or higher education (based on zip codes) was 23.0% and 23.5% for MTX and B/T patients, respectively, and the median average household income (based on zip codes) was $42,248 and $41,972 for MTX and B/T patients, respectively. In the MTX cohort, 19.5% of patients recorded healthy BMI (18.5–24.9), the mean count of active drug ingredients was 7.9, and the median number of days between RA diagnosis and index MTX was

90. Pharmacy-based previously treated musculoskeletal/inflammatory conditions (MUSx030), which include RA, were seen in 83.4% of B/T patients, indicating a high treatment rate for these conditions among B/T patients before index prescription. Note that patients previously treated with conventional DMARDs were allowed in the B/T cohort.

Table 2 also compares baseline characteristics between patients who initiated treatment and those who did not. Compared to treatment initiators, noninitiators tended to be older, more likely to be white, less likely to have commercial insurance, and to have lower prevalence of the pharmacy-based RxMG conditions in both cohorts. Compared to MTX initiators, MTX noninitiators appeared to have a lower active drug ingredient count, longer wait time between RA diagnosis and index prescription, higher prevalence of the diagnosis-based EDC conditions, and a somewhat different geographic distribution.

Table 3 presents details of index B/T prescriptions and their filling/administration status. In most cases (240 out of 258 index prescriptions), the first B/T filled or administered after the index was the same drug as the index B/T prescription. Adalimumab and etanercept accounted for 73.7% of all index B/T prescriptions. In total, 86.9% of index B/T prescriptions were anti-TNFs, 9.9% were non-anti-TNF biologics, and 3.2% were tofacitinib; and 82.7% were subcutaneous injection, 14.1% were intravenous infusion, and 3.2% were oral. After collapsing the index prescriptions into the three types of drugs and the three routes of administration, a chi-square test revealed that the percentage of patients with primary nonadherence

Table 2 Baseline characteristics of patients at index or during 12 months before index prescription

	Methotrexate (MTX)			Biologics/tofacitinib (B/T)		
	Noninitiators (n = 281)	Initiators (n = 482)	Total (n = 763)	Noninitiators (n = 176)	Initiators (n = 258)	Total (n = 434)
Age at index prescription, mean (SD)	67.6 (12.7)	59.5 (13.5)	62.5 (13.8)	63.0 (13.7)	54.0 (13.4)	57.7 (14.2)
Female (%)	73.3	71.6	72.2	74.4	77.1	76.4
Race (%)						
White	87.5	78.4	81.8	83.0	80.2	81.3
African American	5.7	8.1	7.2	5.1	7.4	6.5
Asian	2.1	2.1	2.1	0.6	1.2	0.9
Other/unknown	4.6	11.4	8.9	11.4	11.2	11.3
Geographic division (%)[a]						
East North Central	14.2	23.2	19.9			
East South Central	1.8	0.8	1.2			
Middle Atlantic	5.7	10.0	8.4			
Mountain	2.1	2.9	2.6			
New England	16.7	3.1	8.1			
Other/unknown	1.8	2.5	2.2			
Pacific	8.2	8.9	8.7			
South Atlantic/West South Central	24.2	36.9	32.2			
West North Central	25.3	11.6	16.6			
Commercial insurance (vs Medicare) at index (%)[a,b]	29.9	58.5	47.7	34.1	79.5	61.5
Body mass index during 12 months before index (from EHRs) (%)[a]						
Underweight (< 18.5)	1.4	2.1	1.8			
Healthy weight (18.5–24.9)	16.4	21.4	19.5			
Overweight (25.0–29.9)	20.6	23.9	22.7			
Obesity I (30.0–34.9)	11.7	18.5	16.0			
Obesity II (35.0–39.9)	6.4	8.5	7.7			
Obesity III (40.0+)	5.3	7.9	6.9			
Missing	38.1	17.8	25.3			
Active ingredient counts during 12 months before index (from claims)[a], mean (SD)	3.4 (6.4)	10.5 (6.8)	7.9 (7.5)			
Number of days between RA diagnosis (from claims) and first prescription (from EHRs)[a], median; mean (SD)	371	39	90			
	602	279	398			
	(698)	(502)	(602)			
Diagnosis-based comorbidity indicators (EDCs) during 12 months before index (based on claims) (%)						
ADM05: administrative concerns and nonspecific laboratory abnormalities[a]	70.5	60.0	63.8			
GUR11: incontinence[a]	6.0	1.2	3.0			
Pharmacy-based comorbidity indicators (RxMGs) during 12 months before index (based on claims) (%)						
MUSx020: musculoskeletal/inflammatory conditions[b]				71.6	91.5	83.4
ALLx030: allergy/immunology/chronic inflammatory[a,b]	14.2	66.6	47.3	47.2	76.0	64.3
CARx030: cardiovascular/high blood pressure[a]	13.5	45.4	33.7			
GSIx020: general signs and symptoms/pain[a]	17.8	59.1	43.9			
GSIx030: general signs and symptoms/pain and inflammation[a]	12.5	56.4	40.2			
INFx020: infections/acute minor[a]	18.1	61.2	45.3			
ENDx040: endocrine/diabetes without insulin[a]	0.7	11.0	7.2			

SD standard deviation, *EHR* electronic health record, *RA* rheumatoid arthritis, *EDC* Expanded Diagnosis Cluster, *RxMG* Rx-defined Morbidity Group
[a]Important predictors selected by LASSO logistic regression for predicting MTX primary nonadherence
[b]Important predictors selected for predicting B/T primary nonadherence; age, sex, and race were added to the predictive models regardless

Table 3 Biologics/tofacitinib index prescriptions, filling/administration status, and discrepancies between index prescription and first filling/administration post index

Index prescription drug	Total number of patients (a + b)	Number of patients with no B/T filled/administered within 3 months, n (%) (a)		Number of patients with ≥1 B/T filled/administered within 3 months, n (%) (b)		First B/T filled/administered after index that was different from the index prescription (among b)
Anti-TNF biologics						
Adalimumab (SC)	118	56	(47.5)	62	(52.5)	10 etanercept
Certolizumab (SC)	11	6	(54.5)	5	(45.5)	1 certolizumab IV
Etanercept (SC)	202	65	(32.2)	137	(67.8)	1 adalimumab
Golimumab (SC)	17	8	(47.1)	9	(52.9)	None
Golimumab (IV)	1	–		1	(100.0)	None
Infliximab (IV)	28	14	(50.0)	14	(50.0)	None
Non-anti-TNF biologics						
Abatacept (IV)	23	8	(34.8)	15	(65.2)	5 abatacept SC
Abatacept (SC)	9	5	(55.6)	4	(44.4)	None
Anakinra (SC)	1	–		1	(100.0)	None
Rituximab (IV)	7	4	(57.1)	3	(42.9)	1 abatacept SC
Tocilizumab (IV)	2	1	(50.0)	1	(50.0)	None
Tocilizumab (SC)	1	1	(100.0)	–		–
New synthetic DMARD						
Tofacitinib (oral)	14	8	(57.1)	6	(42.9)	None
Total	434	176	(40.6)	258	(59.4)	18 discrepancies

B/T biologics/tofacitinib, *TNF* tumor necrosis factor, *SC* subcutaneous, *IV* intravenous infusion, *DMARD* disease-modifying anti-rheumatic drug

was not significantly different across the drug types ($p = 0.368$) or across routes of administration ($p = 0.335$).

Table 4 presents regular logistic regression model estimates for predicting primary nonadherence in the training samples. For MTX, older age, certain regions (e.g., New England and West North Central), having higher/missing BMI, and certain diagnosis-based EDC conditions (incontinence, administrative concerns, and nonspecific laboratory abnormality) were associated with a higher probability of MTX primary nonadherence. Being other/unknown in race compared to white was significantly associated with a higher probability of filling MTX. So was more active drug ingredients and having previously treated RxMG conditions such as allergy/immunology/chronic inflammatory, general signs and symptoms/pain and inflammation, diabetes without insulin, and cardiovascular/high blood pressure.

For B/T, older age was associated with a higher probability of B/T primary nonadherence. Having commercial insurance and having previously treated RxMG conditions such as allergy/immunology/chronic inflammatory, and musculoskeletal/inflammatory were highly significantly associated with filling or administration of B/T.

The logistic regression estimated with the training samples was applied to the independent test samples. The estimated AUC was 0.86 and 0.78 for predicting MTX and B/T primary nonadherence, respectively (Fig. 1). Figure 2 shows the calibration plot of predicted vs observed

probability of primary nonadherence in the MTX and B/T test samples, with the 45° line indicating perfect calibration. The Hosmer–Lemeshow test yields $p = 0.014$ for MTX primary nonadherence prediction and $p = 0.484$ for B/T, indicating acceptable calibration under $\alpha = 0.01$. Visual inspection of the predicted vs observed adherence behavior suggested that the prediction model yielded reasonable accuracy, especially in identifying patients who were not adherent (high end of the x axis of Fig. 2).

Discussion

This study estimated the primary nonadherence rate using integrated EHRs and claims data. It confirmed serious primary nonadherence to biologic and new synthetic DMARDs in RA patients, with 41% of patients failing to initiate a new prescription within 3 months, and the primary nonadherence rate did not differ significantly across the types of B/T drugs or routes of administration. Primary nonadherence to methotrexate was also serious, with 37% of patients failing to initiate within 2 months. This high primary nonadherence across RA drugs may not have been fully recognized by practicing physicians.

The predictive models for MTX and B/T primary nonadherence were validated in independent test samples with satisfactory discriminatory power according to the AUC (0.86 for MTX and 0.78 for B/T). Calibration of the two models was good throughout the range of predicted

Table 4 Logistic regression for predicting primary nonadherence in the MTX and B/T training samples

	Methotrexate (MTX) ($n = 584$)			Biologics/tofacitinib (B/T) ($n = 323$)		
	Odds Ratio	2.5%	97.5%	Odds Ratio	2.5%	97.5%
Intercept	2.68	0.44	17.38	5.36**	1.70	17.81
Age at index prescription (vs 18–44 years)						
45–54 years	1.87	0.71	5.25	2.33#	0.97	5.90
55–64 years	0.87	0.32	2.46	1.48	0.60	3.76
65–69 years	2.30	0.56	9.87	2.32	0.64	8.65
70–74 years	1.90	0.44	8.26	2.87	0.81	10.65
75–79 years	2.24	0.50	10.18	1.78	0.46	6.94
80+ years	4.92*	1.03	24.81	2.45	0.55	11.50
Male (vs female)	0.69	0.35	1.35	1.37	0.73	2.58
Race (vs white)						
African American	1.20	0.44	3.18	0.50	0.17	1.37
Asian	0.21	0.02	1.44	1.66	0.07	20.14
Other/unknown	0.27*	0.09	0.73	1.20	0.47	2.95
Geographic division (vs East North Central)[a]						
East South Central	1.83	0.17	21.00			
Middle Atlantic	1.21	0.40	3.59			
Mountain	2.46	0.39	14.75			
New England	3.76#	0.89	16.55			
Other/unknown	0.90	0.14	5.46			
Pacific	1.74	0.56	5.24			
South Atlantic/West South Central	1.69	0.78	3.79			
West North Central	2.44#	0.94	6.43			
Commercial vs Medicare at index[a,b]	1.17	0.45	3.09	0.19***	0.08	0.43
Body mass index (vs healthy weight)[a]						
Underweight (< 18.5)	0.98	0.08	6.96			
Overweight (25.0–29.9)	1.03	0.44	2.42			
Obesity I (30.0–34.9)	1.08	0.43	2.67			
Obesity II (35.0–39.9)	1.11	0.34	3.41			
Obesity III (40.0+)	1.64	0.51	5.07			
Missing	3.28**	1.47	7.51			
Active drug ingredient count during 12 months before index (vs 0)[a]						
1–5	0.13***	0.04	0.37			
6–10	0.06***	0.02	0.24			
11–15	0.08**	0.02	0.36			
16+	0.06**	0.01	0.35			
Time between RA diagnosis and first prescription (years)[a]	1.13	0.95	1.34			
Diagnosis-based comorbidity indicators (EDCs) during 12 months before index						
ADM05: administrative concerns and nonspecific laboratory abnormalities[a]	2.21*	1.22	4.10			
GUI11: incontinence[a]	7.96**	1.92	35.40			
Pharmacy-based comorbidity indicators (RxMGs) during 12 months before index						

Table 4 Logistic regression for predicting primary nonadherence in the MTX and B/T training samples *(Continued)*

	Methotrexate (MTX) (n = 584)			Biologics/tofacitinib (B/T) (n = 323)		
	Odds Ratio	2.5%	97.5%	Odds Ratio	2.5%	97.5%
MUSx020: musculoskeletal/inflammatory conditions[b]				0.28**	0.12	0.63
ALLx030: allergy/immunology/chronic inflammatory[a,b]	0.27***	0.14	0.50	0.34***	0.19	0.60
CARx030: cardiovascular/high blood pressure[a]	0.40*	0.18	0.84			
GSIx020: general signs and symptoms/pain[a]	0.63	0.32	1.22			
GSIx030: general signs and symptoms/pain and inflammation[a]	0.40**	0.21	0.74			
INFx020: infections/acute minor[a]	0.88	0.43	1.79			
ENDx040: endocrine/diabetes without insulin[a]	0.15#	0.01	0.86			

RA rheumatoid arthritis, *EDC* Expanded Diagnosis Cluster, *RxMG* Rx-defined Morbidity Group
*p < 0.05
**p < 0.01
***p < 0.001
#p < 0.1
[a]Important predictors selected by LASSO logistic regression for predicting MTX primary nonadherence
[b]Important predictors selected for predicting B/T primary nonadherence; age, sex, and race were added to the predictive models regardless

probabilities, which is important for real-world prediction to effectively differentiate both low and high risk. This level of predictive performance was achieved with a relatively small number of simple predictors commonly available through any EHR data sources, demonstrating the feasibility of applying the models in the routine clinical setting for identifying patients with varying levels of risk of primary nonadherence.

Older age was associated with a higher probability of primary nonadherence to both MTX and B/T. Insurance stood out as a highly significant predictor for B/T primary nonadherence. This is consistent with the finding that the higher the out-of-pocket cost, the less likely a member of a Medicare Advantage and Prescription Drug plan is to initiate a biologic DMARD therapy for RA [22] and the finding that the vast majority of Medicare prescription drug plans require sufficiently high cost sharing for biologic DMARDs to risk significant financial burden to RA patients [23]. Previous treatment experience in terms of a larger number of all active drug ingredients taken (for MTX) and certain previously treated pharmacy-based conditions (for both MTX and B/T as presented in Table 4) appeared to be associated with a higher probability of initiating the first RA prescription. Thus, it may be fruitful

to target patients with a lack of previous treatment experience with the comorbid conditions identified in the model for interventions to improve primary adherence. In addition, incontinence had a large impact on MTX primary nonadherence (odds ratio = 7.96), due possibly to the fact that urinary incontinence is most prevalent and strongly associated with frailty in the elderly population [24], turning it into a proxy for frailty. In fact, the mean age of MTX patients with incontinence is 69.1 years vs 62. 3 years for those without incontinence.

It is important to note that variables that were not selected as important predictors are equally as informative of primary nonadherence behavior as those selected. Overall disease burden such as the count of chronic diseases at baseline did not turn out to be an important predictor. RA-related clinical characteristics such as pain, swelling, tenderness, anxiety, depression, fatigue, and weakness did not appear to be important predictors. These binary indicators may be missing for many patients and may not capture enough granularity such as severity. However, one exception is the 0–10 pain score from clinical observations which is available to the majority (∼ 65%) of patients in both the cohorts. Moderate differences in mean pain scores were observed between noninitiators (1.48 for B/T and 1.25 for

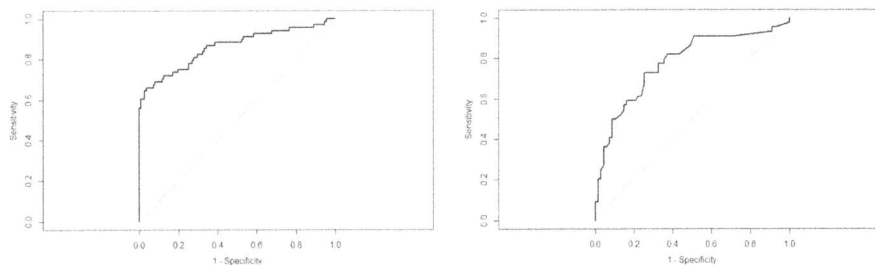

Fig. 1 Receiver operating characteristic curve of predicting primary nonadherence in methotrexate and biologics/tofacitinib test samples. Receiver operating characteristic curve for (left) methotrexate (n = 179, area under the curve (AUC) = 0.86) and (right) biologics/tofacitinib (n = 111, AUC = 0.78)

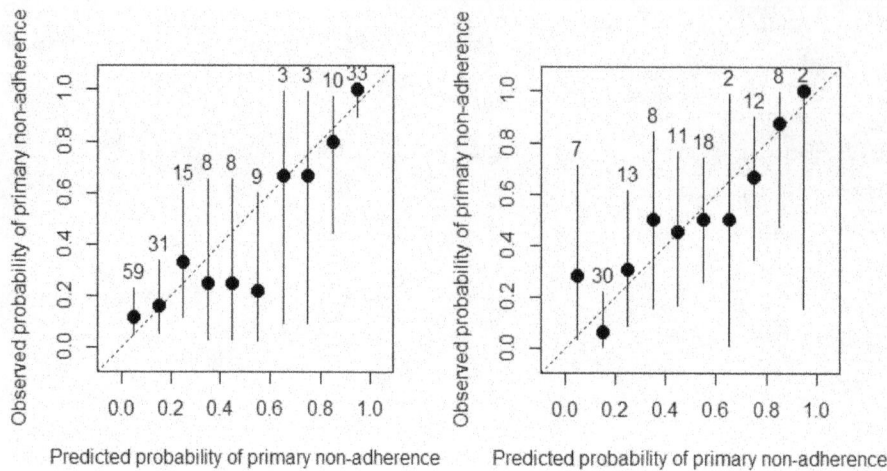

Fig. 2 Calibration of predicted vs observed probability of primary nonadherence in methotrexate and biologics/tofacitinib test samples. Calibration plot for (left) methotrexate ($n = 179$, Hosmer–Lemeshow test $p = 0.014$) and (right) biologics/tofacitinib ($n = 111$, Hosmer–Lemeshow test $p = 0.484$). Numbers above each line of calibration plot refer to number of patients in each decile of predicted probability in the test sample. The 45° line indicates perfect calibration

MTX) and initiators (1.59 for B/T and 1.61 for MTX). In a sensitivity analysis, we added the pain score into the regular logistic regression models, and it did not turn out to be significant in either cohort. In addition, drug-related characteristics such as route of administration for B/T and combination prescription of MTX and B/T did not turn out to be important predictors. Income and education, imputed based on zip codes patients resided in, also did not appear to be important predictors.

Biologics/tofacitinib primary nonadherence was harder to predict compared to MTX as indicated by its lower AUC score, possibly because B/T risk–benefit profiles are more complex to be communicated to and understood by patients, whereas MTX risk benefit may be better understood by patients and the need for any RA treatment may be more compelling, making prior treatment experience and behavior with certain comorbid conditions more predictive of MTX primary adherence. Another possible explanation is that most patients prescribed B/T are likely to have already experienced or been prescribed MTX, and thus have already accepted the concept of disease-modifying therapy for RA, which may have impacted their beliefs and expectations for subsequent treatments and, consequently, their treatment-related behavior.

RA continues to rank as one of the costliest specialty therapy classes [25]. Although it is critical to identify appropriate patients to treat, it is equally important to proactively promote optimal primary and secondary adherence among appropriate patients at risk of nonadherence. Patients with a high predicted probability of primary nonadherence may be appropriate targets of multifaceted system, provider, and patient-level interventions to promote treatment initiation and improve treatment outcomes [26].

Limitations

Our definition of primary nonadherence was based on identifying filling/administration of MTX or B/T in claims data. Although the current data system does not allow direct linkage of a drug filled/administered to a specific prescription, attribution can be inferred based on the temporal relationship since, in most cases, the first B/T filled/administered was the same as the index B/T prescription. We speculate that the few discrepancies observed between the index B/T prescription and the first filled/administered drug, the majority of which involved etanercept and adalimumab, could be due to insurance and other reasons.

Although we aimed to find patients in the earliest stage of RA allowable by the data, it is possible that some of them may have had a RA diagnosis before the first recorded RA diagnosis found in claims due to left-censoring in incomplete claims data. This was suggested in the B/T cohort by the small number of patients prescribed non-anti-TNF biologics or tofacitinib as the seemingly first-line therapy. These drugs typically are not used as first-line therapy after MTX failure, suggesting left-censoring. However, it is noteworthy that the mean age at first RA diagnosis in our sample is not drastically different from that of incident cohorts from other claims-based studies [27]. Despite the fact that all of the RA patients may not have been incident cases, index prescriptions were "incident" in the sense of virtually all of them being new prescriptions after RA diagnosis and no filling or administration of corresponding drugs recorded in claims for at least 12 months prior to index prescription. This study focused on filling and administration of new prescriptions rather than new prescriptions among strictly defined incident RA cases.

Another limitatoin is that filling a drug does not necessarily mean taking the drug by the patient. Note that this, however, is not an issue for infused biologics since actual administration was recorded in medical claims. Nevertheless, it is interesting to study whether a prescription was even filled and picked up by the patient since this is a necessary action to take the medication. Since this study focused on patient adherence behavior, we tried to identify as many patient-reported variables as possible. However, formal instruments for patient-reported outcomes such as the Health Assessment Questionnaire and RAPID3 were not available for a large enough sample through the current NLP processed free text data. We believe that patient-reported factors including their beliefs and perceptions of treatments are important for understanding primary adherence behavior and worth more research in the future.

Finally, the automatic variable selection procedure implemented via LASSO logistic regression cannot necessarily recover the true set of underlying parameters for an outcome. We used clinical judgment in selecting the initial pool of potential predictors and included demographic variables such as age, sex, and race regardless of the LASSO regression results. Although the emphasis of our regression model is more on prediction than explanation [28], the final selected variables generally do seem to make clinical sense. Some of them may be proxies for other unmeasured factors or latent constructs (e.g., incontinence as a proxy for frailty). The final set of predictors was also validated in a separate independent test sample. The relationship found between the predictors and outcome can only be interpreted as associative rather than causal.

Conclusions

This study confirmed serious primary nonadherence not only to biologics/tofacitinib but also to methotrexate. With a small number of simple predictors including age, sex, race, BMI, insurance, region, prior drug count, and certain previously diagnosed and treated conditions, it is feasible to predict patients with high risk of primary nonadherence to biologics/tofacitinib and to methotrexate. Models developed in this study are potentially useful for providers to identify patients at high risk of primary nonadherence when prescribing a new RA medication in clinical care and allow the implementation of targeted interventions to improve drug initiation. How much improved primary adherence may result in improved patient outcomes and cost savings is an interesting topic for future research.

Abbreviations

ACG®: Johns Hopkins Adjusted Clinical Groups®; ADG: Aggregated Diagnosis Group; AUC: Area under the curve of receiver operating characteristic; B/T: Biologic DMARDs or tofacitinib; BMI: Body mass index; CI: Confidence interval; DMARD: Disease-modifying anti-rheumatic drug; EDC: Expanded Diagnosis Cluster; EHR: Electronic health record; ICD-9-CM: International Classification of Diseases, Ninth Revision, Clinical Modification; MTX: Methotrexate; NDC: National Drug Code; NLP: Natural language processing; NSAID: Nonsteroidal anti-inflammatory drug; RA: Rheumatoid arthritis; RxMG: Rx-defined Morbidity Groups; SD: Standard deviation; TNF: Tumor necrosis factor

Acknowledgements

The authors thank Optum for providing the data for this study.

Funding

The authors were fully responsible for all of the content and editorial decisions and received no financial support or other form of compensation related to the study and the development of this manuscript.

Authors' contributions

HJK, KD, PS, SS, HK, DB, CTM, and JRC contributed to study conceptualization and protocol design. HJK, KD, and PS contributed to acquisition and preparation of study data and conducted programming and statistical analysis in R. All authors were involved in data analysis and interpretation. HJK drafted the work. All authors read and approved the final manuscript to be submitted for publication.

Competing interests

HJK, KD, PS, SS, HK, DB, and CTM declare that they have no competing interests. JRC receives salary support from the nonprofit Patient Centered Outcomes Research Institute (PCORI) for unrelated work.

Author details

[1]Center for Population Health IT, Department of Health Policy and Management, Johns Hopkins Bloomberg School of Public Health, Hampton House HH502, 624 N. Broadway, Baltimore, MD 21205, USA. [2]Cortica US, 425 Broadway, New York, NY 10013, USA. [3]Computer Science Department, Johns Hopkins University, 3400 N Charles Sreett, Baltimore, MD 21218, USA. [4]Main Line Rheumatology, Lankenau Medical Center, 100 Lancaster Avenue, Wynnewood, PA 19096, USA. [5]Division of Clinical Immunology and Rheumatology, University of Alabama at Birmingham, 510 20th Street South, Birmingham, AL 35294, USA.

References

1. Curtis JR, Bykerk VP, Aassi M, Schiff M. Adherence and persistence with methotrexate in rheumatoid arthritis: a systematic review. J Rheumatol. 2016;43:1997–2009.
2. Sauer BC, Teng CC, Tang D, Leng J, Curtis JR, Mikuls TR, et al. Persistence with conventional triple therapy versus a tumor necrosis factor inhibitor and methotrexate in U.S. veterans with rheumatoid arthritis. Arthritis Care Res (Hoboken). 2017;69(3):313–22. https://doi.org/10.1002/acr.22944.
3. Blum MA, Koo D, Doshi JA. Measurement and rates of persistence with and adherence to biologics for rheumatoid arthritis: a systematic review. Clin Ther. 2011;33:901–13.
4. Vangeli E, Bakhshi S, Baker A, Fisher A, Bucknor D, Mrowietz U, et al. A systematic review of factors associated with non-adherence to treatment for immune-mediated inflammatory diseases. Adv Ther. 2015;32:983–1028.
5. Hope HF, Bluett J, Barton A, et al. Psychological factors predict adherence to methotrexate in rheumatoid arthritis; findings from a systematic review of rates, predictors and associations with patient-reported and clinical outcomes. RMD Open. 2016;2:e000171. https://doi.org/10.1136/rmdopen-2015-000171.
6. Bluett J, Morgan C, Thurston L, Plant D, Hyrich KL, Morgan AW, et al. Impact of inadequate adherence on response to subcutaneously administered anti-tumour necrosis factor drugs: results from the Biologics in Rheumatoid Arthritis Genetics and Genomics Study Syndicate cohort. Rheumatology (Oxford). 2015;54:494–9.
7. Pasma A, Schenk CV, Timman R, et al. Non-adherence to disease-modifying antirheumatic drugs is associated with higher disease activity in early arthritis patients in the first year of the disease. Arthritis Res Ther. 2015;17: 281. https://doi.org/10.1186/s13075-015-0801-4.
8. Horne R, Chapman SCE, Forbes A, Parham R, Freemantle N, Cooper V. Understanding patients' adherence-related beliefs about prescribed medicines: a meta-analytic review of the Necessity-Concerns Framework. PLoS One. 2013;8(12) https://doi.org/10.1371/journal.pone.0080633

9. McHorney CA, Spain CV. Frequency of and reasons for medication non-fulfillment and non-persistence among American adults with chronic disease in 2008. Health Expect. 2011;14:307–20. https://doi.org/10.1111/j.1369-7625.2010.00619.x.

10. Curtis JR, Xie F, Mackey D, Gerber N, Bharat A, Beukelman T, Saag KG, Chen L, Nowell B, Ginsberg S. Patient's experience with subcutaneous and oral methotrexate for the treatment of rheumatoid arthritis. BMC Musculoskelet Disord. 2016;17(1):405.

11. Singh JA, Christensen R, Wells GA, Suarez-Almazor ME, Buchbinder R, Lopez-Olivo MA, Tanjong Ghogomu E, Tugwell P. Biologics for rheumatoid arthritis: an overview of Cochrane reviews. Cochrane Database Syst Rev. 2009;4:CD007848. https://doi.org/10.1002/14651858.CD007848.pub2.

12. Yelin E, Tonner C, Kim SC, Katz JN, Ayanian JZ, Brookhart MA, Solomon DH. Sociodemographic, disease, health system, and contextual factors affecting the initiation of biologic agents in rheumatoid arthritis: a longitudinal study. Arthritis Care Res (Hoboken). 2014;66:980–9.

13. Harnett J, Wiederkehr D, Gerber R, Gruben D, Bourret J, Koenig A. Primary nonadherence, associated clinical outcomes, and health care resource use among patients with rheumatoid arthritis prescribed treatment with injectable biologic disease-modifying antirheumatic drugs. J Manag Care Spec Pharm. 2016;22:209–18.

14. Kim SY, Servi A, Polinski JM, et al. Validation of rheumatoid arthritis diagnoses in health care utilization data. Arthritis Res Ther 2011;13(1):R32. https://doi.org/10.1186/ar3260.

15. Greenapple R. Trends in biologic therapies for rheumatoid arthritis: results from a survey of payers and providers. Am Health Drug Benefits. 2012;5(2):83–92.

16. Fronstin P, Sepúlveda MJ, Roebuck MC. Consumer-directed health plans reduce the long-term use of outpatient physician visits and prescription drugs. Health Aff (Millwood). 2013;32:1126–34.

17. Johns Hopkins Bloomberg School of Public Health. The Johns Hopkins ACG® System, Version 11.0. https://www.hopkinsacg.org/. Accessed Oct 2016.

18. Hastie T, Tibshirani R, Friedman J. The Elements of Statistical earning; Data Mining, Inference and Prediction. 2nd ed. New York: Springer Verlag; 2009.

19. R Core Team. R: A language and environment for statistical computing. Vienna: R Foundation for Statistical Computing; 2015. https://www.r-project.org/. Accessed 1 Oct 2016.

20. Wickham H, Francois R. dplyr: A Grammar of Data Manipulation. R package version 0.4.3. 2015. https://CRAN.R-project.org/package=dplyr. Accessed 1 Oct 2016.

21. Friedman J, Hastie T, Tibshirani R. Regularization Paths for Generalized Linear Models via Coordinate Descent. 2010. https://www.jstatsoft.org/article/view/v033i01. Accessed 1 Oct 2016.

22. Hopson S, Saverno K, Liu LZ, AL-Sabbagh A, Orazem J, Costantino ME, et al. Impact of out-of-pocket costs on prescription fills among new initiators of biologic therapies for rheumatoid arthritis. J Manag Care Spec Pharm. 2016;22:122–30.

23. Yazdany J, Dudley RA, Chen R, Lin GA, Tseng CW. Coverage for high-cost specialty drugs for rheumatoid arthritis in Medicare Part D. Arthritis Rheumatol. 2015;67:1474–80.

24. Wagg A, Gibson W, Ostaszkiewicz J, Johnson T, Markland A, Palmer MH, et al. Urinary incontinence in frail elderly persons: Report from the 5th International Consultation on Incontinence. Neurourol Urodyn. 2015;34:398–406.

25. Gleason PP, Alexander GC, Starner CI, Ritter ST, Van Houten HK, Gunderson BW, et al. Health plan utilization and costs of specialty drugs within 4 chronic conditions. J Manag Care Pharm. 2013;19(7):542–8.

26. Galo JS, Mehat P, Rai SK, Avina-Zubieta A, De Vera MA. What are the effects of medication adherence interventions in rheumatic diseases: a systematic review. Ann Rheum Dis. 2016;75(4):667–73. https://doi.org/10.1136/annrheumdis-2014-206593.

27. Crane MM, Juneja M, Allen J, Kurrasch RH, Chu ME, Quattrocchi E, et al. Epidemiology and treatment of new-onset and established rheumatoid arthritis in an insured US population. Arthritis Care Res (Hoboken). 2015; 67(12):1646–55.

28. Shmueli G. To explain or to predict? Stat Sci. 2010;3(25):289–310.

12

Presence of hepatitis B virus in synovium and its clinical significance in rheumatoid arthritis

Yu-Lan Chen[1], Jun Jing[1], Ying-Qian Mo[1], Jian-Da Ma[1], Li-Juan Yang[1], Le-Feng Chen[1], Xiang Zhang[2], Tao Yan[3], Dong-Hui Zheng[1], Frank Pessler[4,5*] and Lie Dai[1*]

Abstract

Background: Previous studies have revealed that hepatitis B virus (HBV) infection may be related to rheumatoid arthritis (RA), but there are no studies on the presence of HBV antigens or nucleic acid in synovium from patients with RA with HBV infection. In the present study, we investigated the presence of HBV in the synovium and its clinical significance in RA.

Methods: Fifty-seven consecutive patients with active RA (Disease Activity Score 28-joint assessment based on C-reactive protein ≥ 2.6) and available synovial tissue who had completed 1 year of follow-up were recruited from a prospective cohort. The patients were divided into chronic HBV infection (CHB, $n = 11$) and non-CHB groups according to baseline HBV infection status. Clinical data were collected at baseline and at 1-, 3-, 6-, and 12-month follow-up. Radiographic changes of hand/wrist at baseline and month 12 were assessed with the Sharp/van der Heijde-modified Sharp score (mTSS). HBV in synovium was determined by immunohistochemical staining for hepatitis B virus surface antigen and hepatitis B virus core antigen (HBcAg) and by nested PCR for the HBV S gene.

Results: HBcAg was found in the synovium of patients with RA with CHB (7 of 11, 64%), which was confirmed by PCR for the HBV S gene. Compared with the non-CHB group, more CD68-positive macrophages, CD20-positive B cells, and CD15-positive neutrophils infiltrated the synovium in the CHB group (all $p < 0.05$). There were smaller improvements from baseline in most disease activity indicators mainly at month 12, and a significantly higher percentage of CHB patients experienced 1-year radiographic progression (ΔmTSS ≥ 0.5 unit/yr, 64% vs. 26%, $p = 0.024$). Multivariate logistic regression analysis showed that CHB status (OR 14.230, 95% CI 2.213–95.388; $p = 0.006$) and the density of synovial CD68-positive macrophages (OR 1.002, 95% CI 1.001–1.003; $p = 0.003$) were independently associated with 1-year radiographic progression.

Conclusions: The presence of HBV in RA synovium may be involved in the pathogenesis of local lesions and exacerbate disease progression in RA.

Keywords: Hepatitis B virus, Rheumatoid arthritis, Radiographic progression, Synovium, Synovial biopsy

* Correspondence: frank.pessler@helmholtz-hzi.de; dailie@mail.sysu.edu.cn
[4]TWINCORE Center for Experimental and Clinical Infection Research, Hannover, Germany
[1]Department of Rheumatology, Sun Yat-Sen Memorial Hospital, Sun Yat-Sen University, Guangzhou, People's Republic of China
Full list of author information is available at the end of the article

Background

Rheumatoid arthritis (RA) is a chronic systemic autoimmune disorder characterized by synovitis and bone/cartilage destruction [1]. Even though the etiology of RA remains unknown, there is evidence that it results from a combination of genetic predisposition and environmental factors, especially infectious agents such as Epstein-Barr virus, cytomegalovirus, and *Proteus mirabilis* [2]. Molecular mimicry on the basis of amino acid similarities shared by viral and self-antigens has long been proposed as a pathogenic mechanism for RA [3]. However, the pathogenicity of other infectious agents linked to RA remains to be identified.

Hepatitis B virus (HBV) infection is a major cause of chronic liver diseases, such as liver cirrhosis and hepatocellular carcinoma. The genome of this DNA virus encompasses four partially overlapping open reading frames, of which the *pre-S/S* region encodes the viral surface antigen (HBsAg) and the *pre-core/core* gene encodes the e antigen (HBeAg) and the core antigen (HBcAg) [4]. HBV infects not only human hepatocytes but also diverse extrahepatic tissues such as lymph nodes, kidney, skin, colon, stomach and pancreas, which leads to extrahepatic manifestations in patients with HBV infection or HBV-related diseases such as glomerulonephritis and polyarteritis nodosa [5]. Some patients with symptoms induced by recombinant hepatitis B vaccination were reported to fulfil the 1987 revised criteria of the American College of Rheumatology (ACR) for RA and required disease-modifying anti-rheumatic drug (DMARD) therapy [6]. The serum HBsAg positivity reported in our previous study was 11.2% in Chinese patients with RA, compared with 8.7% in the age-matched Chinese general population [7]. In agreement with this, a recent study revealed a higher HBV period prevalence in 38,969 patients with RA than in 701,476 non-RA control subjects in Taiwan [8], which further supported the hypothesis that HBV infection has a subtle association with RA. In the 1970s, Schumacher et al. first reported the presence of HBV in the synovium of two patients with arthritis with HBV infection using direct immunofluorescence, and they also found virus particles mainly in synovial lining cells and vascular endothelium by electron microscopy [9]. A case report published in 2006 described a patient with knee osteoarthritis who had positive serum HBsAg and HBeAg experienced rapidly destructive knee arthropathy; in that report, immunohistochemical staining revealed diffuse HBsAg expression in the patient's synovium [10]. Nevertheless, no study regarding the presence of HBV in the synovium from patients with RA has been reported. The aim of this study was to investigate the frequency of HBV infection in the synovium of patients with coexisting RA and to determine its influence on histopathological characteristics of synovitis as well as clinical and radiographic outcomes in RA.

Methods

Study patients

Consecutive patients with RA who fulfilled the 1987 ACR revised criteria [11] or the 2010 ACR/European League Against Rheumatism (EULAR) criteria [12] for RA classification were retrospectively recruited from a prospective RA cohort ($n = 239$) in the Department of Rheumatology at Sun Yat-Sen Memorial Hospital from June 2013 to August 2016. The inclusion criteria in this study also included the following: active disease, defined as the Disease Activity Score in 28 joints with four variables including C-reactive protein (DAS28-CRP) ≥ 2.6; availability of synovial tissue at baseline passing quality criteria (at least six pieces containing lining layer and sublining area to a depth of at least 1 high-power microscopic field, 400× magnification); and completion of at least 1 year of follow-up. The exclusion criteria were as follows: overlap with other autoimmune diseases (e.g., systemic lupus erythematosus, scleroderma, dermatomyositis, polyarteritis nodosa); presence of liver cirrhosis or hepatocellular carcinoma, Wilson's disease, steatohepatitis, hemochromatosis, or schistosomiasis japonica; concomitant infection with hepatitis C virus, hepatitis D virus, human immunodeficiency virus, or other serious infection, organ dysfunction, or malignancy; and being lactating, pregnant, or planning to become pregnant. All participants gave their written informed consent before clinical data collection. The study was approved by the Medical Ethics Committee of Sun Yat-Sen Memorial Hospital (identifier SYSEC-2009-06).

Serology and virology of HBV infection and patient grouping

Serological markers of HBV infection, including HBsAg, antibodies to hepatitis B surface antigen (anti-HBs), HBeAg, antibodies to hepatitis B e antigen (anti-HBe), and antibodies to hepatitis B core antigen (anti-HBc), were tested in all patients with RA by electrochemiluminescence immunoassay (Roche Diagnostics, Mannheim, Germany). Serum HBV DNA level was measured with a commercially available qRT-PCR kit (Da An Gene Co., Ltd. of Sun Yat-Sen University, Guangdong, China), with a limit of detection of 500 IU/ml. The diagnosis of HBV infection fulfilled the Chinese guidelines for prevention and treatment of chronic hepatitis B [13]. Chronic hepatitis B virus infection (CHB) was defined as positive HBsAg and (or) HBV DNA persisting in serum for ≥ 6 months. Resolved HBV infection was defined as negative HBsAg and HBV DNA in serum but positive anti-HBc. Non-HBV infection was defined as negative HBsAg, HBeAg, anti-HBe, anti-HBc, and HBV

DNA in serum, regardless of anti-HBs status. According to the baseline HBV infection status, all patients were divided into a CHB group and a non-CHB group (resolved HBV and non-HBV).

Clinical data collection

Demographic and clinical data were collected at baseline and at 1-, 3-, 6-, and 12-month follow-up as in our previous report and modified according to the 2017 EULAR recommendations [14], including the 28-joint tender and swollen joint count (28TJC and 28SJC, respectively), patient and provider global assessment of disease activity (PtGA and PrGA, respectively), pain visual analogue scale (Pain VAS), the Stanford Health Assessment Questionnaire Disability Index (HAQ-DI), erythrocyte sedimentation rate (ESR), C-reactive protein (CRP), serum rheumatoid factor (RF), and anti-cyclic citrullinated peptide antibody (ACPA). Disease activity was assessed with DAS28-CRP, the Disease Activity Score in 28 joints with four variables including ESR (DAS28-ESR), the Simplified Disease Activity Index (SDAI), the Clinical Disease Activity Index (CDAI), and the Routine Assessment of Patient Index Data 3 (RAPID3).

HBV serological markers and HBV DNA levels were evaluated in all patients with RA at baseline and every 1-3 months during follow-up in the CHB group. These parameters in the non-CHB group were reexamined if aminotransferase activity was elevated during follow-up. Liver function, including alanine aminotransferase (ALT, U/L, normal range 5–40 U/L) and aspartate transaminase (AST, U/L, normal range 5–40 U/L), as well as bilirubin as clinically indicated, was also tested at each visit.

Radiographic assessments

Radiographic assessments of bilateral hands and wrists (anteroposterior view) were done at baseline and month 12. Joint damage, including joint erosion (JE) and joint space narrowing (JSN), was assessed with the Sharp/van der Heijde modified Sharp score (mTSS) by two experienced observers (JDM from the Department of Rheumatology and XZ from the Department of Radiology) who were blinded to clinical data as we described previously [15]. Reliability and agreement were assessed using an intraclass correlation coefficient (ICC): the mean ICC for interobserver agreement was 0.90. Bony erosion was defined when a cortical break was detected by radiography [16]. Radiographic progression was defined as a change of mTSS (ΔmTSS) $\geq$ 0.5 unit after 1 year [17]. Rapid radiographic progression was defined as ΔmTSS $\geq$ 5 units after 1 year [18].

Immunohistochemical and synovitis assessments

All synovial tissues in this study were obtained by closed Parker-Pearson needle biopsy from actively inflamed knee joints of patients with RA [19, 20]. Samples were fixed in 10% neutral formalin and embedded in paraffin. Serial sections of synovium (3 μm thick) were stained with H&E and immunohistochemically stained according to a three-step immunoperoxidase method. Sections were stained with anti-human HBsAg (Novocastra Laboratories Ltd., Newcastle Upon Tyne, UK; and Maixin Biotechnologies Ltd., Fuzhou, Fujian, China), HBcAg (Dako, Carpinteria, CA, USA), and the following commercial antibody preparations (Life Technologies, Carlsbad, CA, USA; and Novocastra Laboratories Ltd., Newcastle Upon Tyne, UK) according to standard staining protocols: anti-CD20 (clone L26, B cells), anti-CD38 (clone SPC32, plasma cells), anti-CD3 (clone PS1, T cells), anti-CD68 (clone KP1, macrophages), anti-CD15 (clone My1, neutrophils), and anti-CD34 (clone QB End/10, vascular endothelial cells). All antibodies were mouse monoclonal antibodies, except anti-HBcAg (rabbit polyclonal antibodies). Parallel sections were incubated with irrelevant, isotype, and concentration-matched monoclonal antibodies as a negative control, and liver tissues from patients with HBV-related hepatocellular carcinoma were used as a positive control. Histopathological changes in H&E-stained sections were graded according to the Krenn synovitis score [21–23]. The densities of cells with positive staining for CD3, CD15, CD20, CD38, and CD68 and the microvessel count (MVC; confirmed by the presence of CD34-positive endothelial cells in vessels with diameter $\leq$ 8 erythrocytes) were determined using manual counting by two independent trained investigators (LFC from the Department of Rheumatology and TY from Zhongshan School of Medicine) who were blinded to the clinical data. The densities are given as cells per square millimeter [20, 24].

Detection of HBV DNA in the synovium

The HBV *S* gene was detected by nested PCR as described previously [25]. HBV DNA was extracted from about 30 mg (obtained from approximately 20 sections, 5 μm thick, not attached to glass slides) of paraffin-embedded synovium with the RecoverAll™ total nucleic acid isolation kit (Life Technologies). Liver tissue from patients with HBV-related hepatocellular carcinoma was included as a positive control. Amplification was carried out in a 50-μl reaction volume containing 3 μl of forward and reverse primers (10 μM), 40 ng of DNA template, and 25 μl of 2 × KAPA HiFi HotStart ReadyMix (Kapa Biosystems, Wilmington, MA, USA). The following thermocycles were used: 95 °C for 3 minutes, followed by 35 cycles of 98 °C for 20 seconds, 65 °C for 15 seconds, and 72 °C for 1 minute, with a final extension at 72 °C for 1 minute. The PCR products were then resolved by gel electrophoresis (Life Technologies). DNA bands were visualized by ultraviolet fluorescence. PCR products were sequenced in both directions on an ABI 3730 XL Automated DNA Sequencer with the ABI BigDye Terminator v3.1 cycle sequencing kit (Applied Biosystems, Foster City, CA, USA). The sequences were aligned using the Basic Local Alignment Search Tool (National Center for Biotechnology Information website https://blast.ncbi.nlm.nih.gov/Blast.cgi) to confirm the identity of the HBV S gene.

Statistical analysis
IBM SPSS Statistics 20.0 for Windows software (IBM, Armonk, NY, USA) was used for statistical analyses. For continuous variables, the Mann-Whitney U test or Kruskal-Wallis analysis of variance on ranks between two groups or among three groups was used, and descriptive statistics (median, interquartile range (IQR)) were calculated. The Wilcoxon matched-pairs signed-rank sum test was used to compare the differences of continuous variables between disease activity indicators at baseline and each visit. For categorical variables, the Chi-square test or Fisher's exact test was used, and indicators are presented as frequencies and percentages. Spearman's rank-order correlation test was used to assess the relationship between serum levels of HBV DNA and RA disease characteristics in the CHB group. Logistic regression analyses were performed to identify risk factors for 1-year radiological progression by adjusting for confounding factors. Variables were included in the equation when $p < 0.05$ or removed when $p > 0.10$ following the stepwise forward selection rule. A two-tailed $p < 0.05$ was considered statistically significant.

Results
Baseline characteristics
Baseline characteristics of the 57 included patients with RA are shown in Table 1. There were 43 (75%) female patients. The median age of all patients was 51 years and the median disease duration was 24 months. Eighty-four percent of patients had bony erosion at baseline, and 61% of the patients were without glucocorticosteroid or DMARD therapy in the 6 months before entry into the study (treatment-naïve). According to HBV infection status at baseline, there were 11 (19%), 22 (39%), and 24 (42%) patients with CHB, resolved HBV, and non-HBV infection, respectively. In the CHB group, eight patients had detectable serum HBV DNA at baseline, ranging from 5.00×10^2 IU/ml to 6.96×10^7 IU/ml; four patients had positive HBeAg, but only one had abnormal liver function (AST 50 U/L and ALT 66 U/L). All CHB patients showed persistently positive HBsAg in serum during the 1-year follow-up.

HBV detection in synovium
The results of immunohistochemical staining of synovial tissue were negative for HBsAg in all samples from both the CHB and the non-CHB groups, but they were positive for HBcAg in synovial tissues from seven CHB patients, of whom five had detectable serum HBV DNA (ranging from 5.00×10^2 IU/ml to 6.96×10^7 IU/ml) and two had positive serum HBeAg. HBcAg immunoreactivity was observed in CD38-positive plasma cells and CD68-positive macrophages in the sublining area, located mainly in the cytoplasm (Fig. 1a and b). HBcAg was not detected in the other four patients with CHB or in the non-CHB patients.

The presence of the HBV S gene was tested by nested PCR in synovial tissue from four patients with CHB with positive synovial HBcAg immunoreactivity, two patients with resolved HBV infection, and two non-HBV patients. The HBV S gene was detected only in the four CHB samples (Fig. 1c). Further DNA sequencing of PCR products confirmed the specificity of amplification, demonstrating the presence of HBV DNA in the synovium from patients with RA and CHB.

HBV infection and histopathological synovitis
Synovial histopathological features were compared in patients with RA with and without CHB (Table 2). Compared with non-CHB synovium, significantly higher densities of total and sublining CD68-positive macrophages, CD20-positive B cells, and CD15-positive neutrophils were observed in the CHB specimens (all $p < 0.05$). Further comparison was performed between CHB synovium with and without positive HBcAg. Remarkably, compared with CHB synovium with negative HBcAg ($n = 4$), there were significantly more MVC, sublining CD68-positive macrophages and CD20-positive B cells infiltrating the CHB synovium with positive HBcAg ($n = 7$), with a higher subscore of synovial stroma activation (all $p < 0.05$).

Clinical responses
All patients were treated according to the "treat-to-target" strategy, the patient's willingness, and the patient's HBV infection status [26, 27]. Ten (91%) patients in the CHB group accepted antiviral prophylaxis, including entecavir ($n = 4$), lamivudine ($n = 4$), and adefovir ($n = 2$). Compared with the non-CHB group, patients with RA with CHB showed significantly lower levels of most disease activity indicators at baseline, including TJC28, PtGA, PrGA, Pain VAS, DAS28-CRP, DAS28-ESR, SDAI, CDAI, and RAPID3 (all $p < 0.05$) (Table 1). During 1-year follow-up, significant improvement from baseline was observed in disease activity indicators at each visit (all $p < 0.001$) (Additional file 1). However, compared with the non-CHB group, patients with RA with CHB experienced smaller improvements from baseline in most disease activity indicators, mainly at month 12, including PtGA, PrGA, Pain VAS, HAQ-DI, DAS28-CRP, SDAI, and CDAI, especially RAPID3 at almost each point except month 3 (all $p < 0.05$) (Fig. 2). There were no significant differences in baseline characteristics, initial therapy, or improvements of disease

Table 1 Baseline characteristics of patients

Parameters	All patients (n = 57)	CHB group (n = 11)	Non-CHB group (n = 46)	p Value[a]
Demographic characteristics				
Female, n (%)	43 (75)	7 (64)	36 (78)	0.311
Age, yr	51 (45–59)	49 (41–53)	52 (46–60)	0.311
Disease duration, mo	24 (7–102)	120 (6–120)	24 (7–72)	0.345
Smoking, n (%)	12 (21)	2 (18)	10 (22)	0.795
Disease activity indicators				
TJC28	9 (5–16)	5 (2–9)	11 (5–16)	**0.021**
SJC28	6 (3–9)	5 (2–8)	6 (4–10)	0.300
PtGA	6 (5–8)	5 (3–6)	6 (5–8)	**0.007**
PrGA	6 (4–7)	5 (3–6)	6 (5–8)	**0.006**
Pain VAS	5 (4–6)	4 (2–5)	6 (4–7)	**0.023**
CRP, mg/L	32.0 (14.8–61.0)	24.9 (15.4–66.8)	32.6 (14.2–55.6)	0.656
ESR, mm/h	68 (45–98)	63 (37–105)	70 (49–93)	0.627
Positive RF, n (%)	49 (86)	10 (91)	39 (85)	0.599
Positive ACPA, n (%)	52 (91)	11 (100)	41 (89)	0.252
DAS28-CRP	5.3 (4.6–6.1)	4.7 (4.2–5.8)	5.6 (5.0–6.3)	**0.024**
DAS28-ESR	6.2 (5.4–7.0)	5.4 (4.7–6.2)	6.4 (5.6–7.0)	**0.019**
SDAI	31.8 (21.8–42.3)	22.1 (17.5–34.2)	33.0 (26.9–43.7)	**0.026**
CDAI	27 (19–39)	19 (10–27)	30 (22–41)	**0.009**
RAPID3	12.7 (8.8–14.8)	7.1 (5.5–12.4)	13.1 (10.6–15.1)	**0.001**
HAQ-DI	1.3 (0.6–1.9)	0.5 (0.1–1.4)	1.4 (0.9–2.0)	**0.014**
Liver function				
AST, U/L	16 (14–23)	22 (17–28)	16 (14–18)	**0.027**
ALT, U/L	15 (11–21)	19 (14–31)	15 (11–19)	0.087
Radiographic status				
Bony erosions, n (%)	48 (84)	9 (82)	39 (85)	0.809
JSN subscore	4 (0–17)	1 (0–11)	5 (1–18)	0.331
JE subscore	7 (2–20)	2 (1–23)	9 (2–19)	0.447
mTSS	12 (4–34)	9 (1–34)	13 (4–35)	0.352
Previous medications, n (%)				
Treatment-naïve[b]	35 (61)	5 (46)	30 (65)	0.226
Glucocorticosteroids	21 (37)	4 (36)	17 (37)	0.971
Methotrexate	10 (18)	3 (27)	7 (15)	0.345
Leflunomide	10 (18)	0	10 (22)	NA
Sulfasalazine	6 (11)	2 (18)	4 (9)	0.357
Hydroxychloroquine	5 (9)	3 (27)	2 (4)	**0.016**
Biologic DMARDs	1 (2)	0	1 (2)	NA
Initial medications, n (%)				
Glucocorticosteroids	44 (77)	8 (73)	36 (78)	0.694
Methotrexate	54 (95)	10 (91)	44 (96)	0.527
Leflunomide	39 (68)	0	39 (85)	**< 0.001**
Sulfasalazine	10 (18)	9 (82)	1 (2)	**< 0.001**
Hydroxychloroquine	12 (21)	10 (91)	2 (4)	**< 0.001**

Table 1 Baseline characteristics of patients *(Continued)*

Parameters	All patients (n = 57)	CHB group (n = 11)	Non-CHB group (n = 46)	p Value[a]
Biologic DMARDs	25 (44)	3 (27)	22 (48)	0.217

Abbreviations: ACPA Anti-cyclic citrullinated peptide antibody, *ALT* Alanine aminotransferase, *AST* Aspartate transaminase, *CDAI* Clinical Disease Activity Index, *CHB* Chronic hepatitis B virus infection, *CRP* C-reactive protein, *DAS28* Disease Activity Score 28-joint assessment, *DMARD* Disease-modifying anti-rheumatic drug, *ESR* Erythrocyte sedimentation rate, *HAQ-DI* Stanford Health Assessment Questionnaire Disability Index, *JE* Joint erosion, *JSN* Joint space narrowing, *mTSS* Modified total Sharp score, *NA* Not applicable, *Pain VAS* Pain visual analogue scale, *PrGA* Provider global assessment of disease activity, *PtGA* Patient global assessment of disease activity, *RA* Rheumatoid arthritis, *RAPID3* Routine Assessment of Patient Index Data 3, *RF* Rheumatoid factor, *SDAI* Simplified Disease Activity Index, *SJC28* 28-joint swollen joint count, *TJC28* 28-joint tender joint count
[a]Comparison between the CHB and non-CHB groups. Data correspond to number (percent) or median (interquartile range) unless stated otherwise. Bold *p* values indicate statistically significant levels
[b]Without glucocorticosteroid or disease-modifying anti-rheumatic drug therapy in the 6 months before entry into the study

activity indicators between the resolved HBV group and the non-HBV group.

Spearman's rank-order correlation test was used to assess the relationship between baseline serum HBV DNA levels and clinical outcomes in the CHB group. The results revealed positive correlations between HBV DNA titers and RAPID3 at month 1 ($r = 0.671$, $p = 0.024$) and month 3 ($r = 0.713$, $p = 0.014$). Significant correlations were also observed between a level of HBV DNA $\geq 10^4$ IU/ml and PtGA at month 12 ($r = 0.645$, $p = 0.032$),

SDAI at month 6 ($r = 0.635$, $p = 0.036$), and RAPID3 at month 1 ($r = 0.637$, $p = 0.035$), month 6 ($r = 0.637$, $p = 0.035$), and month 12 ($r = 0.638$, $p = 0.035$).

Radiographic progression

No significant difference was found in JE subscore, JSN subscore, or mTSS between the CHB and non-CHB groups at baseline (all $p > 0.05$) (Table 1). Thirty-three percent of patients with RA had 1-year radiographic progression. Compared with the non-CHB group, a

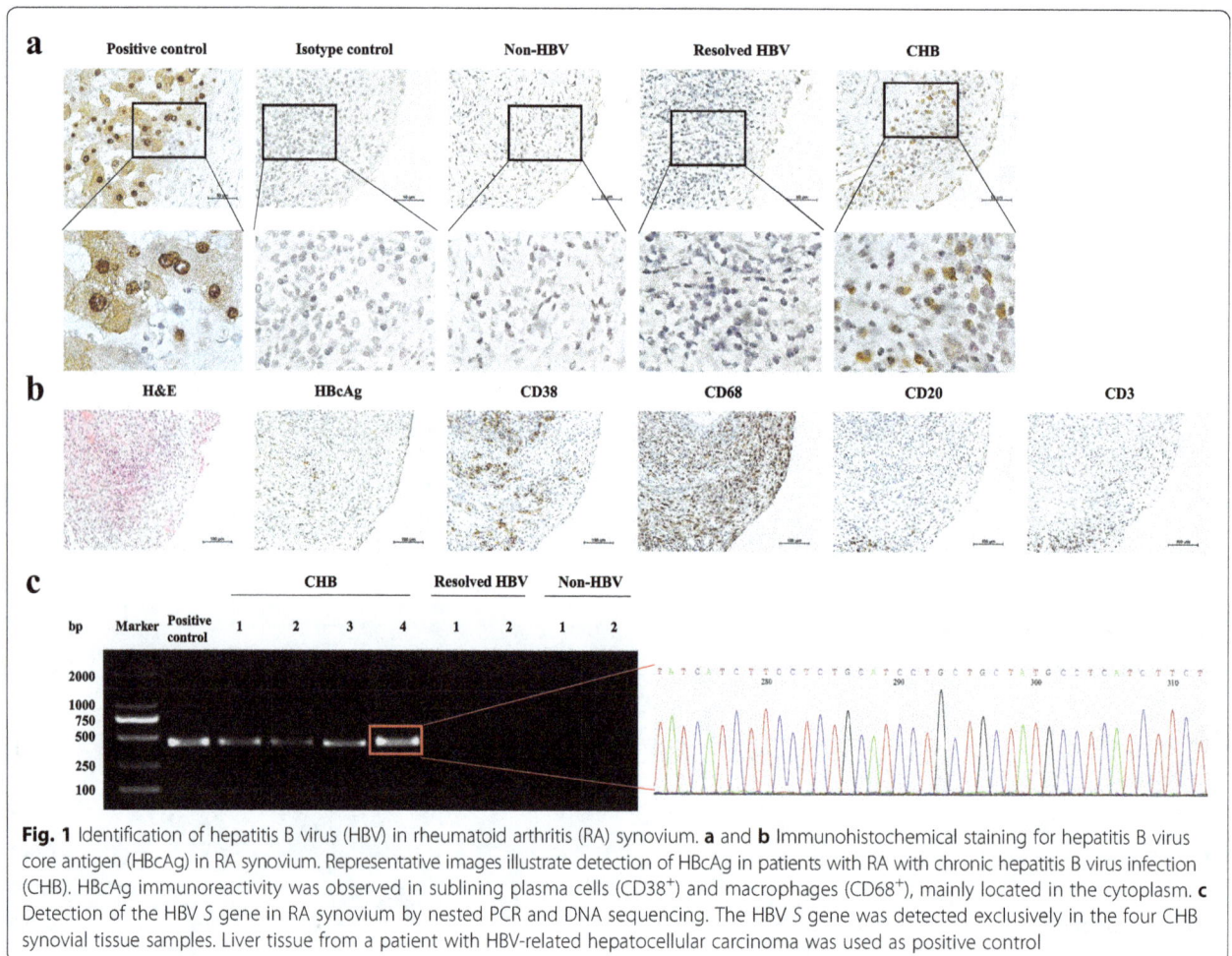

Fig. 1 Identification of hepatitis B virus (HBV) in rheumatoid arthritis (RA) synovium. **a** and **b** Immunohistochemical staining for hepatitis B virus core antigen (HBcAg) in RA synovium. Representative images illustrate detection of HBcAg in patients with RA with chronic hepatitis B virus infection (CHB). HBcAg immunoreactivity was observed in sublining plasma cells (CD38+) and macrophages (CD68+), mainly located in the cytoplasm. **c** Detection of the HBV *S* gene in RA synovium by nested PCR and DNA sequencing. The HBV *S* gene was detected exclusively in the four CHB synovial tissue samples. Liver tissue from a patient with HBV-related hepatocellular carcinoma was used as positive control

Table 2 Comparison of synovial histopathological features

Parameters	CHB group[a] (n = 11)	Non-CHB group[a] (n = 46)	p Value[b]	HBcAg(+)[c] (n = 7)	HBcAg(−)[c] (n = 4)	p Value[d]
MVCs, /mm^2	145 (102–216)	140 (118–177)	0.473	133–286	93–145	**0.023**
CD3$^+$ T cells, /mm^2	1141 (560–1751)	639 (473–1131)	0.124	0–2103	425–1934	0.571
CD15$^+$ neutrophils, /mm^2	638 (297–897)	229 (149–389)	**0.010**	63–1367	16–1484	0.850
CD20$^+$ B cells, /mm^2	1216 (472–2834)	340 (122–753)	**0.001**	773–4695	267–1940	**0.038**
CD38$^+$ plasma cells, /mm^2	1594 (380–2223)	815 (269–1346)	0.124	519–4486	120–1795	0.059
CD68$^+$ macrophages[e], /mm^2	1873 (1016–2304)	923 (622–1310)	**< 0.001**	1016–2806	968–2826	0.257
Sublining CD68$^+$ macrophages	1686 (871–2075)	659 (449–1005)	**< 0.001**	991–2496	784–1345	**0.023**
Lining CD68$^+$ macrophages	202 (158–238)	212 (126–266)	0.911	158–330	193–480	0.450
Krenn synovitis score	4 (2–7)	5 (4–6)	0.682	2–7	1–4	0.071
Hyperplasia of lining layer	2 (1–2)	2 (1–2)	0.808	1–3	1–2	0.308
Inflammatory infiltration	1 (1–2)	1 (1–2)	0.514	0–3	0–1	0.072
Synovial stroma activation	1 (1–2)	2 (1–2)	0.278	1–3	0–1	**0.025**

Abbreviations: CHB Chronic HBV infection, *HBcAg* Hepatitis B virus core antigen, *MVC* Microvessel count, *RA* Rheumatoid arthritis
[a]Data correspond to median (interquartile range) unless stated otherwise. Bold p values indicate statistically significant levels
[b]Comparison between the CHB and non-CHB groups
[c]Data correspond to minimum - maximum
[d]Comparison of HBcAg-positive vs. HBcAg-negative synovial specimens from patients with CHB
[e]CD68-positive macrophages included lining and sublining CD68-positive macrophages

significantly higher percentage of patients with RA with CHB experienced 1-year radiographic progression (64% vs. 26%, $p = 0.024$), together with greater increases in JE subscore (1.5 [IQR 0–4.0] vs. 0 [IQR 0–0], $p = 0.024$) and mTSS (1.5 [IQR 0–4.0] vs. 0 [IQR 0–0.9], $p = 0.024$). The cumulative probability distribution of radiographic change in mTSS from baseline to month 12 for patients with RA in the CHB and non-CHB groups is shown in Fig. 3, where the space between the curves indicates that a higher percentage of patients with RA with CHB experienced 1-year radiographic progression. There were no significant differences in all these indicators between the resolved HBV group and the non-HBV group (all $p > 0.05$).

Spearman's rank-order correlation test was used to assess the relationship between baseline serum HBV DNA levels and radiographic outcomes in the CHB group. The results revealed positive correlations between HBV DNA titers and increases in JSN subscore ($r = 0.606$, $p = 0.048$) and rapid radiographic progression ($r = 0.677$, $p = 0.022$).

Risk factors for 1-year radiographic progression

To determine risk factors for 1-year radiographic progression, univariate logistic regression analysis was performed, including baseline characteristics and initial therapies after enrollment as variables. The results showed that CHB status, female sex, smoking status, and treatment-naïve status as well as higher baseline mTSS were significantly associated with 1-year radiographic progression (all $p < 0.05$) (Table 3). In bivariate analyses that were adjusted for the significant confounding factors in univariate logistic regression analysis, CHB status was always positively associated with 1-year

radiographic progression (OR 4.632–7.069, all $p < 0.05$). Furthermore, multivariate logistic regression analysis that was adjusted for all significant factors in univariate analyses revealed that CHB status (OR 14.230, 95% CI 2.213–95.388, $p = 0.006$) and the count of CD68-positive macrophages (OR 1.002, 95% CI 1.001–1.003, $p = 0.003$) were independently associated with 1-year radiographic progression.

Discussion

This study was performed using a prospective cohort of consecutive patients with RA with available synovium. The results of immunohistochemical staining and nested PCR revealed the presence of HBcAg and HBV *S* gene in the synovium from patients with RA with CHB. Of note, this is the first report, to our knowledge, of the presence of HBV in RA synovium. Synovial tissue is the primary target of disturbed immunomodulatory pathways in RA. Our previous study revealed HBV DNA in synovial fluid from patients with RA with CHB, but it failed to demonstrate positive HBsAg staining by immunohistochemistry in the synovium from patients with RA with either current or resolved HBV infection [7]. In the present study, even though results of HBsAg staining were negative using two different commercial antibodies against HBsAg, HBV was detected in the synovium of patients with RA with CHB, as evidenced by positive HBcAg immunoreactivity and further confirmation by nested PCR for the HBV *S* gene. HBcAg is a reliable marker for HBV infection and viral replication. Full-length HBc capsids could induce tumor necrosis factor-α (TNF-α), interleukin (IL)-6, and IL-12p40 via

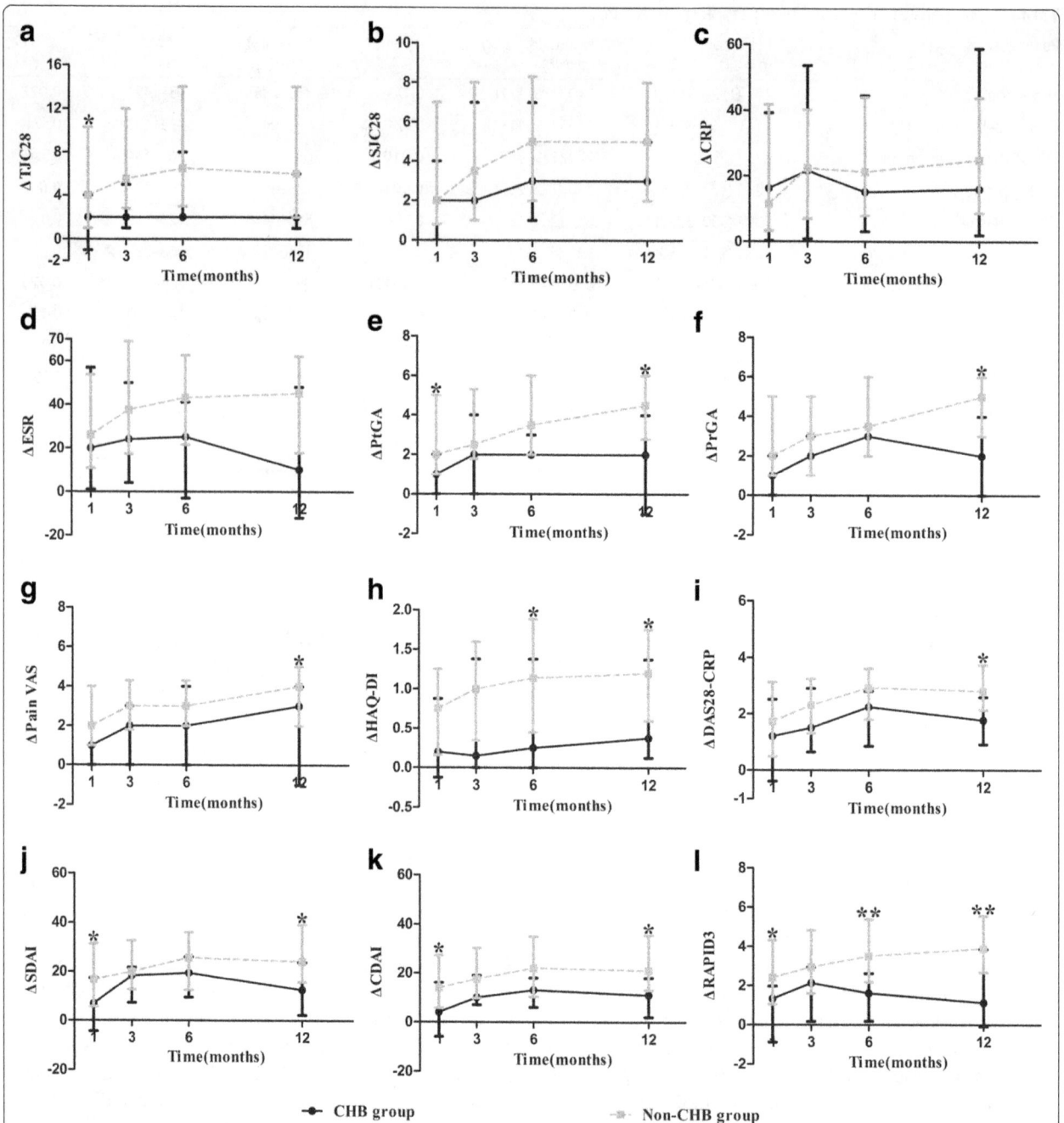

Fig. 2 Comparison of improvements in disease activity indicators between patients with rheumatoid arthritis (RA) with and without chronic hepatitis B virus infection (CHB). **a–l** Compared with the non-CHB group, patients with RA in the CHB group experienced significantly smaller improvements from baseline in most disease activity indicators mainly at month 12 (including PtGA, PrGA, Pain VAS, HAQ-DI, DAS28-CRP, SDAI, and CDAI), in TJC28 at month 1, and especially RAPID3 at almost each point except month 3, but no significant improvements were observed in SJC28, CRP, or ESR. *$p < 0.05$, **$p < 0.01$. *CDAI* Clinical Disease Activity Index, *CRP* C-reactive protein, *DAS28* Disease Activity Score 28-joint assessment, *ESR* Erythrocyte sedimentation rate, *HAQ-DI* Stanford Health Assessment Questionnaire Disability Index, *Pain VAS* Pain visual analogue scale, *PrGA* Provider global assessment of disease activity, *PtGA* Patient global assessment of disease activity, *RAPID3* Routine Assessment of Patient Index Data 3, *SDAI* Simplified disease activity index, *SJC28* 28-joint swollen joint count, *TJC28* 28-joint tender joint count

activation of nuclear factor kappa-B (NF-κB), extracellular signal-regulated protein kinases 1/2, and p38 mitogen-activated protein kinase in macrophages [28]. The distribution of HBcAg could be generally classified as cytoplasmic, nuclear, or mixed in expression [29]. Cytoplasmic HBcAg is more likely to be recognized by CD4$^+$ T cells and acts as a target antigen of immune-mediated cytolysis, which implicates its role in

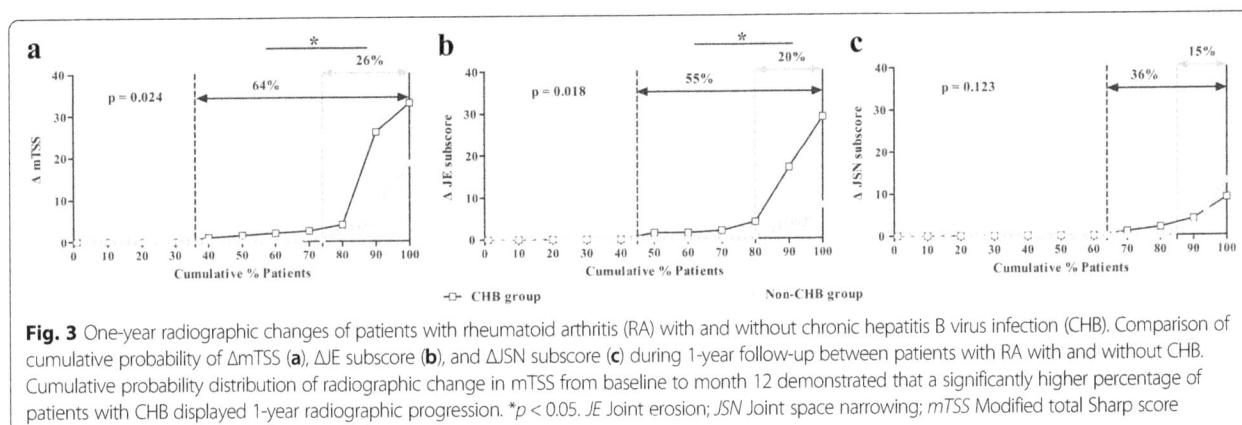

Fig. 3 One-year radiographic changes of patients with rheumatoid arthritis (RA) with and without chronic hepatitis B virus infection (CHB). Comparison of cumulative probability of ∆mTSS (**a**), ∆JE subscore (**b**), and ∆JSN subscore (**c**) during 1-year follow-up between patients with RA with and without CHB. Cumulative probability distribution of radiographic change in mTSS from baseline to month 12 demonstrated that a significantly higher percentage of patients with CHB displayed 1-year radiographic progression. *p < 0.05. *JE* Joint erosion; *JSN* Joint space narrowing; *mTSS* Modified total Sharp score

the pathogenesis of liver damage caused by HBV infection [30, 31]. HBV DNA replicative intermediates and viral proteins can be detected in peripheral blood mononuclear cells (PBMCs) of patients with CHB, with monocytes and B cells being the most frequently infected cells [32]. Studies on vertical transmission revealed the presence of HBsAg and HBcAg in CD68+ cells of villous stroma and blood capillaries in placenta from mothers with HBV-positive PBMCs, which may serve as a vector for maternal-fetal transmission of HBV [33]. In our study, HBcAg was located mainly in the cytoplasm of plasma cells and sublining macrophages in the synovium, which may result partially from migration and differentiation of HBV-infected PBMCs. However, studies have suggested that the severity of extrahepatic disease in patients with HBV infection might be related to viral burden, which may need to reach a certain threshold before extrahepatic HBV syndromes become clinically evident [5, 34]. In this study, higher baseline serum HBV DNA levels were observed to be positively correlated with poorer clinical and radiographic outcomes, indicating that higher levels of HBV DNA may contribute to more pronounced disease progression. However, our results showed that not all patients with RA with CHB had HBV markers in the synovium and that the intensity of HBcAg expression was not completely in line with serum HBV DNA level. Owing to confounding factors such as different antiviral therapies and anti-RA regimens among different patients, it may not suffice to simply investigate the relationship between serum HBV DNA levels and RA clinical characteristics. Future studies should feature larger numbers of patients with RA with CHB and thus provide sufficient statistical power for further multivariate logistic regression analyses.

Further analyses of the influence of HBV infection on histopathological characteristics of synovitis showed more pronounced CD68-positive macrophages, CD20-positive B cells, and CD15-positive neutrophils infiltrating CHB synovium. Despite the small number of CHB specimens,

this group seemed to have a higher synovial stroma activation subscore, more MVCs, and more pronounced sublining CD68-positive macrophages as well as CD20-positive B cells in CHB synovium with positive HBcAg than without it. Synovial macrophages are the main source of proinflammatory cytokines, including TNF-α and IL-1. Their density (cell count per unit area) is associated with synovial inflammation and joint destruction in RA, and it has a predictive role in evaluating the clinical efficacy of RA treatment [35]. Increased CD20-positive B cells infiltrating RA synovium could promote disease progression by producing autoantibodies and cytokines such as TNF-α, IL-6, and receptor activator of NF-κB ligand [36], enhancing osteoclastogenesis. B-cell-targeted therapy such as rituximab can alleviate such abnormalities and improve disease prognosis. Neutrophils have been a focus of RA research since the discovery of neutrophil extracellular traps (NETs), and increased components of NETs have been found in RA sera [37]. NETs are highly enriched in specific autoantigens such as citrullinated proteins targeted by ACPA in patients with RA [38, 39], but they also provide stimuli to fibroblast-like synoviocytes [40], dendritic cells [41], macrophages [42], and lymphocytes [43, 44], which promote systemic and local (synovial) autoimmune responses. However, although no significant difference was found in CD3+ T-cell count between CHB synovium with and without positive HBcAg, there was a trend of more CD3+ T cells infiltrating CHB synovium than non-CHB synovium (1141 [560–1751]/mm^2 vs. 639 [473–1131]/mm^2, p = 0.124). The small number of RA synovial tissues may have precluded us from obtaining a statistically significant difference. In the present study, we only used CD3 to stain for T cells in RA synovium. Therefore, we cannot rule out the possibility of an increased count or an enhanced activity of some T-cell subsets in the CHB synovium. Further explorations on the topic and the potential mechanism are needed. In total, HBV infection—especially its presence in synovium—may play a role in the pathogenesis of local lesions of synovitis in RA.

Table 3 Logistic regression analyses for risk factors of 1-year radiographic progression

Parameters	OR	95% CI	p Value[a]
Univariate analyses			
Female	0.258	(0.073–0.910)	**0.035**
Age	0.965	(0.922–1.010)	0.128
Disease duration	1.008	(1.000–1.017)	0.050
Smoking status	3.850	(1.024–14.473)	**0.046**
CHB status	4.958	(1.231–19.980)	**0.024**
TJC28	0.958	(0.885–1.126)	0.293
SJC28	1.017	(0.918–1.126)	0.752
PtGA	1.122	(0.853–1.476)	0.411
PrGA	1.031	(0.766–1.387)	0.841
Pain VAS	1.093	(0.824–1.448)	0.537
CRP	1.008	(0.991–1.025)	0.342
ESR	0.993	(0.997–1.010)	0.441
Positive RF	4.065	(0.462–35.752)	0.206
Positive ACPA	0.729	(0.111–4.778)	0.741
DAS28-CRP	0.975	(0.571–1.664)	0.926
HAQ-DI	0.724	(0.359–1.463)	0.369
mTSS	1.024	(1.004–1.044)	**0.021**
Treatment-naïve[b]	0.296	(0.094–0.935)	**0.038**
Glucocorticosteroids[c]	1.164	(0.307–4.412)	0.823
Methotrexate[c,£]	1.000	(0.085–11.778)	0.999
Leflunomide[c]	0.397	(0.125–1.259)	0.117
Sulfasalazine[c]	1.905	(0.497–7.294)	0.347
Hydroxychloroquine[c]	3.111	(0.868–11.149)	0.081
Biological DMARDs[c]	0.357	(0.107–1.189)	0.093
MVCs	1.005	(0.996–1.014)	0.302
CD3-positive T cells[d]	1.000	(0.999–1.001)	0.982
CD15-positive neutrophils	1.001	(0.999–1.002)	0.393
CD20-positive B cells[e]	1.000	(1.000–1.001)	0.389
CD38-positive plasma cells[f]	1.000	(1.000–1.001)	0.396
CD68-positive macrophages	1.002	(1.000–1.003)	**0.006**
Bivariate models			
CHB status adjusted for gender	4.632	(1.089–19.697)	**0.038**
CHB status adjusted for smoking status	6.097	(1.397–26.616)	**0.016**
CHB status adjusted for treatment-naïve status	4.958	(1.231–19.980)	**0.024**
CHB status adjusted for baseline mTSS	7.069	(1.539–32.480)	**0.012**

Table 3 Logistic regression analyses for risk factors of 1-year radiographic progression (Continued)

Parameters	OR	95% CI	p Value[a]
Multivariate models[g]			
CHB status adjusted for gender, smoking status, treatment-naïve status, and baseline mTSS	14.230	(2.123–95.388)	**0.006**
CD68-positive macrophages adjusted for gender, smoking status, treatment-naïve status, and baseline mTSS	1.002	(1.001–1.003)	**0.003**

Abbreviations: ACPA Anti-cyclic citrullinated peptide antibody, *CHB* Chronic hepatitis B virus infection, *CRP* C-reactive protein, *DAS28* Disease Activity Score 28-joint assessment, *ESR* Erythrocyte sedimentation rate, *HAQ-DI* Stanford Health Assessment Questionnaire Disability Index, *mTSS* Modified total Sharp score, *MVC* Microvessel count, *Pain VAS* Pain visual analogue scale, *PrGA* Provider global assessment of disease activity, *PtGA* Patient global assessment of disease activity, *RA* Rheumatoid arthritis, *RF* Rheumatoid factor, *SJC28* 28-joint swollen joint count, *TJC28* 28-joint tender joint count
[a]Calculated using logistic regression analysis. Bold *p* values indicate statistically significant levels
[b]Without glucocorticosteroid or disease-modifying anti-rheumatic drug therapy since 6 months before enrollment
[c]Initial medications after enrollment
[£]Methotrexate: OR: 1.000000, 95% CI: 0.084904–11.778006, *p* = 0.999
[d]CD3-positive T cells: OR: 1.000011, 95% CI: 0.999047–1.000976, *p* = 0.982
[e]CD20-positive B cells: OR: 1.000272, 95% CI: 0.999653–1.000892, *p* = 0.389
[f]CD38-positive plasma cells: OR: 1.000261, 95% CI: 0.999658–1.000865, *p* = 0.396
[g]Owing to the multicollinearity between CHB status and the total count of CD68-positive macrophages, two multivariate models were established, respectively, by adjusting for all significant univariate factors

Previous studies have indicated that HBV infection was more likely to be an exacerbating factor in the pathogenicity and progression of RA. Arthritis of several patients with HBV infection who fulfilled the ACR diagnostic criteria for RA could be resolved by anti-HBV therapy [45, 46]. An acute case of seropositive RA was reported in a woman 24 hours after receiving the first dose of hepatitis B vaccine. She showed a steady improvement after receiving glucocorticosteroids and sulfasalazine, but x-rays of both hands showed erosions with minimal periarticular osteoporosis 10 months later [47]. In the present study, analysis of the influence of HBV infection on clinical and radiographic outcomes showed smaller improvements from baseline in most disease activity indicators at month 12, with a significantly higher percentage of patients with CHB experiencing 1-year radiographic progression, and multivariate logistic regression analysis revealed that CHB status was an independent risk factor for 1-year radiographic progression in RA. These results were consistent with the aforementioned hypothesis and further implied that HBV infection might exacerbate disease progression, causing poor clinical response and subsequent radiographic progression in patients with RA with CHB. With the results of histopathological characteristics of synovitis, we speculated that RA concurrent with HBV infection, especially its presence in synovium, may be classified as a new phenotype of HBV-induced RA that may need adjusted and specific treatment regimens to obtain a satisfactory therapeutic response.

There are several limitations of this study. First, the small number of patients with RA with CHB and synovial tissue of adequate quality clearly limits its statistical power. There was no significant difference in disease activity or 1-year radiographic progression between patients with CHB with and without HBcAg expression in synovium. Despite the small number of CHB synovial samples, patients with positive HBcAg in synovium seemed to have more pronounced synovitis than those without it. Second, compared with the non-CHB group, a tendency of longer disease duration (120 [6–120] vs. 24 [7–72], $p = 0.345$) and a smaller percentage of medication-naïve patients (46% vs. 65%, $p = 0.226$) were observed in the CHB group, which may lead to significantly lower levels of most disease activity indicators at baseline and subsequent analyses at each visit. Further prospective cohort studies of RA with more patients with CHB, especially treatment-naïve patients with early disease, are needed. The potential mechanism of HBV infection in RA progression, the possibility of a new phenotype of HBV-induced RA, and the method of choosing DMARDs and antiviral therapy for these patients merit further exploration.

Conclusions

This study reveals the presence of HBV in the synovium of patients with RA with CHB. HBV may be involved in the pathogenesis of local lesions and exacerbate disease progression, including disease activity and joint destruction.

Abbreviations

ACPA: Anti-cyclic citrullinated peptide antibody; ACR: American College of Rheumatology; ALT: Alanine aminotransferase; AST: Aspartate transaminase; CDAI: Clinical Disease Activity Index; CHB: Chronic hepatitis B virus infection; CRP: C-reactive protein; DAS28: Disease Activity Score 28-joint assessment; DMARD: Disease-modifying anti-rheumatic drug; ESR: Erythrocyte sedimentation rate; EULAR: European League Against Rheumatism; HAQ-DI: Stanford Health Assessment Questionnaire Disability Index; HBcAg: Hepatitis B virus core antigen; HBeAg: Hepatitis B virus e antigen; HBsAg: Hepatitis B virus surface antigen; HBV: Hepatitis B virus; ICC: Intraclass correlation coefficient; IL: Interleukin; IQR: Interquartile range; JE: Joint erosion; JSN: Joint space narrowing; mTSS: Modified total Sharp score; MVC: Microvessel count; NA: Not applicable; NET: Neutrophil extracellular trap; NF-κB: Nuclear factor-κB; PBMC: Peripheral blood mononuclear cell; PrGA: Provider global assessment of disease activity; PtGA: Patient global assessment of disease activity; RA: Rheumatoid arthritis; RAPID3: Routine Assessment of Patient Index Data 3; RF: Rheumatoid factor; SDAI: Simplified Disease Activity Index; SJC28: 28-joint swollen joint count; TJC28: 28-joint tender joint count; TNF-α: Tumor necrosis factor-α; VAS: Visual analogue scale

Acknowledgements

The authors thank the patients and medical staff for their contributions to the study and Yan-Fang Ye of Sun Yat-Sen Memorial Hospital for her statistical assistance. This paper is dedicated to the memory of Prof. H. Ralph Schumacher Jr., pioneer of the closed-needle synovial biopsy technique.

Funding

This work was supported by the National Natural Science Foundation of China (nos. 81471597, 81671612, and 81601427), Guangdong Natural Science Foundation (nos. 2016A030313307, 2017A030313576, and 2017A030310236), and Fundamental Research Funds for the Central Universities (no. 17ykjc12).

Authors' contributions

YLC conceived of and designed the study, analyzed the data, and drafted the manuscript. LD and FP conceived of and participated in the study, read and analyzed documents, and revised the manuscript. JJ, YQM, LJY, and DHZ participated in clinical assessment at each visit during the follow-up. LFC and TY performed synovitis assessments and cell counting. JDM and XZ performed the radiographic assessment. All authors contributed to the final manuscript. All authors read and approved the final manuscript.

Competing interests

The authors declare that they have no competing interests relating to the conduct of the study or the publication of this report.

Author details

[1]Department of Rheumatology, Sun Yat-Sen Memorial Hospital, Sun Yat-Sen University, Guangzhou, People's Republic of China. [2]Department of Radiology, Sun Yat-Sen Memorial Hospital, Sun Yat-Sen University, Guangzhou, People's Republic of China. [3]Zhongshan School of Medicine, Sun Yat-sen University, Guangzhou, People's Republic of China. [4]TWINCORE Center for Experimental and Clinical Infection Research, Hannover, Germany. [5]Helmholtz Center for Infection Research, Braunschweig, Germany.

References

1. McInnes IB, Schett G. Pathogenetic insights from the treatment of rheumatoid arthritis. Lancet. 2017;389:2328–37.
2. Ebringer A, Wilson C. HLA molecules, bacteria and autoimmunity. J Med Microbiol. 2000;49:305–11.
3. Alam J, Jantan I, Bukhari SNA. Rheumatoid arthritis: recent advances on its etiology, role of cytokines and pharmacotherapy. Biomed Pharmacother. 2017;92:615–33.
4. Neuveut C, Yu W, Buendia MA. Mechanisms of HBV-related hepatocarcinogenesis. J Hepatol. 2010;52:594–604.
5. Mason A, Theal J, Bain V, Adams E, Perrillo R. Hepatitis B virus replication in damaged endothelial tissues of patients with extrahepatic disease. Am J Gastroenterol. 2005;100:972–6.
6. Pope JE, Stevens A, Howson W, Bell DA. The development of rheumatoid arthritis after recombinant hepatitis B vaccination. J Rheumatol. 1998;25:1687–93.
7. Zou CJ, Zhu LJ, Li YH, Mo YQ, Zheng DH, Ma JD, et al. The association between hepatitis B virus infection and disease activity, synovitis, or joint destruction in rheumatoid arthritis. Clin Rheumatol. 2013;32:787–95.
8. Hsu CS, Lang HC, Huang KY, Lin HH, Chen CL. Association of rheumatoid arthritis and hepatitis B infection: a nationwide nested case-control study from 1999 to 2009 in Taiwan. Medicine (Baltimore). 2016;95:e3551.
9. Schumacher HR, Gall EP. Arthritis in acute hepatitis and chronic active hepatitis: pathology of the synovial membrane with evidence for the presence of Australia antigen in synovial membranes. Am J Med. 1974;57:655–64.
10. Momohara S, Okamoto H, Tokita N, Tomatsu T, Kamatani N. Rapidly destructive knee arthropathy associated with hepatitis B. Clin Exp Rheumatol. 2006;24:111–2.
11. Arnett FC, Edworthy SM, Bloch DA, McShane DJ, Fries JF, Cooper NS, et al. The American Rheumatism Association 1987 revised criteria for the classification of rheumatoid arthritis. Arthritis Rheum. 1988;31:315–24.
12. Aletaha D, Neogi T, Silman AJ, Funovits J, Felson DT, Bingham CR, et al. 2010 Rheumatoid arthritis classification criteria: an American College of Rheumatology/European League Against Rheumatism collaborative initiative. Ann Rheum Dis. 2010;69:1580–8.
13. Hou JL, Lai W. The guideline of prevention and treatment for chronic hepatitis B: a 2015 update. Zhonghua Gan Zang Bing Za Zhi. 2015;23:888–905.
14. Radner H, Chatzidionysiou K, Nikiphorou E, Gossec L, Hyrich KL, Zabalan C, et al. 2017 EULAR recommendations for a core data set to support observational research and clinical care in rheumatoid arthritis. Ann Rheum Dis. 2018;77:476–9.

15. Ma J, Wei X, Zheng D, Mo Y, Chen L, Zhang X, et al. Continuously elevated serum matrix metalloproteinase-3 for 3 ~ 6 months predict one-year radiographic progression in rheumatoid arthritis: a prospective cohort study. Arthritis Res Ther. 2015;17:289.

16. van der Heijde D, van der Helm-van MA, Aletaha D, Bingham CO, Burmester GR, Dougados M, et al. EULAR definition of erosive disease in light of the 2010 ACR/EULAR rheumatoid arthritis classification criteria. Ann Rheum Dis. 2013;72:479–81.

17. Takeuchi T, Yamanaka H, Ishiguro N, Miyasaka N, Mukai M, Matsubara T, et al. Adalimumab, a human anti-TNF monoclonal antibody, outcome study for the prevention of joint damage in Japanese patients with early rheumatoid arthritis: the HOPEFUL 1 study. Ann Rheum Dis. 2014;73:536–43.

18. Meyer M, Sellam J, Fellahi S, Kotti S, Bastard JP, Meyer O, et al. Serum level of adiponectin is a surrogate independent biomarker of radiographic disease progression in early rheumatoid arthritis: results from the ESPOIR cohort. Arthritis Res Ther. 2013;15:R210.

19. Schumacher HJ, Kulka JP. Needle biopsy of the synovial membrane—experience with the Parker-Pearson technic. N Engl J Med. 1972;286:416–9.

20. Ma JD, Zhou JJ, Zheng DH, Chen LF, Mo YQ, Wei XN, et al. Serum matrix metalloproteinase-3 as a noninvasive biomarker of histological synovitis for diagnosis of rheumatoid arthritis. Mediators Inflamm. 2014;2014:179284.

21. Slansky E, Li J, Haupl T, Morawietz L, Krenn V, Pessler F. Quantitative determination of the diagnostic accuracy of the synovitis score and its components. Histopathology. 2010;57:436–43.

22. Krenn V, Morawietz L, Burmester GR, Kinne RW, Mueller-Ladner U, Muller B, et al. Synovitis score: discrimination between chronic low-grade and high-grade synovitis. Histopathology. 2006;49:358–64.

23. Krenn V, Perino G, Rüther W, Krenn VT, Huber M, Hügle T, et al. 15 years of the histopathological synovitis score, further development and review: a diagnostic score for rheumatology and orthopaedics. Pathol Res Pract. 2017; 213:874–81.

24. Chen LF, Mo YQ, Ma JD, Luo L, Zheng DH, Dai L. Elevated serum IgG4 defines specific clinical phenotype of rheumatoid arthritis. Mediators Inflamm. 2014;2014:635293.

25. Livingston SE, Simonetti JP, McMahon BJ, Bulkow LR, Hurlburt KJ, Homan CE, et al. Hepatitis B virus genotypes in Alaska native people with hepatocellular carcinoma: preponderance of genotype F. J Infect Dis. 2007; 195:5–11.

26. Saag KG, Teng GG, Patkar NM, Anuntiyo J, Finney C, Curtis JR, et al. American College of Rheumatology 2008 recommendations for the use of nonbiologic and biologic disease-modifying antirheumatic drugs in rheumatoid arthritis. Arthritis Rheum. 2008;59:762–84.

27. Singh JA, Furst DE, Bharat A, Curtis JR, Kavanaugh AF, Kremer JM, et al. 2012 Update of the 2008 American College of Rheumatology recommendations for the use of disease-modifying antirheumatic drugs and biologic agents in the treatment of rheumatoid arthritis. Arthritis Care Res (Hoboken). 2012;64:625–39.

28. Cooper A, Tal G, Lider O, Shaul Y. Cytokine induction by the hepatitis B virus capsid in macrophages is facilitated by membrane heparan sulfate and involves TLR2. J Immunol. 2005;175:3165–76.

29. Kim CW, Yoon SK, Jung ES, Jung CK, Jang JW, Kim MS, et al. Correlation of hepatitis B core antigen and β-catenin expression on hepatocytes in chronic hepatitis B virus infection: relevance to the severity of liver damage and viral replication. J Gastroenterol Hepatol. 2007;22:1534–42.

30. Hsu HC, Su IJ, Lai MY, Chen DS, Chang MH, Chuang SM, et al. Biologic and prognostic significance of hepatocyte hepatitis B core antigen expressions in the natural course of chronic hepatitis B virus infection. J Hepatol. 1987;5:45–50.

31. Chu CM, Liaw YF. Intrahepatic distribution of hepatitis B surface and core antigens in chronic hepatitis B virus infection: hepatocyte with cytoplasmic/ membranous hepatitis B core antigen as a possible target for immune hepatocytolysis. Gastroenterology. 1987;92:220–5.

32. Pontisso P, Vidalino L, Quarta S, Gatta A. Biological and clinical implications of HBV infection in peripheral blood mononuclear cells. Autoimmun Rev. 2008;8:13–7.

33. Bai GQ, Li SH, Yue YF, Shi L. The study on role of peripheral blood mononuclear cell in HBV intrauterine infection. Arch Gynecol Obstet. 2011; 283:317–21.

34. Trepo C, Guillevin L. Polyarteritis nodosa and extrahepatic manifestations of HBV infection: the case against autoimmune intervention in pathogenesis. J Autoimmun. 2001;16:269–74.

35. Haringman JJ, Gerlag DM, Zwinderman AH, Smeets TJ, Kraan MC, Baeten D, et al. Synovial tissue macrophages: a sensitive biomarker for response to treatment in patients with rheumatoid arthritis. Ann Rheum Dis. 2005;64:834–8.

36. Yeo L, Toellner KM, Salmon M, Filer A, Buckley CD, Raza K, et al. Cytokine mRNA profiling identifies B cells as a major source of RANKL in rheumatoid arthritis. Ann Rheum Dis. 2011;70:2022–8.

37. Sur CC, Giaglis S, Walker UA, Buser A, Hahn S, Hasler P. Enhanced neutrophil extracellular trap generation in rheumatoid arthritis: analysis of underlying signal transduction pathways and potential diagnostic utility. Arthritis Res Ther. 2014;16:R122.

38. Khandpur R, Carmona-Rivera C, Vivekanandan-Giri A, Gizinski A, Yalavarthi S, Knight JS, et al. NETs are a source of citrullinated autoantigens and stimulate inflammatory responses in rheumatoid arthritis. Sci Transl Med. 2013;5:178ra40.

39. Corsiero E, Bombardieri M, Carlotti E, Pratesi F, Robinson W, Migliorini P, et al. Single cell cloning and recombinant monoclonal antibodies generation from RA synovial B cells reveal frequent targeting of citrullinated histones of NETs. Ann Rheum Dis. 2016;75:1866–75.

40. Carmona-Rivera C, Carlucci PM, Moore E, Lingampalli N, Uchtenhagen H, James E, et al. Synovial fibroblast-neutrophil interactions promote pathogenic adaptive immunity in rheumatoid arthritis. Sci Immunol. 2017;2:1–26.

41. Lande R, Ganguly D, Facchinetti V, Frasca L, Conrad C, Gregorio J, et al. Neutrophils activate plasmacytoid dendritic cells by releasing self-DNA-peptide complexes in systemic lupus erythematosus. Sci Transl Med. 2011;3:73ra19.

42. Kahlenberg JM, Carmona-Rivera C, Smith CK, Kaplan MJ. Neutrophil extracellular trap-associated protein activation of the NLRP3 inflammasome is enhanced in lupus macrophages. J Immunol. 2013;190:1217–26.

43. Puga I, Cols M, Barra CM, He B, Cassis L, Gentile M, et al. B cell-helper neutrophils stimulate the diversification and production of immunoglobulin in the marginal zone of the spleen. Nat Immunol. 2011;13:170–80.

44. Tillack K, Breiden P, Martin R, Sospedra M. T lymphocyte priming by neutrophil extracellular traps links innate and adaptive immune responses. J Immunol. 2012;188:3150–9.

45. Scully LJ, Karayiannis P, Thomas HC. Interferon therapy is effective in treatment of hepatitis B-induced polyarthritis. Dig Dis Sci. 1992;37:1757–60.

46. Csepregi A, Rojkovich B, Nemesanszky E, Poor G, Hejjas M, Horanyi M. Chronic seropositive polyarthritis associated with hepatitis B virus-induced chronic liver disease: a sequel of virus persistence. Arthritis Rheum. 2000;43:232–3.

47. Hepatitis B vaccine recombinant: Rheumatoid arthritis?: case report. Reactions.1994;1:9.

13

A randomized controlled trial comparing PF-06438179/GP1111 (an infliximab biosimilar) and infliximab reference product for treatment of moderate to severe active rheumatoid arthritis despite methotrexate therapy

Stanley B. Cohen[1*], Rieke Alten[2], Hideto Kameda[3], Tomas Hala[4], Sebastiao C. Radominski[5], Muhammad I. Rehman[6], Ramesh Palaparthy[7], Karl Schumacher[8], Susanne Schmitt[8], Steven Y. Hua[7], Claudia Ianos[9] and K. Lea Sewell[10]

Abstract

Background: This double-blind, active-controlled, randomized, multinational study evaluated the efficacy, safety, pharmacokinetics (PK), and immunogenicity of PF-06438179/GP1111 (IxifiTM/Zessly®), an infliximab biosimilar, vs infliximab (Remicade®) reference product sourced from the European Union (infliximab-EU) in biologic-naïve patients with moderate to severe active rheumatoid arthritis (RA) despite methotrexate therapy. This paper reports results from the initial 30-week treatment period.

Methods: Patients ($N = 650$) were stratified by geographic region and randomized 1:1 to PF-06438179/GP1111 or infliximab-EU (3 mg/kg intravenous at weeks 0, 2, and 6, then every 8 weeks). Dose escalation to 5 mg/kg was allowed starting at week 14 for patients with inadequate RA response. The primary endpoint was American College of Rheumatology criteria for ≥ 20% clinical improvement (ACR20) response at week 14. Therapeutic equivalence was declared if the two-sided 95% CI for the treatment difference was within the symmetric equivalence margin of ± 13.5%. Statistical analysis was also performed with a two-sided 90% CI using an asymmetric equivalence margin (− 12.0%, 15.0%).

(Continued on next page)

* Correspondence: arthdoc@aol.com
[1]Metroplex Clinical Research Center, 8144 Walnut Hill Lane, Suite 810, Dallas, TX 75231, USA
Full list of author information is available at the end of the article

(Continued from previous page)

Results: Patients (80.3% female; 79.4% seropositive) had a mean RA duration of 6.9 years, and mean baseline Disease Activity Score in 28 joints, four components based on C-reactive protein was 6.0 in both arms. Week 14 ACR20 in the intention-to-treat population was 62.7% for PF-06438179/GP1111 and 64.1% for infliximab-EU. Week 14 ACR20 using nonresponder imputation was 61.1% for PF-06438179/GP1111 and 63.5% for infliximab-EU, and the 95% (− 9.92%, 5.11%) and 90% (− 8.75%, 4.02%) CIs for the treatment difference (− 2.39%) were entirely contained within the prespecified symmetric and asymmetric equivalence margins, respectively. No differences were observed between arms for secondary efficacy endpoints. Overall postdose antidrug antibody (ADA) rates through week 30 were 48.6% and 51.2% for PF-06438179/GP1111 and infliximab-EU, respectively. Efficacy and immunogenicity were similar between treatments for patients with dose escalation (at or after week 14), as well as between treatments for patients without dose escalation. Safety profiles of PF-06438179/GP1111 and infliximab-EU were similar, with no clinically meaningful differences observed between arms, including after ADA development. Serum drug concentrations were similar between arms at each time point during the initial 30-week treatment period.

Conclusion: PF-06438179/GP1111 and infliximab-EU demonstrated similar efficacy, safety, immunogenicity, and PK with or without dose escalation in patients with moderate to severe active RA on background methotrexate.

Keywords: Infliximab, PF-06438179/GP1111, Biosimilar, Rheumatoid arthritis, Dose escalation

Background

Infliximab (Remicade®; Janssen Biotech, Horsham, PA, USA, and Janssen Biologics B.V., Leiden, The Netherlands) is a chimeric monoclonal antibody specific for human tumor necrosis factor (TNF)-α, a cytokine with a demonstrated role in autoimmune and inflammatory diseases [1, 2]. Infliximab, in combination with methotrexate (MTX), is indicated for the reduction of signs and symptoms of moderate to severe active rheumatoid arthritis (RA) [1, 2]. Among patients with RA, those who receive infliximab plus MTX achieve greater clinical, radiographic, and functional benefits than those who receive MTX alone [3, 4]. Nevertheless, access to infliximab varies. Differences in national reimbursement criteria between European countries have created inequities in access to biologic disease-modifying antirheumatic drugs (DMARDs), such as infliximab, for patients with RA [5]. Furthermore, patients in the United States with RA who are covered by Medicaid are less likely than privately insured patients to receive biologic DMARDs, demonstrating disparities in treatment access by insurance type [6].

A biosimilar is a biologic drug that is highly similar in structure and function to a licensed (i.e., reference or originator) biologic product [7, 8]. In defining a biosimilar, the U.S. Food and Drug Administration further specifies that there must be no clinically meaningful differences in safety, purity, and potency between the biosimilar and the reference products [8]. The European Medicines Agency requires evidence to demonstrate the similar nature of the two products in terms of quality, safety, and efficacy [7]. The introduction of biosimilars has been associated with cost savings and improved access to biologic therapies [9–11]. For example, introduction of epoetin biosimilars in

the European Union (EU) was followed by a 27% decrease in treatment costs and a 16% increase in the use of erythropoietins [9]. Furthermore, a budget impact analysis of switching patients to the infliximab biosimilar CT-P13 projected annual cost savings that could support treatment for an additional 1960 (10% price discount) to 7561 (30% price discount) patients across France, Germany, Italy, the Netherlands, and the United Kingdom [10]. This is complemented by real-world data from the NOR-SWITCH trial, which demonstrated that switching from originator infliximab (Remicade®) to CT-P13 on the basis of cost was not inferior to continued treatment with originator infliximab in patients with chronic inflammatory diseases [12].

PF-06438179/GP1111 (IxifiTM/Zessly®; Pfizer Inc, New York, NY, USA, and Sandoz GmbH, Kundl, Austria) is a biosimilar of infliximab (Remicade®) reference product marketed in the United States (infliximab-US) and the EU (infliximab-EU) [13, 14]. Comparative assessments of protein structure confirmed that PF-06438179/GP1111 and infliximab have an identical primary amino acid sequence and similar posttranslational modifications, charge heterogeneity, and product purity [15]. In vitro characterization of biological activity established functional similarity in the ability of PF-06438179/GP1111 and infliximab to bind TNF and inhibit TNF-induced cell apoptosis [15]. PF-06438179/ GP1111 demonstrated similar toxicokinetic, tolerability, and antidrug antibody (ADA) responses to infliximab in a nonclinical in vivo toxicity study [15]. A phase I pharmacokinetics (PK) clinical study in healthy volunteers demonstrated similarity in PK, safety, and immunogenicity of PF-06438179/GP1111 to infliximab-US and infliximab-EU, as well as between infliximab-EU and infliximab-US reference products [16]. In the present double-blind, active-controlled, randomized, multinational study, we compared the efficacy, safety, PK, and immunogenicity of PF-06438179/GP1111 with infliximab-EU (Remicade®), each with background MTX therapy, as treatment for patients with moderate to severe active RA and inadequate response to MTX therapy. We report the efficacy and safety results from the initial 30-week treatment period.

Methods
Study population
Eligible patients were adults (aged ≥18 years) who met the 2010 American College of Rheumatology/European League Against Rheumatism (ACR/EULAR) classification criteria for RA for ≥ 4 months and ACR classes I–III functional status, based on the 1991 revised criteria [17, 18]. Patients had moderate to severe active RA, with at least six swollen and at least six tender joints at both screening and baseline, and high-sensitivity C-reactive protein (hs-CRP) ≥ 10 mg/L at screening. Patients must have received oral or parenteral MTX (10–25 mg/wk) for ≥ 12 weeks (at stable dose for ≥ 4 weeks) and oral folic/folinic acid (≥ 5 mg/wk) for ≥ 21 days prior to the first dose of study drug. Patients intolerant to 10–25 mg/wk could enroll with an MTX dose as low as 7.5 mg/wk. A dose of 6.0 mg/wk was allowed in geographic regions where specified by local guidance or standard of care.

Patients enrolled under the original protocol could receive concomitant sulfasalazine and/or antimalarial drugs at a stable dose. A protocol amendment later removed these allowable background therapies and required a 4-week washout period prior to the first dose of study drug. Use of other DMARDs also required a washout period prior to the first dose of study drug.

The main exclusion criteria were current infection or infection requiring hospitalization or parenteral antimicrobial therapy judged clinically significant by the investigator ≤ 6 months prior to the first dose of study drug; evidence or history of congestive heart failure, demyelinating disease, untreated or inadequately treated latent or active tuberculosis, or malignancy within the past 5 years; inadequate bone marrow, liver, renal, and immune system function at screening; and positivity for human immunodeficiency virus, hepatitis B virus, or hepatitis C virus. Patients were excluded if they had current or prior treatment with infliximab or lymphocyte-depleting therapies (e.g., rituximab, alemtuzumab); however, they were allowed up to two doses of one nondepleting, noninfliximab biologic if discontinued ≥ 12 weeks or five half-lives (whichever was longer) prior to the first dose of study drug.

Study design and treatments
This double-blind, active-controlled, randomized, multinational study (ClinicalTrials.gov identifier NCT02222493; EudraCT number 2013-004148-49) [19] was initiated at 174 centers in 28 countries. The study consisted of an initial 30-week treatment period (treatment period 1) and two subsequent 24-week treatment periods, during which patients were evaluated following a single transition from infliximab-EU to PF-06438179/GP1111 after 30 (treatment period 2) or 54 (treatment period 3) weeks of treatment (Fig. 1). At the start of treatment period 1, patients were randomized (1:1) to receive blinded treatment with PF-06438179/GP1111 or infliximab-EU, each in combination with MTX, with randomization stratified according to geographic region (North America and Western Europe, Japan, Republic of Korea, Latin America, and the rest of the world). At the start of treatment period 2, patients on infliximab-EU were rerandomized (1:1) to either blinded treatment with continued infliximab-EU or a transition to PF-06438179/GP1111. During treatment period 3, all patients received open-label treatment with PF-06438179/GP1111. This report presents the efficacy and safety results for treatment period 1, which ended with the week 30 predose assessment.

PF-06438179/GP1111 or infliximab-EU solutions for infusion were prepared by the site's pharmacists, who were designated to participate in the study and unblinded with regard to study treatments. Intravenous infliximab (PF-06438179/GP1111 or infliximab-EU) 3 mg/kg was given as an induction regimen at weeks 0, 2, and 6, followed by maintenance treatment with a 3 mg/kg dose starting at week 14 and continuing every 8 weeks thereafter. Dose escalation to 5 mg/kg infliximab was allowed starting at week 14 for patients who failed to achieve ≥ 20% improvement from baseline in both tender (68) and swollen (66) joint counts. Dose escalation to 5 mg/kg infliximab was also allowed for patients who achieved this response at week 14 but subsequently lost response to < 20% improvement from baseline in both joint counts. Patients remained on the escalated dose level for the remainder of the study. Premedication with antihistamines, acetaminophen/paracetamol, and/or corticosteroids could be administered at the investigator's discretion in compliance with local practice, the premedication label, and regulations.

Patients were required to continue their stable background MTX dose (10–25 mg/wk, 7.5 mg/wk if intolerant to higher doses, or 6 mg/wk in geographic regions where specified by local guidance or standard of care), any second DMARD (sulfasalazine/hydroxychloroquine), and folic/folinic acid supplementation throughout the study. If receiving corticosteroid (≤ 10 mg/d prednisone equivalent) and/or a nonsteroidal anti-inflammatory drug/Cox-2 inhibitor, the stable background dose remained the same for the first year, unless toxicity occurred.

Primary and secondary efficacy endpoints
The primary efficacy endpoint was the percentage of patients achieving ACR criteria for ≥ 20% clinical

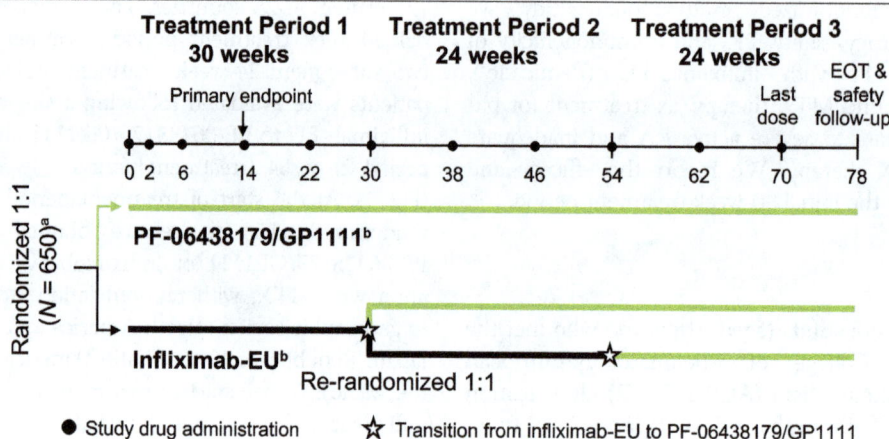

Fig. 1 Study design. [a]A sample size of approximately 614 patients was planned for enrollment; the actual number of patients randomized was 650. [b]Intravenous PF-06438179/GP1111 or infliximab-EU 3 mg/kg was given as an induction regimen at weeks 0, 2, and 6, followed by maintenance treatment with a 3 mg/kg dose starting at week 14 and continuing every 8 weeks thereafter. Dose escalation to 5 mg/kg PF-06438179/GP1111 or infliximab-EU was permitted at or after week 14 for patients with inadequate RA response. *EOT* End of treatment, *Infliximab-EU* Infliximab sourced from the European Union, *RA* Rheumatoid arthritis

improvement (ACR20) at week 14. Evaluation of ACR20 response at this time point reflects the beginning of the therapeutic plateau and provides greater sensitivity to detect possible differences in the rate of response between treatment arms, as compared with later time points [20].

Secondary efficacy endpoints at weeks 2, 4, 6, 12, 14, 22, and 30 included ACR20 (other than week 14), ACR50 ($\geq 50\%$ clinical improvement), and ACR70 ($\geq 70\%$ clinical improvement) response rates; Disease Activity Score in 28 joints, four components based on C-reactive protein (DAS28-CRP); percentages of patients with response defined according to EULAR criteria; the percentages of patients with DAS and ACR/EULAR remission; and changes from baseline for individual ACR parameters, including Health Assessment Questionnaire Disability Index (HAQ-DI). Patients were considered to be in DAS remission when DAS28-CRP was < 2.6, and in ACR/EULAR remission when either scores for tender joint count, swollen joint count, hs-CRP, and patient global assessment were all ≤ 1, or when the Simplified Disease Activity Index score was ≤ 3.3. Joint examinations were performed by an independent assessor who was blinded with regard to study treatments. In addition, pharmacodynamic (PD) response was assessed by the serum hs-CRP concentration (Covance Inc., Princeton, NJ, USA).

Additional secondary endpoints

Safety endpoints included adverse events (AEs) and laboratory abnormalities, characterized by their type, incidence, severity, timing, duration, seriousness, and relatedness to study drug. Other safety measures included electrocardiogram readings, vital signs, and physical examination. AEs were coded using the Medical Dictionary for

Regulatory Activities (MedDRA; version 19.0) classification system, and severity was graded according to the National Cancer Institute Common Terminology Criteria for Adverse Events (version 4.03). Treatment-emergent AEs (TEAEs) were defined as any AE that occurred, or any pre-existing AE that worsened, after the beginning of study treatment. TEAEs of special interest comprised infusion-related reactions (IRRs), hypersensitivity, infections (including tuberculosis and pneumonia), and malignancy (including lymphoma). Hypersensitivity events were identified by applying the MedDRA version 19.0 search criteria, hypersensitivity standardized MedDRA query (broad and narrow), and anaphylactic reactions standardized MedDRA query (broad and narrow), and high-level group terms immunology and allergy investigations.

Immunogenicity endpoints included the incidence and titers of ADAs and neutralizing antibodies (NAbs). Serum samples were first analyzed at ICON Laboratory Services, Inc. (Whitesboro, NY, USA) for the presence of ADAs using a validated electrochemiluminescence assay with a tiered approach of screening, confirmation, and titer/quantitation. ADA-positive samples were those that tested positive at both screening and confirmation, and had an ADA titer ≥ 1.30. Confirmed ADA-positive samples were then tested for NAbs using a validated cell-based bioassay with a tiered approach of screening and titer/quantitation. NAb-positive samples were those that tested positive at screening and had an NAb titer ≥ 0.70. The criteria for defining positive and negative results was established as cut points during method validation against the biosimilar for ADA and NAb assays. Transient ADA response was defined as having treatment-induced ADA detected at at least two sampling time points during treatment (including the follow-up period), where the first and last ADA-positive samples (regardless of any negative samples in between) were separated by < 16 weeks and the patient's last sampling time point was ADA-negative.

PK serum samples were analyzed for PF-06438179/GP1111 and infliximab-EU at ICON Laboratory Services, Inc. using a validated, sensitive, and specific enzyme-linked immunosorbent assay with limits of quantification of 100 ng/ml (lower) and 5000 ng/ml (upper).

Statistical methods

A sample of 614 patients was planned; this provided ≥ 85% power to demonstrate equivalence using a prespecified symmetric margin of ± 13.5% with a two-sided 95% CI when assuming ACR20 response rates of 57.5% at week 14 in both arms. The symmetric equivalence margin (± 13.5%) with a two-sided 95% CI was derived using a meta-analysis of historical published data for infliximab in RA, and > 50% preservation of the historical treatment effect for infliximab as compared with placebo [21–26]. In addition, an asymmetric margin of – 12.0% to 15.0% with a two-sided 90% CI was specifically requested by the U.S. Food and Drug Administration.

Primary analysis of ACR20 response rate at week 14 was performed in the intention-to-treat (ITT) population (all randomized patients) using nonresponder imputation (NRI) for missing data and for patients who discontinued study treatment prior to week 14. Robustness of the primary analysis was confirmed for the per-protocol (PP) population (all patients who received study treatment as planned up to week 14 and had no major protocol deviations). Other sensitivity analyses for the primary endpoint included analysis using observed data, analysis adjusting for the stratification variable geographic region, analysis incorporating one additional responder in the infliximab-EU arm who was identified at site closeout, and tipping point analysis for the asymmetric margin (– 12.0%, 15.0%) based on multiple imputation of missing data (Additional file 1: Supplementary Methods). In addition, repeated measures analysis of ACR20 response rates across all study visits up to week 30 was performed, adjusting for geographic region. The analysis was performed using the original database snapshot for the week 30 clinical study report and an additional sensitivity analysis for the one additional responder identified at site closeout.

Secondary efficacy endpoints were summarized descriptively; no conclusions regarding equivalence were drawn from analyses of secondary endpoints. Safety and immunogenicity endpoints were analyzed descriptively for the safety population (all randomized patients who received at least a portion of at least one dose of study drug). Drug concentration–time data were summarized descriptively for the PK population (all patients from the safety population who provided at least one postdose drug concentration measurement).

Results

Patient disposition and demographics

A total of 1603 patients were screened, of whom 650 were randomized to study treatment. The most common reason for screening failure was low hs-CRP value. The ITT population included 324 and 326 patients in the PF-06438179/GP1111 and infliximab-EU study arms, respectively (Additional file 1: Figure. S1). One patient in the PF-06438179/GP1111 arm was randomized twice; data were not collected for this patient's second randomization. Therefore, the safety population consisted of 323 (99.7%) patients who received PF-06438179/GP1111 and 326 (100%) who received infliximab-EU. A total of 280 (86.4%) patients in the PF-06438179/GP1111 arm and 286 (87.7%) in the infliximab-EU arm completed the 30-week treatment period. Forty-three (13.3%) patients in the PF-06438179/GP1111 arm and 40 (12.3%) in the infliximab-EU arm discontinued treatment, including 23 (7.1%) and 13 (4.0%), respectively, who discontinued before week 14.

Patient demographics and baseline disease characteristics were similar between treatment arms (Tables 1 and 2). Within each geographic region, enrollment in the two study arms was completely balanced or varied by only one patient because randomization was stratified by region. The majority of all patients in the ITT population were

Table 1 Patient demographic characteristics (intention-to-treat population)

	PF-06438179/GP1111 (n = 324)	Infliximab-EU (n = 326)	All patients (N = 650)
Gender, n (%)			
Female	258 (79.4)	264 (81.0)	522 (80.3)
Male	66 (20.4)	62 (19.0)	128 (19.7)
Age, mean (SD), years	52.8 (13.3)	52.8 (12.9)	52.8 (13.1)
Weight, mean (SD), kg	73.3 (19.8)	74.2 (20.0)	73.8 (19.9)
Body mass index, mean (SD), kg/m²	27.2 (6.4)	27.7 (7.0)	27.4 (6.7)
Race, n (%)			
White	257 (79.3)	247 (75.8)	504 (77.5)
Black	5 (1.5)	9 (2.8)	14 (2.2)
Asian	46 (14.2)	45 (13.8)	91 (14.0)
Other	15 (4.6)	25 (7.7)	40 (6.2)
Unspecified	1 (0.3)	0	1 (0.2)
Geographic region, n (%)			
North American and Western Europe	50 (15.4)	51 (15.6)	101 (15.5)
Japan	24 (7.4)	23 (7.1)	47 (7.2)
South Korea	4 (1.2)	5 (1.5)	9 (1.4)
Latin America	22 (6.8)	22 (6.7)	44 (6.8)
Rest of the world	224 (69.1)	225 (69.0)	449 (69.1)

Infliximab-EU Infliximab sourced from the European Union

Table 2 Baseline disease characteristics (intention-to-treat population)

	PF-06438179/GP1111 (n = 324)	Infliximab-EU (n = 326)	All patients (N = 650)
RA duration, mean (SD), years	7.3 (8.6)	6.4 (6.7)	6.9 (7.7)
RF or anti-CCP antibody positive, n (%)	249 (76.9)	267 (81.9)	516 (79.4)
Swollen joint count, mean (SD)	16.1 (9.4)	16.3 (8.7)	16.2 (9.1)
Tender joint count, mean (SD)	24.7 (13.9)	25.7 (12.9)	25.2 (13.4)
hs-CRP, mg/L			
Mean (SD)	25.8 (24.3)	25.3 (28.4)	25.6 (26.4)
Median (range)	17.9 (0.5–135.0)	16.5 (0.8–203.0)	17.4 (0.5–203.0)
DAS28-CRP, mean (SD)	6.0 (1.0)	6.0 (0.9)	6.0 (0.9)
HAQ-DI, mean (SD)	1.6 (0.6)	1.6 (0.7)	NC
Prior use of one biologic drug, n (%)	7 (2.2)[a]	3 (0.9)	10 (1.5)[a]
MTX dose, mean (SD), mg/wk	14.2 (4.5)[b]	14.4 (4.5)	14.3 (4.5)[b]
Corticosteroid use, n (%)	178 (54.9)	192 (58.9)	370 (56.9)
Antimalarial drug use,[c] n (%)	2 (0.6)	5 (1.5)	7 (1.1)
Sulfasalazine drug use,[c] n (%)	2 (0.6)	2 (0.6)	4 (0.6)

Abbreviations: Anti-CCP Anticyclic citrullinated peptide, *DAS28-CRP* Disease Activity Score in 28 joints, four components based on C-reactive protein, *HAQ-DI* Health Assessment Questionnaire Disability Index, *hs-CRP* High-sensitivity C-reactive protein, *Infliximab-EU* Infliximab sourced from the European Union, *MTX* Methotrexate, *NC* not calculated, *RA* Rheumatoid arthritis, *RF* Rheumatoid factor

[a]Includes one patient (PF-06438179/GP1111) who received more than two doses of sarilumab; this patient was not captured as biologic-experienced but was correctly recorded as having an exclusion criterion protocol deviation
[b]Total weekly dose of MTX was 16 mg/wk for one patient (PF-06438179/GP1111) but incorrectly recorded as 32 mg/wk; incorrect dose was the maximum value of the MTX dose range and was used for calculation of mean dose
[c]Use of sulfasalazine and antimalarial drugs was allowed only in the original protocol, but not in subsequent protocol amendments

women (80.3%) and rheumatoid factor- or anticyclic citrullinated peptide antibody-positive (79.4%). Patients were biologic-naïve, defined as receipt of up to two doses of one prior noninfliximab, nondepleting biologic DMARD; only ten (1.5%) had received a biologic DMARD, of whom four exceeded the two doses maximally allowed of one prior biologic. Eleven (1.7%) patients received concomitant sulfasalazine or antimalarial drugs under the original protocol. Patients had a mean RA duration of 6.9 years, with a mean of 16.2 swollen and 25.2 tender joints, a mean DAS28-CRP of 6.0, and a mean hs-CRP of 25.6 mg/L. The mean dose of MTX and the percentage of patients receiving oral corticosteroids were similar between the two arms (Table 2).

Total dose exposure and the percentage of patients with dose escalation to 5 mg/kg at or after week 14 were similar between the two arms. Sixty (18.5%) and 68 (20.9%) patients in the PF-06438179/GP1111 and infliximab-EU arms, respectively, had dose escalation to 5 mg/kg at week 14. An additional 23 (7.1%) and 15 (4.6%) patients in the PF-06438179/GP1111 and infliximab-EU arms, respectively, had dose escalation to 5 mg/kg at week 22.

Efficacy

In the ITT population, 203 (62.7%) patients in the PF-06438179/GP1111 arm and 209 (64.1%) in the infliximab-EU arm achieved ACR20 response at week 14. Using NRI (required for 18 [5.6%] and 12 [3.7%] PF-06438179/GP1111 and infliximab-EU patients, respectively), 198

(61.1%) patients in the PF-06438179/GP1111 arm and 207 (63.5%) in the infliximab-EU arm had a week 14 ACR20 response. The treatment difference was – 2.39%, and the corresponding 95% (– 9.92%, 5.11%) and 90% (– 8.75%, 4.02%) CIs were entirely contained within the prespecified symmetric (± 13.5%) and asymmetric (– 12.0%, 15.0%) equivalence margins, respectively (Fig. 2a and b).

ACR20 response rates at week 14 for the PP population were similar to those reported for the ITT population for both PF-06438179/GP1111 (186 of 279 [66.7%]) and infliximab-EU (195 of 290 [67.2%]). Furthermore, the 95% (– 8.42%, 7.23%) and 90% (– 7.15%, 6.02%) CIs for the treatment difference of – 0.58% were entirely contained within the prespecified symmetric and asymmetric equivalence margins, respectively (Fig. 2a and b). Other sensitivity analyses of the primary endpoint were consistent with the primary analysis results (Additional file 1: Supplementary Results, Table S1, Figure S2).

ACR20, ACR50, and ACR70 response rates were similar between PF-06438179/GP1111 and infliximab-EU at all time points through week 30 (Fig. 2c; Additional file 1: Supplementary Results; Table S2). Mean change from baseline in DAS28-CRP (Fig. 2d) was similar between PF-06438179/GP1111 and infliximab-EU at each study visit. At week 30, a mean decrease of 2.1 in DAS28-CRP from baseline was observed for both arms. Likewise, the percentages of patients in each EULAR response category were similar between treatment arms (Additional file 1:

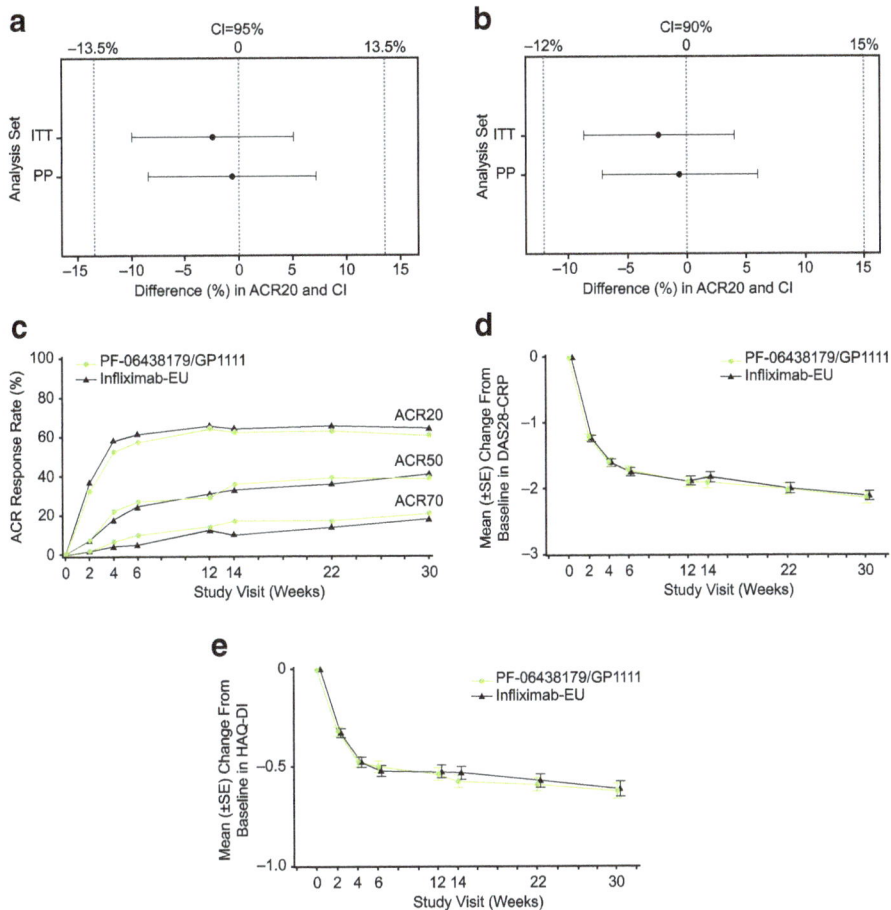

Fig. 2 Efficacy of PF-06438179/GP1111 and infliximab-EU. **a** Difference (95% CI) in week 14 ACR20 response between PF-06438179/GP1111 and infliximab-EU using NRI and symmetric equivalence margin. **b** Difference (90% CI) in week 14 ACR20 response between PF-06438179/GP1111 and infliximab-EU using NRI and asymmetric margin. **c** ACR20, ACR50, and ACR70 response rates by visit (ITT population). **d** Mean (± SE) change from baseline in DAS28-CRP by visit (ITT population). **e** Mean (± SE) change from baseline in HAQ-DI by visit (ITT population). *ACR20/50/70* American College of Rheumatology criteria for ≥ 20%/50%/70% clinical improvement, *DAS28-CRP* Disease Activity Score in 28 joints, four components based on C-reactive protein, *HAQ-DI* Health Assessment Questionnaire Disability Index; *Infliximab-EU* Infliximab sourced from the European Union, *ITT* Intention to treat, *NRI* Nonresponder imputation, *PP* Per protocol

Table S3). At week 30, 31.2% of PF-06438179/GP1111 and 28.8% of infliximab-EU patients a achieved good EULAR response.

Similar percentages of patients in the PF-06438179/GP1111 and infliximab-EU arms achieved DAS or ACR/EULAR remission at each study visit (Additional file 1: Table S4). At week 30, DAS remission was achieved by 19.1% and 16.6% of PF-06438179/GP1111 and infliximab-EU patients, respectively. ACR/EULAR remission was achieved by 9.3% and 7.1% of patients, respectively, including 6.8% and 5.5% using the Boolean definition. Mean values and changes from baseline in HAQ-DI (Fig. 2e) were similar between the two treatment arms at each study visit up to week 30. The maximal decrease in HAQ-DI was observed at week 30, with a mean decrease of 0.6 from baseline observed for both arms. Likewise, mean values and changes from baseline in the

PD marker hs-CRP were similar between the PF-06438179/GP1111 and infliximab-EU arms at each study visit (Additional file 1: Figure S3), with a maximum decrease from baseline at week 2 for both PF-06438179/GP1111 (17.2 mg/L) and infliximab-EU (16.1 mg/L).

ACR20 responses were similar between PF-06438179/GP1111 and infliximab-EU for patients who dose-escalated to 5 mg/wk at week 14 and between arms for patients who did not (Table 3). ACR20 response rates at week 30 for PF-06438179/GP1111 and infliximab-EU patients who dose-escalated at week 14 were 45.0% and 39.7%, respectively, and were 6 of 23 (26.1%) and 7 of 15 (46.7%) respectively, for patients who dose-escalated at week 22.

ACR20 response rates at weeks 14 and 30 trended higher for the patient subset that did not develop an ADA through week 30 (PF-06438179/GP1111, $n = 220$;

Table 3 Descriptive summary of ACR20 response rate at weeks 22 and 30 by dose received at week 14 (intention-to-treat population)

	No dose escalation (3 mg/kg) at week 14			Dose escalation (5 mg/kg) at week 14		
	PF-06438179/GP1111 ($n = 240$), n (%)	Infliximab-EU ($n = 244$), n (%)	Treatment difference, %	PF-06438179/GP1111 ($n = 60$), n (%)	Infliximab-EU ($n = 68$), n (%)	Treatment difference, %
Week 22						
ACR20 response						
Yes	180 (75.0)	185 (75.8)	− 0.82	23 (38.3)	27 (39.7)	− 1.37
No	58 (24.2)	58 (23.8)		36 (60.0)	36 (52.9)	
Missing	2 (0.8)	1 (0.4)		1 (1.7)	5 (7.4)	
Week 30						
ACR20 response						
Yes	169 (70.4)	181 (74.2)	− 3.76	27 (45.0)	27 (39.7)	5.29
No	65 (27.1)	55 (22.5)		29 (48.3)	30 (44.1)	
Missing	6 (2.5)	8 (3.3)		4 (6.7)	11 (16.2)	

ACR20 American College of Rheumatology criteria for ≥ 20% clinical improvement, Infliximab-EU Infliximab sourced from the European Union

infliximab-EU, $n = 222$) as compared with the ADA-positive subset (PF-06438179/GP1111, $n = 100$; infliximab-EU, $n = 103$), but they were similar between the two treatment arms within each subset. At week 14, 152 (69.1%) and 158 (71.2%) patients in the PF-06438179/GP1111 and infliximab-EU ADA-negative subsets, respectively, had ACR20 response, as compared with 51 (51.0%) and 51 (49.5%) patients, respectively, in the ADA-positive subsets.

Safety

A total of 185 (57.3%) patients in the PF-06438179/GP1111 arm and 176 (54.0%) in the infliximab-EU arm reported all-cause TEAEs (Table 4). The MedDRA System Organ Class (SOC) with the highest percentage of patients was infections and infestations in 86 (26.6%) and 72 (22.1%) PF-06438179/GP1111 and infliximab-EU patients, respectively. The most frequently reported TEAE was IRR in 19 (5.9%) and 21 (6.4%) patients in the PF-06438179/GP1111 and infliximab-EU arms, respectively. In the PF-06438179/GP1111 and infliximab-EU arms, respectively, 31 (9.6%) and 28 (8.6%) patients temporarily discontinued, and 23 (7.1%) and 24 (7.4%) patients permanently discontinued, treatment due to AEs. Sixteen (5.0%) and 14 (4.3%) patients, respectively, discontinued study participation because of AEs, including 4 (1.2%) and 3 (0.9%) due to IRR.

TEAEs reported by the investigator as potentially related to study treatment (treatment-related) occurred in 81 (25.1%) and 75 (23.0%) patients in the PF-06438179/GP1111 and infliximab-EU arms, respectively. The SOC with the highest percentage of patients who experienced treatment-related TEAEs was infections and infestations in 28 (8.7%) and 22 (6.7%) PF-06438179/GP1111 and infliximab-EU patients, respectively. The most frequently reported treatment-related TEAE was IRR in 17 (5.3%)

and 20 (6.1%) PF-06438179/GP1111 and infliximab-EU patients, respectively.

Sixteen (5.0%) patients in the PF-06438179/GP1111 arm and 20 (6.1%) in the infliximab-EU arm reported serious adverse events (SAEs) (Table 4). The two SOCs with the highest percentages of patients who experienced all-cause SAEs (PF-06438179/GP1111 vs infliximab-EU) were infections and infestations (six [1.9%] vs nine [2.8%]) and cardiac disorders (four [1.2%] vs three [0.9%]). Two patients in each treatment arm experienced SAEs with a fatal outcome; one death (infliximab-EU) following an SAE that

Table 4 All-cause treatment-emergent adverse events (safety population)[a]

	PF-06438179/GP1111 ($n = 323$)	Infliximab-EU ($n = 326$)
Number of AEs	486	492
Patients with events, n (%)		
AEs	185 (57.3)	176 (54.0)
SAEs	16 (5.0)	20 (6.1)
Grade 3 AEs	34 (10.5)	34 (10.4)
Grade 4 AEs	1 (0.3)	6 (1.8)
Grade 5 AEs	2 (0.6)	1 (0.3)
Temporarily discontinued from treatment due to AEs	31 (9.6)	28 (8.6)
Permanently discontinued from treatment due to AEs	23 (7.1)	24 (7.4)
Discontinued from study due to AEs	16 (5.0)	14 (4.3)

Abbreviations: AE Adverse event, Infliximab-EU Infliximab sourced from the European Union, SAE Serious adverse event
[a]Includes all AEs collected from the first infusion through week 30 study visit for each patient. AEs were graded in accordance with National Cancer Institute Common Terminology Criteria for AEs (version 4.03). Grades 1–5 AEs are defined as mild, moderate, severe, and life-threatening AEs and death related to AEs, respectively

started in treatment period 1 occurred outside the 30-week treatment period.

TEAEs of special interest included the IRRs noted above and hypersensitivity events in 44 (13.6%) and 51 (15.6%) patients in the PF-06438179/GP1111 and infliximab-EU arms, respectively (Additional file 1: Table S5). IRRs and hypersensitivity events occurring on or after the date a patient first tested positive for ADAs were similar between treatment arms, with 11 (7.0%) PF-06438179/GP1111 and 14 (8.4%) infliximab-EU patients experiencing a single IRR and 11 (7.0%) PF-06438179/GP1111 and 19 (11.4%) infliximab-EU patients reporting 14 and 25 hypersensitivity events, respectively. In summary, the majority (25 of 40 patients) of IRR events in both arms appeared to be associated with the development of ADAs, whereas the correlation for the broader category of hypersensitivity events, which included IRRs (30 of 95 patients), appeared to be weaker.

Treatment-emergent infectious AEs were reported by 87 (26.9%) and 73 (22.4%) patients in the PF-06438179/GP1111 and infliximab-EU arms, respectively (Additional file 1: Table S5). Six patients (three [0.9%] per arm) reported pneumonia as follows: two cases of pneumonia and one case of *Pneumocystis jirovecii* pneumonia in the PF-06438179/GP1111 arm, and three cases of pneumonia in the infliximab-EU arm. One (0.3%) patient in the PF-06438179/GP1111 arm reported latent tuberculosis, and one (0.3%) patient in the infliximab-EU arm reported active tuberculosis. One (0.3%) patient in each arm reported malignant tumors (colon cancer). The percentages of patients with laboratory abnormalities and the severity of abnormalities as well as vital sign results were comparable between treatment arms.

Immunogenicity and PK

The incidence of ADA was similar between treatment arms at all measured time points (Fig. 3a; Additional file 1: Table S6). At baseline, nine (2.8%) patients in each of the PF-06438179/GP1111 and infliximab-EU arms tested positive for ADA, with five (55%) and two (22%) of these patients, respectively, also testing positive at week 2. Overall, 157 (48.6%) and 167 (51.2%) patients in the PF-06438179/GP1111 and infliximab-EU arms, respectively, had at least one postdose sample that tested positive for ADA during the 30-week treatment period. Only one patient (0.6%) in each arm had a transient ADA response. The distribution of ADA titers was comparable between arms over the 30-week treatment period (Additional file 1: Figure S4). Of the ADA-positive patients, 124 (79.0%) and 143 (85.6%), in the PF-06438179/GP1111 and infliximab-EU arms, respectively, tested NAb-positive. The incidence of NAb was similar between treatment arms at all measured time points. (Fig. 3b; Additional file 1: Table S6)

Patients qualifying for dose escalation to 5 mg/kg infliximab had higher ADA rates of 38.6% (PF-06438179/GP1111) and 44.6% (infliximab-EU) at week 14, as compared with 26.7% (PF-06438179/GP1111) and 25.9% (infliximab-EU) for patients remaining on 3 mg/kg (Additional file 1: Table S7). Incidence of ADA was similar between PF-06438179/GP1111 and infliximab-EU for patients who dose-escalated, as well as between the two arms for patients who did not (Additional file 1: Table S7). A similar trend was observed for NAb rates between treatment arms for patients who remained at 3 mg/kg infliximab. There were slight numerical differences in NAb rates between treatment arms for patients who dose-escalated to 5 mg/kg infliximab, which could be due to smaller subgroup size. However, these differences are not clinically meaningful, because ACR20 response rates were similar between treatment arms for patients who dose-escalated to 5 mg/kg infliximab.

Trough serum concentrations at weeks 2, 4, 6, 14, 22, and 30 and immediate postdose serum concentrations on day 1 and week 14 were similar between treatment arms (Table 5). The PK of infliximab is known to be affected by the presence of ADA [2], and the serum drug concentrations in this trial were lower in ADA-positive than in ADA-negative patients (Table 5). The presence of ADA affected the disposition of both PF-06438179/GP1111 and infliximab-EU in a similar manner in ADA-positive patients (Table 5; Additional file 1: Figure S5).

Discussion

The availability of biosimilars may expand access to biologic therapies such as infliximab, providing patients with additional safe and efficacious treatment options. Regulatory approval for biosimilars relies on a demonstration of biosimilarity that establishes there are no clinically meaningful differences in safety, purity, or potency between the proposed biosimilar and the originator product [8]. This determination of biosimilarity is made on the basis of the totality of the evidence obtained from all stages of the development process, which begins with comprehensive analytical (i.e., structural and functional) characterization followed by nonclinical testing [7, 8]. Finally, a confirmatory clinical study (or studies) is conducted to demonstrate similarity between the proposed biosimilar and the originator product in terms of their PK, efficacy, safety, and immunogenicity profiles [7, 8].

As the final step in the biosimilarity exercise, this study was conducted to compare the efficacy and safety of PF-06438179/GP1111 and infliximab-EU. The study met its primary objective by demonstrating therapeutic equivalence between PF-06438179/GP1111 and infliximab-EU. The 95% and 90% CIs for the difference between arms in week 14 ACR20 response rates were entirely contained within the prespecified symmetric and asymmetric equivalence margins, respectively. Compared with the symmetric

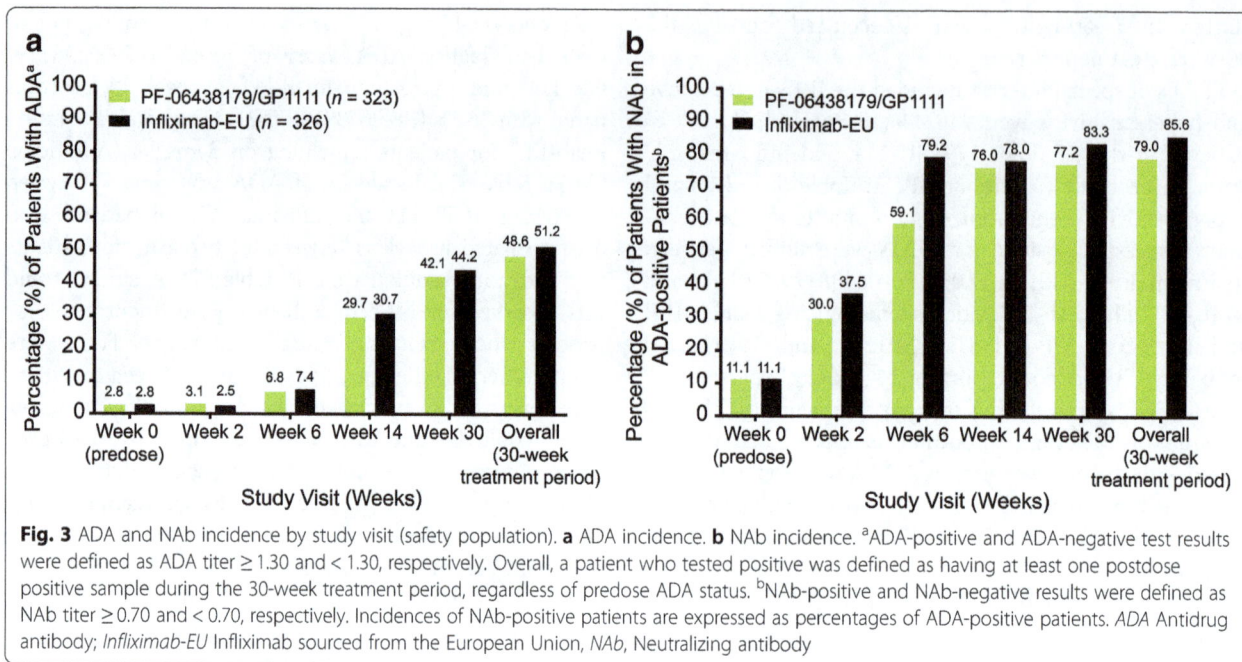

Fig. 3 ADA and NAb incidence by study visit (safety population). **a** ADA incidence. **b** NAb incidence. [a]ADA-positive and ADA-negative test results were defined as ADA titer ≥ 1.30 and < 1.30, respectively. Overall, a patient who tested positive was defined as having at least one postdose positive sample during the 30-week treatment period, regardless of predose ADA status. [b]NAb-positive and NAb-negative results were defined as NAb titer ≥ 0.70 and < 0.70, respectively. Incidences of NAb-positive patients are expressed as percentages of ADA-positive patients. *ADA* Antidrug antibody; *Infliximab-EU* Infliximab sourced from the European Union, *NAb*, Neutralizing antibody

margin, the asymmetric margin applied a smaller lower bound but a larger upper bound for the CI. Although this is less stringent for higher efficacy of the biosimilar, it is more stringent for potential lower efficacy of the biosimilar. Sensitivity analyses confirmed that the comparison of PF-06438179/GP1111 and infliximab-EU in ACR20 response rate at week 14 was robust under different missing data imputation approaches. No differences were observed between PF-06438179/GP1111 and infliximab-EU for secondary efficacy endpoints, supporting the results of the primary endpoint analysis.

The week 14 ACR20 responses observed in this study (62.7% for PF-06438179/GP1111 and 64.1% for infliximab-EU) were within the range of ACR20 response rates reported in historical registration trials for infliximab (Remicade®; 50–76%) [21, 22, 24, 25]. Furthermore, the current study and historical reference trials for infliximab were generally similar in terms of patient enrollment criteria, MTX dosing, and patient demographic and baseline disease characteristics [21, 22, 24, 25]. The primary assessment of ACR20 response was evaluated at week 14, an earlier time point than used in the historical reference studies of infliximab vs placebo in patients with RA [3, 4, 22–25]. Evaluation of ACR20 response early in the therapeutic plateau provides greater sensitivity to detect possible differences in the rate of response between treatment arms, as compared with later time points. This is relevant and appropriate for biosimilarity studies, which are designed to demonstrate there are no clinically meaningful differences between treatments [8, 20].

The safety profiles of PF-06438179/GP1111 and infliximab-EU were similar, with no clinically meaningful

differences observed between arms. The incidence and characteristics of TEAEs of special interest were similar between treatment arms, including IRRs and hypersensitivity events for both arms and for the ADA-positive subsets following ADA onset. The incidence of patients with at least one positive postdose ADA result during the 30-week treatment period (48.6% for PF-06438179/GP1111 and 51.2% for infliximab-EU) and the percentage of ADA-positive patients who tested positive for NAb (79.0% for PF-06438179/GP1111 and 85.6% for infliximab-EU) were similar between the two arms. Incidence of ADAs in both arms was higher than reported in a pivotal infliximab trial ($\sim 22\%$) [24]; however, this is attributed to the higher sensitivity of electrochemiluminescence assays, which result in detection of lower-titer ADA. Evaluation of immunogenicity during the initial 30-week treatment period was supported by the higher sensitivity of current methods to detect the development of ADA. Serum PF-06438179/GP1111 and infliximab-EU concentrations were similar at each time point during the first 30 weeks of dosing.

The current study incorporated dose escalation to 5 mg/kg infliximab, starting at week 14, for patients with an inadequate RA response. Efficacy and immunogenicity profiles were comparable between PF-06438179/GP1111 and infliximab-EU for patients with dose escalation to 5 mg/kg, as well as between the two treatment arms for patients without dose escalation. These data are reassuring because dose optimization is common for infliximab and because patients with RA who experience nonresponse, inadequate response, or loss of response generally demonstrate improvement after a dose increase

Table 5 Serum PF-06438179/GP1111 and infliximab-EU concentrations by study visit and antidrug antibody status (pharmacokinetics population)

	All patients		ADA-positive patients		ADA-negative patients	
	PF-06438179/GP1111	Infliximab-EU	PF-06438179/GP1111	Infliximab-EU	PF-06438179/GP1111	Infliximab-EU
C_{trough} median (5th–95th percentile), ng/ml						
Week 0 (day 1)	$n = 322$ 0 (0–0)	$n = 323$ 0 (0–0)	$n = 156$ 0 (0–0)	$n = 166$ 0 (0–0)	$n = 163$ 0 (0–0)	$n = 156$ 0 (0–0)
Week 2	$n = 316$ 16,830 (6241–28,660)	$n = 323$ 16,070 (6241–27,270)	$n = 155$ 15,540 (5675–26,780)	$n = 166$ 14,230 (5243–26,130)	$n = 161$ 18,230 (6316–28,830)	$n = 157$ 18,020 (9075–29,630)
Week 4	$n = 308$ 23,540 (4300–45,750)	$n = 314$ 21,250 (2258–40,120)	$n = 151$ 17,760 (765–37,420)	$n = 164$ 16,370 (256–32,450)	$n = 157$ 27,850 (10,660–49,180)	$n = 150$ 26,880 (12,980–41,390)
Week 6	$n = 308$ 10,020 (102–26,650)	$n = 315$ 9266 (0–24,180)	$n = 151$ 6159 (0–20,180)	$n = 163$ 5122 (0–17,440)	$n = 157$ 14,030 (3960–29,890)	$n = 152$ 12,790 (4321–26,420)
Week 14	$n = 302$ 1497 (0–10,590)	$n = 310$ 1025 (0–7643)	$n = 154$ 0 (0–4014)	$n = 159$ 0 (0–3428)	$n = 148$ 3351 (492–15,660)	$n = 151$ 3063 (197–8440)
Week 22	$n = 295$ 576 (0–7911)	$n = 303$ 433 (0–6221)	$n = 152$ 0 (0–2262)	$n = 156$ 0 (0–1151)	$n = 143$ 2977 (206–10,640)	$n = 147$ 2489 (0–7577)
Week 30	$n = 281$ 413 (0–7253)	$n = 290$ 279 (0–6017)	$n = 143$ 0 (0–533)	$n = 149$ 0 (0–575)	$n = 138$ 2846 (386–10,050)	$n = 141$ 2385 (192–7580)
C_{max} median (5th–95th percentile), ng/ml						
Week 0 (day 1)	$n = 319$ 64,240 (31,570–102,000)	$n = 322$ 62,200 (23,260–95,990)	$n = 154$ 63,830 (35,630–101,500)	$n = 166$ 59,290 (1603–93,170)	$n = 162$ 65,530 (11,180–102,000)	$n = 155$ 66,080 (29,140–101,200)
Week 14	$n = 297$ 71,250 (1617–150,500)	$n = 299$ 68,450 (3367–144,500)	$n = 149$ 68,280 (0–157,500)	$n = 152$ 62,010 (1091–118,200)	$n = 148$ 75,640 (5633–129,400)	$n = 147$ 75,090 (8857–159,800)

Abbreviations: ADA Antidrug antibody, C_{max} Observed serum drug concentration prior to the end of infusion, C_{trough} Observed predose trough serum concentration, *Infliximab-EU* Infliximab sourced from the European Union

[27–29]. Furthermore, the placebo-adjusted response to infliximab in RA is greater with higher doses of infliximab [3, 4, 30], which increases the sensitivity of RA as a clinical model for detecting potential differences between originator infliximab and proposed infliximab biosimilars [30]. Therefore, evidence for similar efficacy between PF-06438179/GP1111 and infliximab-EU at the 5 mg/kg dose could support its use in other indications (e.g., inflammatory bowel disease, ankylosing spondylitis) for which infliximab is approved.

Conclusions

PF-06438179/GP1111 and infliximab-EU demonstrated similar efficacy, safety, immunogenicity, and PK profiles in patients with moderate to severe active RA on background MTX up to 30 weeks. Furthermore, efficacy and immunogenicity of PF-06438179/GP1111 and infliximab-EU were comparable for patients with dose escalation to 5 mg/kg infliximab, as well as between arms for patients without dose escalation. The results of this study, combined with previous results of an analytical (structural and functional) evaluation [15], demonstrate similarity of PF-06438179/GP1111 to infliximab-EU. This trial will also evaluate clinical efficacy, safety, and immunogenicity after a single transition from infliximab-EU to PF-06438179/GP1111 after 30 or 54 weeks of treatment.

Abbreviations

ACR: American College of Rheumatology; ACR20/50/70: American College of Rheumatology criteria for ≥ 20%/50%/70% clinical improvement; ADA: Antidrug antibody; AE: Adverse event; Anti-CCP: Anticyclic citrullinated peptide; C_{max}: Observed serum drug concentration prior to the end of infusion; C_{trough}: Observed predose trough serum concentration; DAS: Disease Activity Score; DAS28-CRP: Disease Activity Score in 28 joints, four components based on C-reactive protein; DMARD: Disease-modifying antirheumatic drugs; EOT: End of treatment; EU: European Union; EULAR: European League Against Rheumatism; HAQ-DI: Health Assessment Questionnaire Disability Index; hs-CRP: High-sensitivity C-reactive protein; Infliximab-EU/US: Infliximab sourced from the European Union/United States; IRR: Infusion-related reaction; ITT: Intention to treat; MedDRA: Medical Dictionary for Regulatory Activities; MTX: Methotrexate; NAb: Neutralizing antibody; NRI: Nonresponder imputation; PD: Pharmacodynamics; PK: Pharmacokinetics; PP: Per protocol; RA: Rheumatoid arthritis; RF: Rheumatoid factor; SAE: Serious adverse event; SOC: System Organ Class; TEAE: Treatment-emergent adverse event; TNF: Tumor necrosis factor

Acknowledgements

Professional medical writing and editorial assistance was provided by Elyse Smith, PhD, at Engage Scientific Solutions and was funded by Sandoz Inc. and Pfizer Inc.

Funding

This study was funded by Pfizer Inc.

Availability of data and materials

Pfizer's policies on the provision of clinical trial data are set out on its website: http://www.pfizer.com/research/clinical_trials/trial_data_and_results. In addition to posting clinical trial results on the clinicaltrials.gov registry, Pfizer will provide access to anonymized patient-level data in response to scientifically valid research protocols. Data from Pfizer-sponsored global interventional clinical studies are available from trials conducted for medicines, vaccines, and medical devices for indications that have been approved in the United States and/or by the European Union and from trials conducted for medicines, vaccines, and medical devices that have been terminated (i.e., development for all indications has been discontinued). Data from these trials will be made available 24 months after study completion. Pfizer will make reasonable efforts to fulfill all data requests for legitimate research purposes, but there may be instances in which retrieval or delivery of data is not feasible (e.g., if Pfizer does not have legal authority to provide the data, if costs of retrieval of older or preelectronic data are prohibitive; see page 5 at the following link: https://www.pfizer.com/files/research/research_clinical_trials/A_Guide_to_Requesting_Pfizer_Patient-Level_Clinical_Trial_Data_2017.pdf). Further details can be found at: http://www.pfizer.com/research/clinical_trials/trial_data_and_results/data_requests. Pfizer's practices adhere to the principles for responsible data sharing laid out by the European Federation of Pharmaceutical Industries and Associations (EFPIA) and the Pharmaceutical Research and Manufacturers of America (PhRMA); see http://phrma.org/sites/default/files/pdf/PhRMAPrinciplesForResponsibleClinicalTrialDataSharing.pdf.

Authors' contributions

MIR, KLS, and SYH made substantial contributions to study conception and design. SYH analyzed the data and provided statistical support. RP contributed to study design and analyses of pharmacokinetic and immunogenicity data. KS contributed to analysis of efficacy data, and SS and CI contributed to analysis of safety data. SBC, RA, HK, TH, and SCR contributed to acquisition of data. SBC reviewed for investigator approval all study data in the clinical study report, which was written by KLS. All authors made substantial contributions to interpretation of data, were involved in drafting the manuscript and/or revising it critically for important intellectual content, and read and approved the final manuscript for submission.

Competing interests

SBC has received consulting fees from Amgen, Boehringer-Ingelheim, Coherus, Merck, Pfizer, and Sandoz and has received research grants from Amgen, Boehringer-Ingelheim, Coherus, Merck, and Pfizer. RA has received honoraria and research grants from Pfizer. HK has received consulting fees, speaking fees, and/or honoraria from AbbVie GK, Bristol-Myers Squibb, Chugai Pharmaceutical Co. Ltd., Eli Lilly Japan K.K., Janssen Pharmaceutical K.K., Mitsubishi Tanabe Pharma, Novartis Pharma K.K., Pfizer Japan Inc., and Sanofi K.K. and has received research grants from AbbVie GK, Astellas Pharma Inc., Chugai Pharmaceutical Co. Ltd., Eisai Co. Ltd., Mitsubishi Tanabe Pharma, and Takeda Pharmaceutical Co. Ltd. SCR has received research grants and consulting fees, speaking fees, and/or honoraria from Pfizer Inc. TH has no competing interests to disclose. KS and SS are employees of Hexal AG, a Sandoz company. MIR, RP, and KLS are full-time employees of and declare having stock holdings and/or stock options from Pfizer Inc. SYH and CI were employees of and had stock holdings and/or stock options from Pfizer Inc. at the time of the study.

Author details

[1]Metroplex Clinical Research Center, 8144 Walnut Hill Lane, Suite 810, Dallas, TX 75231, USA. [2]Schlosspark-Klinik University Medicine, Heubnerweg 2, 14059 Berlin, Germany. [3]Toho University Ohashi Medical Center, 2-17-6, Ohashi Muguro-ku, Tokyo 153-8515, Japan. [4]Center for Clinical and Basic Research, Trida Miru 2800, 530 02 Pardubice, Czech Republic. [5]Universidade Federal do Paraná, Rua General Carneiro, 181 - Alto da Glória, Curitiba, PR 80.060-900, Brazil. [6]Pfizer Inc., 1 Burtt Road, Andover, MA 01810, USA. [7]Pfizer Inc., 10777 Science Center Drive, CB1/2103, San Diego, CA 92121, USA. [8]Hexal AG, Industriestraße 25, D-83607 Holzkirchen, Germany. [9]Pfizer UK, Discovery Park, Ramsgate Road, Sandwich CT13 9ND, UK. [10]Pfizer Inc., 300 Technology Square, Cambridge, MA 02139, USA.

References

1. European Medicines Agency (EMA). Remicade (infliximab) summary of product characteristics. London: EMA; 2017. http://www.ema.europa.eu/docs/en_GB/document_library/EPAR_-_Product_Information/human/000240/WC500050888.pdf. Accessed 14 Aug 2017.
2. Janssen Biotech Inc. Remicade (infliximab) US prescribing information. Horsham, PA: Janssen Biotech, Inc.; 2017. https://www.accessdata.fda.gov/drugsatfda_docs/label/2017/761072s000lbl.pdf. Accessed 14 Aug 2017.
3. Lipsky PE, van der Heijde DM, St Clair EW, Furst DE, Breedveld FC, Kalden JR, et al. Infliximab and methotrexate in the treatment of rheumatoid arthritis: anti-tumor necrosis factor trial in rheumatoid arthritis with concomitant therapy study group. N Engl J Med. 2000;343:1594–602.
4. St Clair EW, van der Heijde DM, Smolen JS, Maini RN, Bathon JM, Emery P, et al. Combination of infliximab and methotrexate therapy for early rheumatoid arthritis: a randomized, controlled trial. Arthritis Rheum. 2004;50:3432–43.
5. Kalo Z, Voko Z, Ostor A, Clifton-Brown E, Vasilescu R, Battersby A, et al. Patient access to reimbursed biological disease-modifying antirheumatic drugs in the European region. J Mark Access Health Policy. 2017;5:1345580.
6. Cifaldi M, Renaud J, Ganguli A, Halpern MT. Disparities in care by insurance status for individuals with rheumatoid arthritis: analysis of the medical expenditure panel survey, 2006-2009. Curr Med Res Opin. 2016;32:2029–37.
7. Committee for Medicinal Products for Human Use (CHMP), European Medicines Agency (EMA). Guideline on similar biological medicinal products. London: EMA; 2014. http://www.ema.europa.eu/docs/en_GB/document_library/Scientific_guideline/2014/10/WC500176768.pdf. Accessed 14 Aug 2017.
8. US Food and Drug Administration (FDA). Scientific considerations in demonstrating biosimilarity to a reference product. Guidance for industry. Silver Spring, MD: FDA; 2015. http://www.fda.gov/downloads/Drugs/GuidanceComplianceRegulatoryInformation/Guidances/UCM291128.pdf. Accessed 14 Aug 2017.
9. IMS Institute for Healthcare Informatics. Delivering on the potential of biosimilar medicines: the role of functioning competitive markets. Parsippany, NJ: IMS Health and the IMS Institute for Healthcare Informatics; March 2016. https://www.medicinesforeurope.com/wp-content/uploads/2016/03/IMS-Institute-Biosimilar-Report-March-2016-FINAL.pdf. Accessed 21 Aug 2017.
10. Jha A, Upton A, Dunlop WC, Akehurst R. The budget impact of biosimilar infliximab (Remsima®) for the treatment of autoimmune diseases in five European countries. Adv Ther. 2015;32:742–56.
11. Singh SC, Bagnato KM. The economic implications of biosimilars. Am J Manag Care. 2015;21(16 Suppl):s331–40.
12. Jorgensen KK, Olsen IC, Goll GL, Lorentzen M, Bolstad N, Haavardsholm EA, et al. Switching from originator infliximab to biosimilar CT-P13 compared with maintained treatment with originator infliximab (NOR-SWITCH): a 52-week, randomised, double-blind, non-inferiority trial. Lancet. 2017;389:2304–16.
13. Pfizer Inc. Ixifi (infliximab-qbtx) US prescribing information. Pfizer Inc. 2017. https://www.accessdata.fda.gov/drugsatfda_docs/label/2017/761072s000lbl.pdf. Accessed 2 July 2018.
14. European Medicines Agency. Zessly (infliximab) summary of product characteristics. 2018. http://www.ema.europa.eu/docs/en_GB/document_library/EPAR_-_Product_Information/human/004647/WC500249647.pdf. Accessed 2 July 2018.
15. Derzi M, Johnson TR, Shoieb AM, Conlon HD, Sharpe P, Saati A, et al. Nonclinical evaluation of PF-06438179: a potential biosimilar to Remicade® (infliximab). Adv Ther. 2016;33:1964–82.
16. Palaparthy R, Udata C, Hua SY, Yin D, Cai CH, Salts S, et al. A randomized study comparing the pharmacokinetics of the potential biosimilar PF-06438179/GP1111 with Remicade® (infliximab) in healthy subjects (REFLECTIONS B537-01). Expert Rev Clin Immunol. 2018;14:329–36.
17. Aletaha D, Neogi T, Silman AJ, Funovits J, Felson DT, Bingham CO 3rd, et al. 2010 rheumatoid arthritis classification criteria: an American College of Rheumatology/European League Against Rheumatism collaborative initiative. Ann Rheum Dis. 2010;69:1580–8.
18. Hochberg MC, Chang RW, Dwosh I, Lindsey S, Pincus T, Wolfe F. The American College of Rheumatology 1991 revised criteria for the classification of global functional status in rheumatoid arthritis. Arthritis Rheum. 1992;35:498–502.
19. ClinicalTrials.gov. A study of PF-06438179 (infliximab-Pfizer) and infliximab in combination with methotrexate in subjects with active rheumatoid arthritis (REFLECTIONS B537–02). Registered on 21 Aug 2014. https://clinicaltrials.gov/ct2/show/NCT02222493. Accessed 14 Aug 2017.
20. US Food and Drug Administration (FDA). Guidance for industry. Rheumatoid arthritis: developing drug products for treatment. Rockville, MD: U.S. Department of Health and Human Services, FDA, Center for Drug Evaluation and Research (CDER); 2013. https://www.fda.gov/downloads/drugs/guidancecomplianceregulatoryinformation/guidances/ucm354468.pdf. Accessed 22 Aug 2017.
21. Abe T, Takeuchi T, Miyasaka N, Hashimoto H, Kondo H, Ichikawa Y, et al. A multicenter, double-blind, randomized, placebo controlled trial of infliximab combined with low dose methotrexate in Japanese patients with rheumatoid arthritis. J Rheumatol. 2006;33:37–44.
22. Maini R, St Clair EW, Breedveld F, Furst D, Kalden J, Weisman M, et al. Infliximab (chimeric anti-tumour necrosis factor α monoclonal antibody) versus placebo in rheumatoid arthritis patients receiving concomitant methotrexate: a randomised phase III trial. ATTRACT study group. Lancet. 1999;354:1932–9.
23. Schiff M, Keiserman M, Codding C, Songcharoen S, Berman A, Nayiager S, et al. Efficacy and safety of abatacept or infliximab vs placebo in ATTEST: a phase III, multi-centre, randomised, double-blind, placebo-controlled study in patients with rheumatoid arthritis and an inadequate response to methotrexate. Ann Rheum Dis. 2008;67:1096–103.
24. Westhovens R, Yocum D, Han J, Berman A, Strusberg I, Geusens P, et al. The safety of infliximab, combined with background treatments, among patients with rheumatoid arthritis and various comorbidities: a large, randomized, placebo-controlled trial. Arthritis Rheum. 2006;54:1075–86.
25. Zhang F-C, Hou Y, Huang F, Wu D-H, Bao C-D, Ni L-Q, et al. Infliximab versus placebo in rheumatoid arthritis patients receiving concomitant methotrexate: a preliminary study from China. APLAR J Rheumatol. 2006;9:127–30.
26. Hua SY, Xu S, Barker KB, Liao SM, Li S. Bayesian methods to assess bioequivalence and biosimilarity with case studies. In: Barker KB, Menon SM, D' Agostino RB, Xu S, Jin B, editors. Biosimilar clinical development: scientific considerations and new methodologies. Boca Raton, FL: CRC Press; 2017. p. 181–98.
27. Alten R, van den Bosch F. Dose optimization of infliximab in patients with rheumatoid arthritis. Int J Rheum Dis. 2014;17:5–18.
28. Ariza-Ariza R, Navarro-Sarabia F, Hernandez-Cruz B, Rodriguez-Arboleya L, Navarro-Compan V, Toyos J. Dose escalation of the anti-TNF-α agents in patients with rheumatoid arthritis: a systematic review. Rheumatology (Oxford). 2007;46:529–32.
29. Wu E, Chen L, Birnbaum H, Yang E, Cifaldi M. Retrospective claims data analysis of dosage adjustment patterns of TNF antagonists among patients with rheumatoid arthritis. Curr Med Res Opin. 2008;24:2229–44.
30. Lee H. Is extrapolation of the safety and efficacy data in one indication to another appropriate for biosimilars? AAPS J. 2014;16:22–6.

14

The effect of the cholinergic anti-inflammatory pathway on collagen-induced arthritis involves the modulation of dendritic cell differentiation

Di Liu, Tong Li, Hui Luo, Xiaoxia Zuo, Sijia Liu[*] and Shiyao Wu[*]

Abstract

Background: The cholinergic anti-inflammatory pathway (CAP) has a strong anti-inflammatory effect on collagen-induced arthritis (CIA), a classic animal model of rheumatoid arthritis (RA). However, the underlying immune regulatory mechanism remains unclear. Here, we investigated the effect of the CAP on arthritis development and the involvement of dendritic cells (DCs).

Methods: Forty DBA/1 mice were randomly divided into five groups: a control group (sham vagotomy+ phosphate-buffered saline; shamVGX+PBS), a CIA group (shamVGX+CIA + PBS), a vagotomy group (VGX + CIA + PBS), a GTS-21 (4 mg/kg) group (shamVGX+CIA + GTS-4), and a GTS-21 (8 mg/kg) group (shamVGX +CIA + GTS-8). The vagotomy group underwent left cervical vagotomy 4 days before arthritis induction, whereas the sham-vagotomy group underwent vagus nerve exposure. Mice were pretreated with GTS-21 by intraperitoneal injection on the day of surgery. The degree of arthritis was measured by using the arthritis score, hematoxylin and eosin staining, and TRAP (tartrate-resistant acid phosphatase) staining. Flow cytometry was used to detect the expression of CD80 and major histocompatibility complex II (MHC II) on CD11c[+] DCs in the spleen. Luminex was used to detect the serum concentration of interleukin-6 (IL-6), tumor necrosis factor-alpha (TNFα), and IL-10. Immunohistochemistry was used to detect CD11c expression in the synovium. The effects of GTS-21 on DC differentiation and maturation were examined *in vitro* by treating bone marrow–derived DCs with GTS-21 and assessing differentiation and maturation. Flow cytometry was used to analyze CD80 and MHC II expression on the surface of DCs.

Results: GTS-21 treatment ameliorated clinical arthritis in a mouse model of CIA *in vivo*, decreasing the secretion of pro-inflammatory cytokines in the serum and downregulating CD80 and MHC II expression on DCs in the spleen of CIA mice. GTS-21 treatment strongly suppressed the infiltration of DCs into the synovium. Vagotomy itself did not exacerbate the severity of arthritis in CIA mice. *In vitro*, GTS-21 (10 μmol/L) significantly downregulated CD80 and MHC II in bone marrow–derived immature DCs and this effect was blocked by the α7-nicotinic acetylcholine receptor antagonist methyllycaconitine (MLA). However, GTS-21 had no effects on mature DCs.

Conclusions: The present study provides new insight into the mechanism underlying the effects of the CAP on RA and indicates that the immunosuppressive effect of GTS-21 may be mediated by the inhibition of DC differentiation.

Keywords: Rheumatoid arthritis, Dendritic cells, Cholinergic anti-inflammatory pathway, GTS-21

* Correspondence: celialiu@csu.edu.cn; wushiyao1985@yeah.net
Department of Rheumatology and Immunology, Xiangya Hospital, Central South University, Hunan Province, Changsha 410008, People's Republic of China

Introduction

Rheumatoid arthritis (RA) is a chronic autoimmune disease characterized by synovial inflammation and cartilage and bone destruction. Although the pathogenesis is unknown, it is believed that inflammatory cell infiltration into the synovium is the main cause of persisting synovitis [1]. Dendritic cells (DCs) are important innate immune cells and professional antigen-presenting cells that play an important role in immunologic priming. DCs contribute to the pathogenesis of RA. Mature DCs in the synovium and secondary lymphoid organs can present antigens to naïve T cells and induce T-cell activation [2, 3]; DCs secrete inflammatory cytokines such as interleukin-12 (IL-12), IL-23, IL-6, tumor necrosis factor-alpha (TNF-α), and IL-1 to induce Th1, Th2, and Th17 differentiation, aggravating the inflammation of the synovium [4–7]. In addition, DCs produce B cell–activating factor, thus promoting the proliferation of antibody-producing B cells [8]. Studies indicate that DC-based immunotherapy may be effective for the treatment of RA. In a mouse model of collagen-induced arthritis (CIA), DCs with tolerogenic characteristics suppressed the progression of established CIA [9–11]. DC differentiation into a tolerogenic state is an attractive tool to restore self-tolerance in RA and other autoimmune disorders [12]. Moreover, clinical trials confirmed that the strategy is safe, feasible, and acceptable [13, 14]. These data suggest that DCs are a promising target for the treatment of RA.

The cholinergic anti-inflammatory pathway (CAP) is an endogenous anti-inflammatory pathway that links the nervous system and the immune system via the vagus nerve [15]. Activation of the CAP can be achieved by vagus nerve stimulation or cholinergic agonists [16]. GTS-21, a classic cholinergic agonist, can bind to the $\alpha 7$ subunit of the nicotinic acetylcholine receptor ($\alpha 7$nAChR) of inflammatory cells to induce an anti-inflammatory response [17]. A previous study showed that the CAP is involved in the reduction of inflammation in experimental sepsis, acute lung injury, ischemia/reperfusion injury, and pancreatitis [18].

Accumulating evidence indicates that the CAP suppresses inflammation in RA. Stimulation of nicotinic acetylcholine receptors attenuates CIA in mice, whereas knockdown of the $\alpha 7$nAChR aggravates CIA [19]. Previous work from our group confirmed that the CAP inhibits arthritis development by regulating immune cells, such suppressing the TNF-α–dependent inflammatory pathway in synoviocytes and Th1 cells, Th17 cell differentiation, and macrophage migration [20–24]. The $\alpha 7$nAChR is also expressed on the surface of DCs [25]. However, the effects of CAP on DCs remain unclear in RA. Here, we investigated the anti-inflammatory effect of the cholinergic agonist GTS-21 on RA and examined the role of DCs.

Materials and methods

Animals

Five-week-old C57BL/6 J male mice and 5-week-old DBA/1 male mice were purchased from the Shanghai Institute of Experimental Animals. The mice were fed adaptively for 1 week. The experiment was approved by the Ethics Committee for Laboratory Animals of Central South University.

Experimental groups

Forty DBA/1 male mice were randomly divided into five groups: a control group (sham vagotomy + phosphate-buffered saline, sham VGX + PBS), a model group (sham VGX + PBS + CIA), a vagotomy group (VGX + PBS + CIA), a GTS-21 4 mg/kg group (sham VGX + GTS-21 4 mg/kg + CIA), and a GTS-21 8 mg/kg group (sham VGX + GTS-21 8 mg/kg + CIA). To block the CAP, mice in the vagotomy group underwent left cervical vagotomy 4 days before CIA induction, whereas the left vagus nerve was exposed but not cut in the sham operation group. To activate the CAP, mice received different doses of GTS-21 (4 and 8 mg/kg) from 4 days before the induction of CIA to 45 days after the first immunization, and the other group received an equal volume of phosphate buffer by intraperitoneal injection at the same time points.

CIA induction

Bovine type II collagen (Chondrex, Redmond, WA, USA) was diluted to 2 mg/mL with 10 mM acetic acid and emulsified with an equal volume of Freund's complete adjuvant (Chondrex). The CIA model mice were injected with 0.1 mL of fully emulsified bovine collagen intradermally at the tail base. At 21 days after the first immunization, CIA mice were injected with the same amount of bovine type II collagen emulsified with Freund's incomplete adjuvant (Chondrex) as the second immunization.

Evaluation of arthritis

Starting on the day of the second immunization, each digit and paw were assessed every 3 days by two investigators until day 45. The arthritis index scoring criteria were as follows: 0, normal; 1, slight redness or swelling of the joint; 2, moderate swelling; 3, obvious swelling; and 4, severe swelling and inability to bear weight.

Histopathological examination and immunohistochemistry

Mice were sacrificed on day 45. The joints were removed, fixed in formalin for 48 h, decalcified in 10% ethylenediaminetetraacetic acid, and embedded in paraffin. The sections were stained with hematoxylin and eosin (HE) and tartrate-resistant acid phosphatase (TRAP) for histopathological analysis. The severity of inflammatory cell infiltration (grade 0–4) and synovial hyperplasia (grade 0–3) were scored as previously described in joints of ankle and knee [26, 27]. TRAP$^+$ osteoclasts were counted manually in joints of the ankle and knee. The CD11c expression level in the synovium was examined with immunohistochemistry by using a rabbit anti-mouse CD11c antibody (1:200; Servicebio, Wuhan, China) in accordance with the instructions of the manufacturer. The integrated optical density (IOD) values of tissue sections in each group were measured by Image-Pro Plus 6.0 software (Media Cybernetics, Inc., Rockville, MD, USA) after tissue images were captured under an optical microscope (100×). Five views were randomly selected to determine the positive IOD values and the mean of these values was considered the relative expression of CD11c [28, 29].

Cytokine analysis
Sera were collected from the blood of all mice on day 45; the content of cytokines (TNF-a, IL-6, and IL-10) was measured by using the mouse magnetic Luminex screening assay (R&D Systems, Minneapolis, MN, USA).

Analysis of DC phenotypes in the spleen
On day 45, spleen single-cell suspensions were collected from the five groups of mice, filtered with a cell strainer, and stained with PerCP/Cy5.5 anti-mouse CD11c, PE anti-mouse CD80, APC anti-mouse I-A/I-E (major histocompatibility complex II, or MHC II), or the corresponding isotype control (BioLegend, San Diego, CA, USA) for 25 min at 4 °C. After washing with wash buffer, cells were analyzed by using flow cytometry.

Preparation of bone marrow–derived DCs
Bone marrow–derived DCs (BMDCs) were generated from the tibias and femurs of 6-week-old male C57BL/6 J mice as described previously [30, 31]. Cells were cultured in complete RPMI 1640 medium (HyClone, part of GE Healthcare, Chicago, IL, USA) supplemented with 10% fetal bovine serum, 20 ng/mL recombinant mouse granulocyte-macrophage colony-stimulating factor (rmGM-CSF), and 10 ng/mL rmIL-4 (PeproTech, Rocky Hill, NJ, USA) at a density of 5×106 cells/mL in six-well plates. After 1 day, non-adherent cells were washed off and new complete medium supplemented with 10% fetal bovine serum, 20 ng/mL rmGM-CSF, and 10 ng/mL rmIL-4 was added. New complete medium and cytokines were added every 3 days. On day 6 of culture, immature BMDCs were collected. Immature BMDCs were matured by further culturing in the presence of 1 µg/mL lipopolysaccharide (Sigma-Aldrich, Munich, Germany) for 24 h, and mature BMDCs were harvested.

Phenotyping of BMDCs
BMDCs prepared as described earlier were harvested and stained with PerCP/Cy5.5 anti-mouse CD11c, PE anti-mouse CD80, APC anti-mouse I-A/I-E (MHC II), FITC anti-mouse F4/80, or the corresponding isotype control (BioLegend) for 25 min at 4 °C. After washing, cells were analyzed with flow cytometry. Data analysis was performed by using FlowJo software (Tree Star, Ashland, OR, USA), and the results were reported as mean fluorescence intensity.

Statistical analysis
Statistical analysis was performed with GraphPad Prism software (GraphPad Software, La Jolla, CA, USA). Data were expressed as the mean ± standard deviation. Intergroup comparisons were performed by using one-way analysis of variance. If the data did not satisfy normal distribution, the rank sum test was used. A P value of less than 0.05 was considered significant.

Results

GTS-21 attenuates the inflammatory response in CIA mice
To determine whether the CAP regulates the inflammatory response in RA, the left vagus nerve was sectioned to inhibit the pathway, and GTS-21 was injected into the peritoneal cavity to activate the pathway 4 days before CIA induction. The degree of paw swelling was evaluated by using the arthritis index score every 3 days starting on day 21 after the first immunization. No paw swelling was observed in the control group, whereas the first signs of swelling appeared on day 24 in other groups. Joint swelling in the model and vagotomy groups reached a peak on days 42 and 39, respectively. The GTS-21 4 and 8 mg/kg groups showed mild joint swelling, and the arthritis scores were significantly lower than those in the model and vagotomy groups ($P <0.05$) (Fig. 1a and b).

The ameliorating effect of GTS-21 on CIA was confirmed by HE staining and TRAP staining of joints. The model and vagotomy groups showed infiltration of numerous inflammatory cells, osteoclasts, and synovial hyperplasia in the ankle and knee joints compared with the control group. The abnormalities were significantly alleviated in CIA mice after administration of GTS-21 (4 and 8 mg/kg) (Fig. 1c–h).

GTS-21 reduces the levels of serum TNF-α and IL-6, but not IL-10, in CIA mice
To examine the effect of GTS-21 and vagotomy on inflammatory factors in the serum of DBA/1 mice, Luminex was used to detect the levels of IL-6, TNF-α, and IL-10. The serum levels of TNF-α and IL-6 were significantly higher in the model and vagotomy groups than in the control group, whereas GTS-21 (4 and 8 mg/kg)

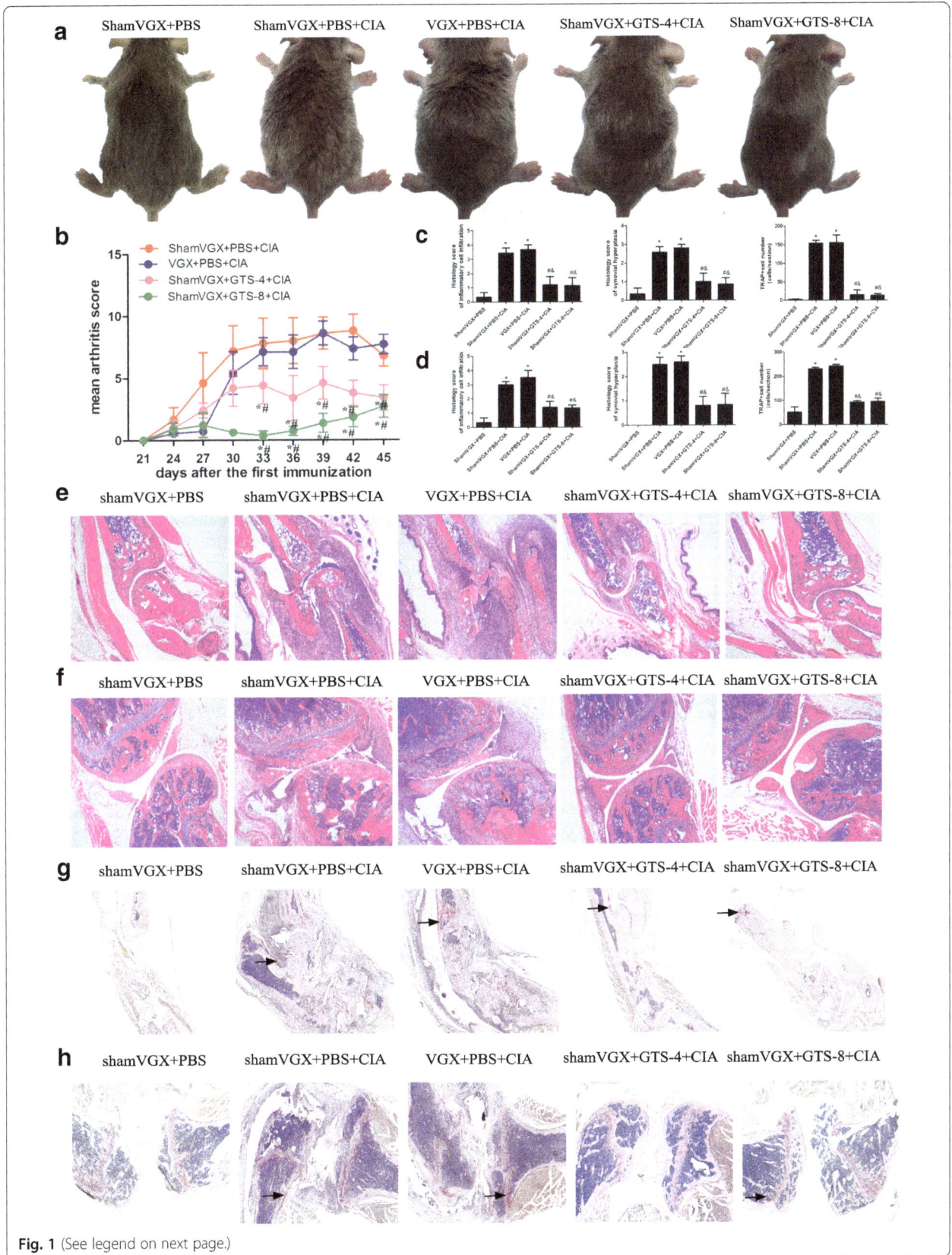

Fig. 1 (See legend on next page.)

(See figure on previous page.)
Fig. 1 GTS-21 ameliorated inflammation in collagen-induced arthritis (CIA) mice. **a** The CIA model in DBA/1 mice was successfully established. GTS-21 decreased the redness and swelling of joints in CIA mice. **b** The arthritis score index was used to assess the severity of arthritis. GTS-21–treated CIA mice showed a dramatic decrease in arthritis scores compared with those in mice in the model group and vagotomy group. **c** and **d** The score of inflammatory cell infiltration (grade 0–4), synovial hyperplasia (grade 0–3), and tartrate-resistant acid phosphatase–positive (TRAP$^+$) cells in the ankle (**c**) and knee (**d**). **e** and **f** GTS-21 decreased the infiltration of inflammatory cells and synovial proliferation in the ankle (e, 40×) and knee (f, 40×) in CIA mice. **g** and **h** GTS-21 decreased the infiltration of osteoclasts in the ankle (g, 40×) and knee (h, 40×) in CIA mice (the arrows point to TRAP$^+$ cells). Data are expressed as the mean ± standard deviation ($n = 8$). *P <0.05 versus the model group; #P <0.05 versus the vagotomy group

treatment markedly decreased the levels of these cytokines. There was no significant difference in the level of IL-10 between the five groups (Fig. 2a–c).

GTS-21 downregulates the surface molecules CD80 and MHC II in DCs in the spleen of CIA mice

On day 45 after the first immunization, DBA/1 mice were humanely killed, and spleen single-cell suspensions were prepared. The expression of the co-stimulatory molecule CD80 and the antigen-presenting molecule MHC II on CD11c$^+$ DCs was detected by using flow cytometry. The expression of CD80 and MHC II in DCs in the spleen was significantly higher in the CIA group and vagotomy group than in the control group, and treatment with GTS-21 (4 and 8 mg/kg) significantly downregulated CD80 and MHC II expression compared with that in the model and vagotomy groups (Fig. 3).

GTS-21 decreases DC infiltration into the synovium in CIA mice

To further evaluate the effect of GTS-21 on DCs, the expression of the DC-specific marker CD11c was assessed in joint synovial tissues by immunohistochemistry. Few cells expressed CD11c in the control group. CD11c expression was significantly upregulated in the

model and vagotomy groups. GTS-21 downregulated CD11c expression compared with that in the model and vagotomy groups (Fig. 4).

GTS-21 inhibits BMDC differentiation

To examine the direct effects of GTS-21 on DC differentiation, BMDCs were generated from C57BL/6 J mice. GTS-21 (0.1, 1, 10, or 100 μmol/L) was added to BMDCs (except the control group) cultured under DC differentiation conditions. CD11c is a relatively specific marker for BMDCs, and F4/80 is considered a macrophage marker [32]. To ensure that BMDCs and CD11c$^+$ F4/80$^-$ cells were gated (Additional file 1), within this population, the expression of CD80 and MHC II on DCs was measured with flow cytometry. The results showed that GTS-21 (1, 10, or 100 μmol/L) significantly inhibited the expression of the surface molecules MHC II (Fig. 5a and b) and CD80 (Fig. 5c and d) in DCs. The effect of GTS-21 (10 μmol/L) on inhibiting the expression of these molecules was significant and antagonized by the selective α7nAChR antagonist methyllycaconitine (MLA) (10 μmol/L) (Fig. 5e–h).

GTS-21 has no obvious effect on BMDC maturation

To induce BMDC maturation, lipopolysaccharide (LPS) (1 μg/mL) was added to BMDCs cultured under

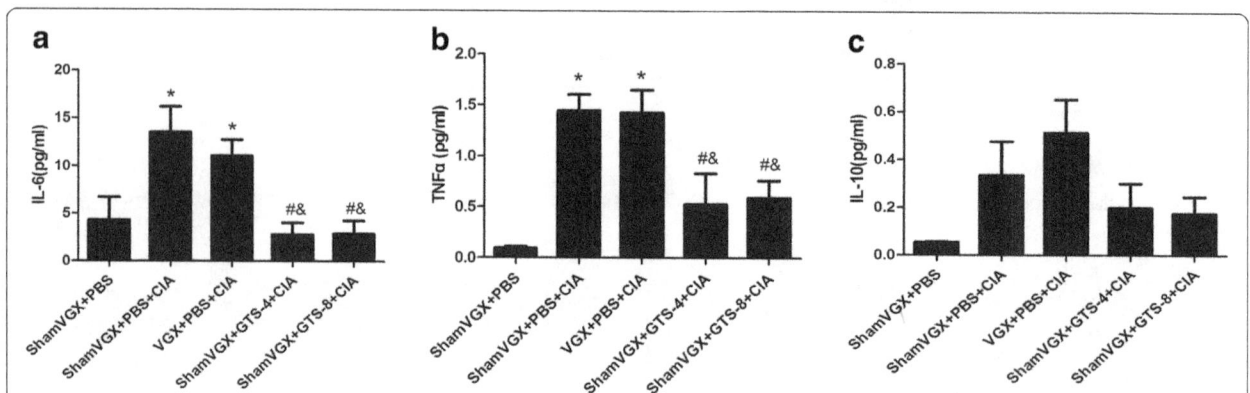

Fig. 2 Analysis of cytokine levels in the serum of DBA/1 mice. On day 45 after the initial immunization, the serum was collected. Luminex was used to detect the levels of tumor necrosis factor-alpha (TNF-α), interleukin-6 (IL-6), and IL-10. GTS-21 reduced the levels of IL-6(**a**) and TNF-α(**b**) but had no effect on IL-10. Data are expressed as the mean ± standard deviation ($n = 8$). *P <0.05 versus the control group; #P <0.05 versus the model group; &P <0.05 versus the vagotomy group

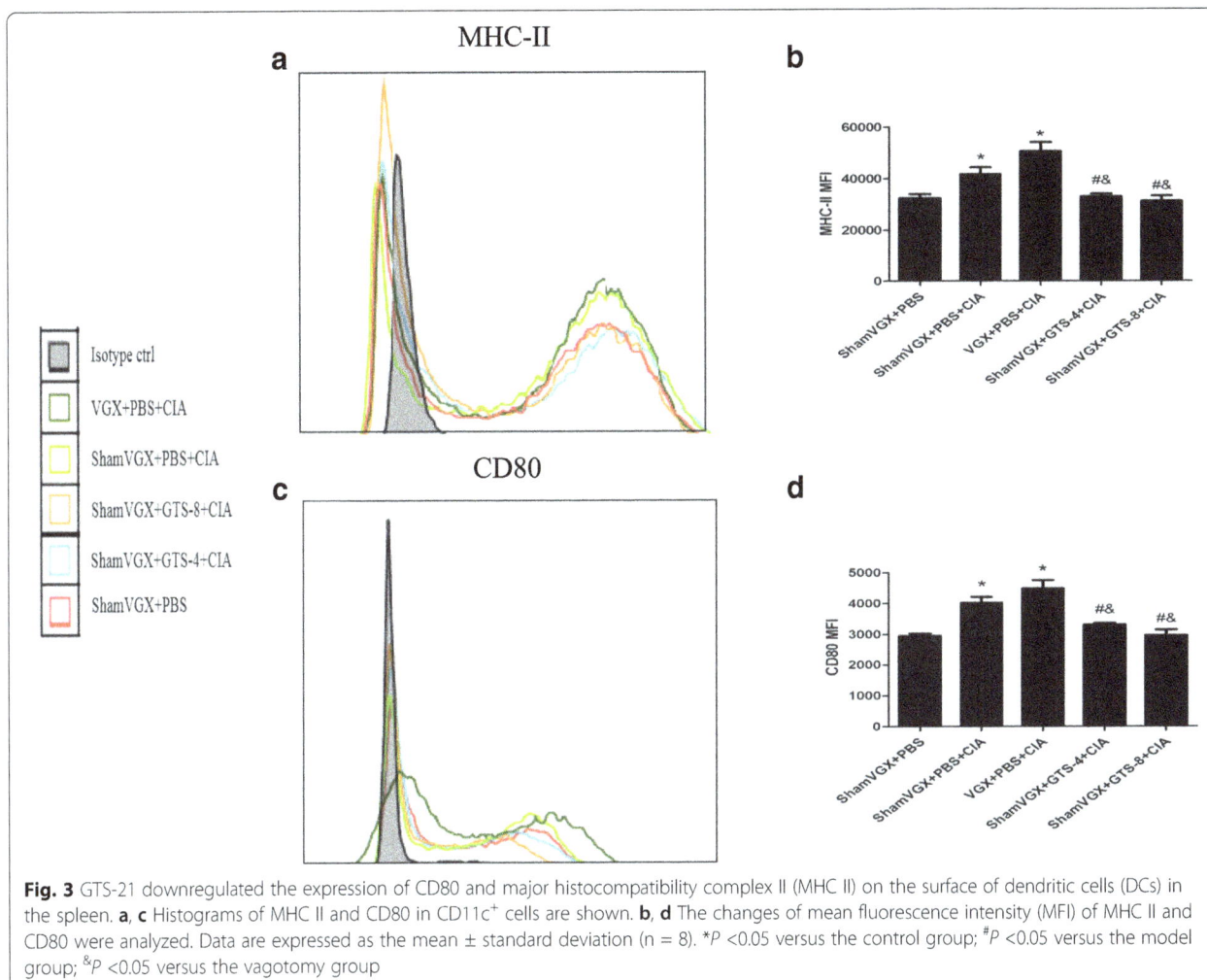

Fig. 3 GTS-21 downregulated the expression of CD80 and major histocompatibility complex II (MHC II) on the surface of dendritic cells (DCs) in the spleen. **a**, **c** Histograms of MHC II and CD80 in CD11c$^+$ cells are shown. **b**, **d** The changes of mean fluorescence intensity (MFI) of MHC II and CD80 were analyzed. Data are expressed as the mean ± standard deviation (n = 8). *P <0.05 versus the control group; #P <0.05 versus the model group; &P <0.05 versus the vagotomy group

differentiation conditions on day 6. GTS-21 (0.1, 1, 10, or 100 µmol/L) was added to inhibit the maturation process. The expression of CD80 and MHC II on BMDCs was detected with flow cytometry on day 7. Compared with the BMDCs on day 6, LPS upregulated the expression of the surface molecules CD80 and MHC II, and GTS-21 had no obvious effect on CD80 and MHC II expression (Fig. 6).

Discussions

DCs are potent antigen-presenting cells that play a major role in the regulation of immune responses in RA. Rheumatoid synovial fluid and synovial tissues are enriched in mature DCs, which participate in the inflammatory cascade by secreting specific T cell–attracting chemokines and through the ongoing presentation of antigen to autoreactive T cells [33–35]. In animal models, administration of collagen-pulsed mature DCs is sufficient to induce arthritis [36]. This suggests that DCs are a valuable target for the management of RA. Here, we explored whether the anti-inflammatory pathway can

prevent the development of RA through the modulation of DCs.

First, we investigated the effects of the cholinergic agonist GTS-21 on the pathogenesis of RA in a CIA model. Activation of the CAP with GTS-21 markedly reduced clinical arthritis, inflammatory cell infiltration, synovial hyperplasia, and bone damage. TNF-α and IL-6 are key pro-inflammatory cytokines in RA [37, 38]. Therefore, TNFα and IL-6 levels were detected in the serum of CIA mice. The results showed that treatment with GTS-21 decreased the levels of the two cytokines. These data indicated that the CAP exerted strong anti-inflammatory effects in CIA mice. However, vagotomy did not exacerbate the inflammation in CIA mice, indicating that the contralateral vagus nerve may have a compensatory role. Further study is necessary to clarify this issue [19, 21]. Moreover, a study showed that denervation protected limbs from arthritis using the K/BxN serum-transfer system by affecting the microvasculature [39]. More research is needed to explore the link between the nervous and immune systems.

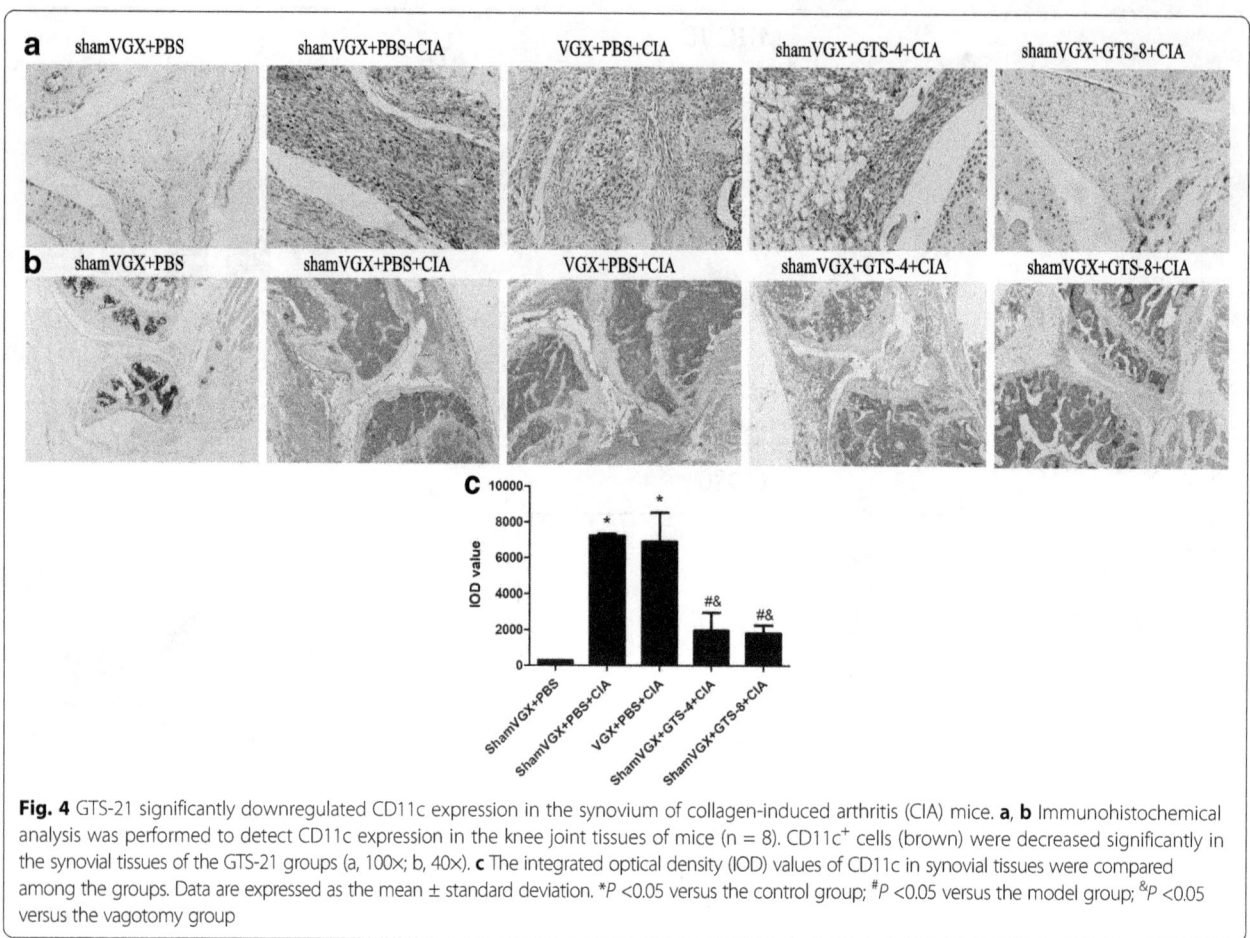

Fig. 4 GTS-21 significantly downregulated CD11c expression in the synovium of collagen-induced arthritis (CIA) mice. **a**, **b** Immunohistochemical analysis was performed to detect CD11c expression in the knee joint tissues of mice (n = 8). CD11c+ cells (brown) were decreased significantly in the synovial tissues of the GTS-21 groups (a, 100×; b, 40×). **c** The integrated optical density (IOD) values of CD11c in synovial tissues were compared among the groups. Data are expressed as the mean ± standard deviation. *P <0.05 versus the control group; #P <0.05 versus the model group; &P <0.05 versus the vagotomy group

The immunologic mechanism underlying the effect of the CAP on protecting against CIA remains unclear. The results of this study demonstrated that the expression of the co-stimulatory molecules CD80 and MHC II in CD11c+ DCs in the spleen was upregulated in the CIA group, which is consistent with the results of a previous study [40]. We confirmed that DCs are involved in inflammation associated with CIA. GTS-21, a selective α7nAChR agonist, has been used in clinical trials and is less toxic than nicotine [41, 42]. GTS-21 (4 mg/kg) significantly improves survival in murine models of endotoxemia, severe sepsis, and burns [43, 44]. Our data firstly confirmed the immunomodulatory effects of GTS-21 on DCs in CIA mice. GTS-21 (4 and 8 mg/kg) significantly downregulated the expression of MHC II and CD80 on the surface of DCs in the spleen of CIA mice. CD80 and MHC II are important surface molecules involved in the activation of Ag-specific CD4+ T cells [40], which suggests that the anti-inflammatory activity of the CAP in RA may be mediated, at least in part, by the modulation of DCs. CD11c is a relatively specific marker of DCs in mice [45, 46]. The present results showed that CD11c was upregulated in the joint synovium of CIA mice and that GTS-21 treatment downregulated

CD11c. This suggests that the anti-inflammatory pathway can directly affect the infiltration of DCs into the synovium.

DCs are derived from hematopoietic stem cells or peripheral blood mononuclear cells [47, 48]. The expression of related specific markers such as HLA-DR on the surface of DCs increases during differentiation [49]. Immature DCs have a strong capacity for antigen uptake. Once activated, DCs are converted into mature DCs, which express high levels of the co-stimulatory molecules CD80/86 and the antigen-presenting molecule MHC II, and stimulate T-cell proliferation [50–52]. To determine whether GTS-21 suppressed the infiltration of DCs into the synovium by affecting DC differentiation or maturation, we performed a follow-up experiment. BMDCs were generated from mouse bone marrow progenitor cells through stimulation with GM-CSF and IL-4 *in vitro* [53], and LPS can induce the mutation of BMDCs. Our results showed that GTS-21 inhibited the differentiation of BMDCs from progenitor cells but had no effect on the maturation of BMDCs, which indicated that GTS-21 exerts an anti-inflammatory effect by inhibiting the differentiation of DCs. The effects of GTS-21 on BMDC differentiation were counteracted by the

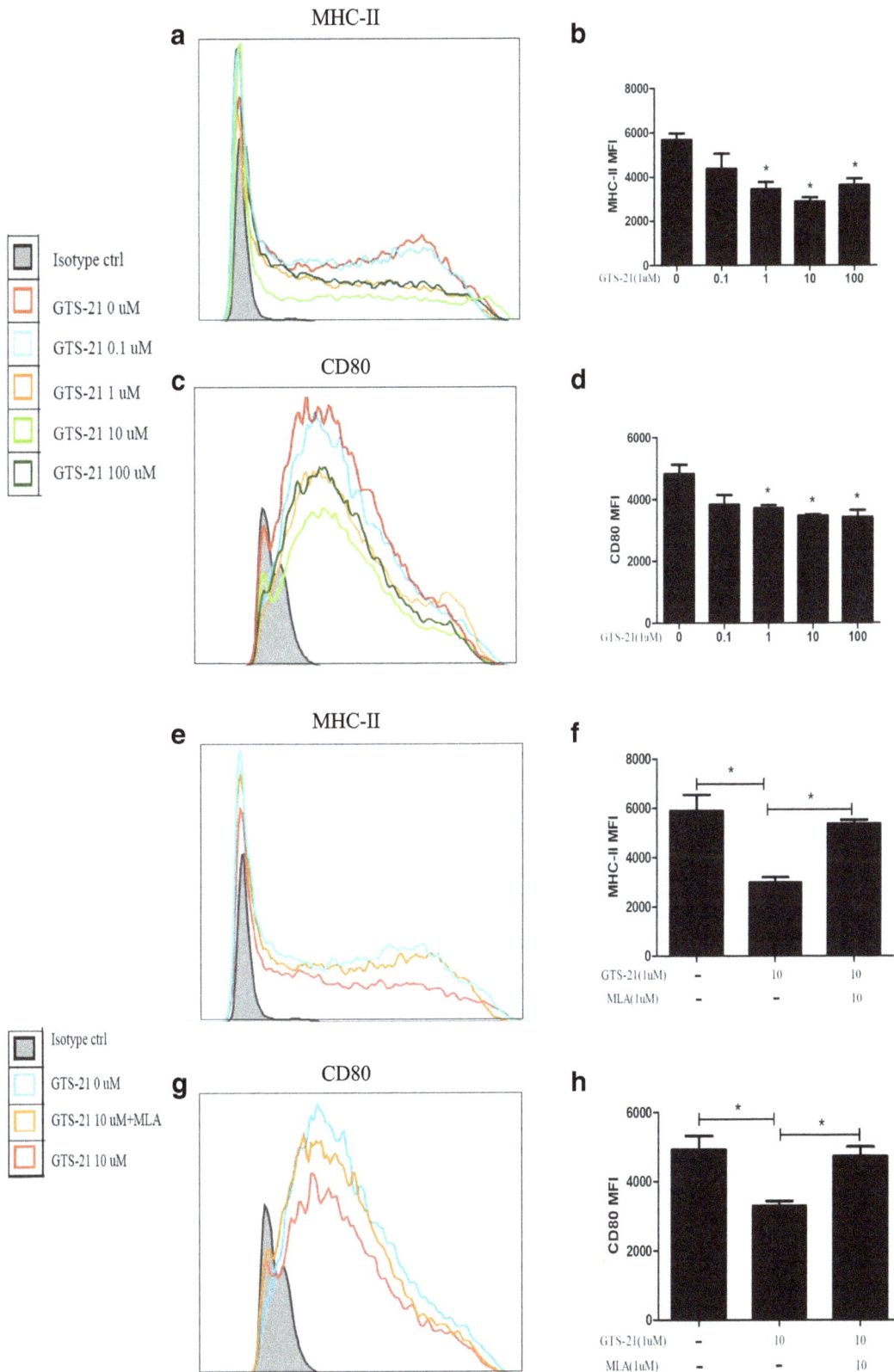

Fig. 5 (See legend on next page.)

(See figure on previous page.)

Fig. 5 GTS-21 efficiently inhibited the expression of CD80 and major histocompatibility complex II (MHC II) on the surface of dendritic cells (DCs) during DC differentiation. Bone marrow–derived DCs were stimulated with GTS-21 (0.1, 1, 10, or 100 μmol/L) for 6 days. The expression levels of MHC II and CD80 were detected by using flow cytometry. All data shown were gated on CD11c$^+$ F4/80$^-$ cells. **a**, **c**, **e**, **g** Histograms of MHC II and CD80 in CD11c$^+$ F4/80$^-$ cells are shown. **b**, **d**, **f**, **h** The changes of mean fluorescence intensity (MFI) of MHC II and CD80 were analyzed. (b, d) GTS-21 (1, 10, or 100 μmol/L) decreased the MFI of CD80 and MHC II. (f, h) GTS-21 (10 μmol/L) significantly decreased the MFI of CD80 and MHC II, and methyllycaconitine (MLA) reversed this effect. Data are expressed as the mean ± standard deviation. *P <0.05 versus the control ("ctrl") group. All data are representative of three independent experiments

acetylcholine receptor antagonist MLA, confirming that GTS-21 affected DC differentiation by activating the α7nAchR.

The mechanism underlying the suppression of DCs by GTS-21 remains unclear. GM-CSF, a critical factor for DC development, can target multiple intracellular signaling pathways to affect DC differentiation, including the Janus kinase/signal transducer and activator of transcription (JAK/STAT) pathway, the mitogen-activated protein kinase (MAPK) pathway, and the phosphatidylinositol 3-kinase (PI3K) pathway [54]. Inhibition of JAK2/STAT5, among these pathways, suppresses terminal DC differentiation [55, 56]. The MAPK and nuclear factor kappa-light-chain-enhancer of activated B cells (NF-κB) signaling pathways are involved in the maturation of DCs. Further experiments are needed to determine whether GTS-21 can regulate GM-CSF–related DC differentiation pathways.

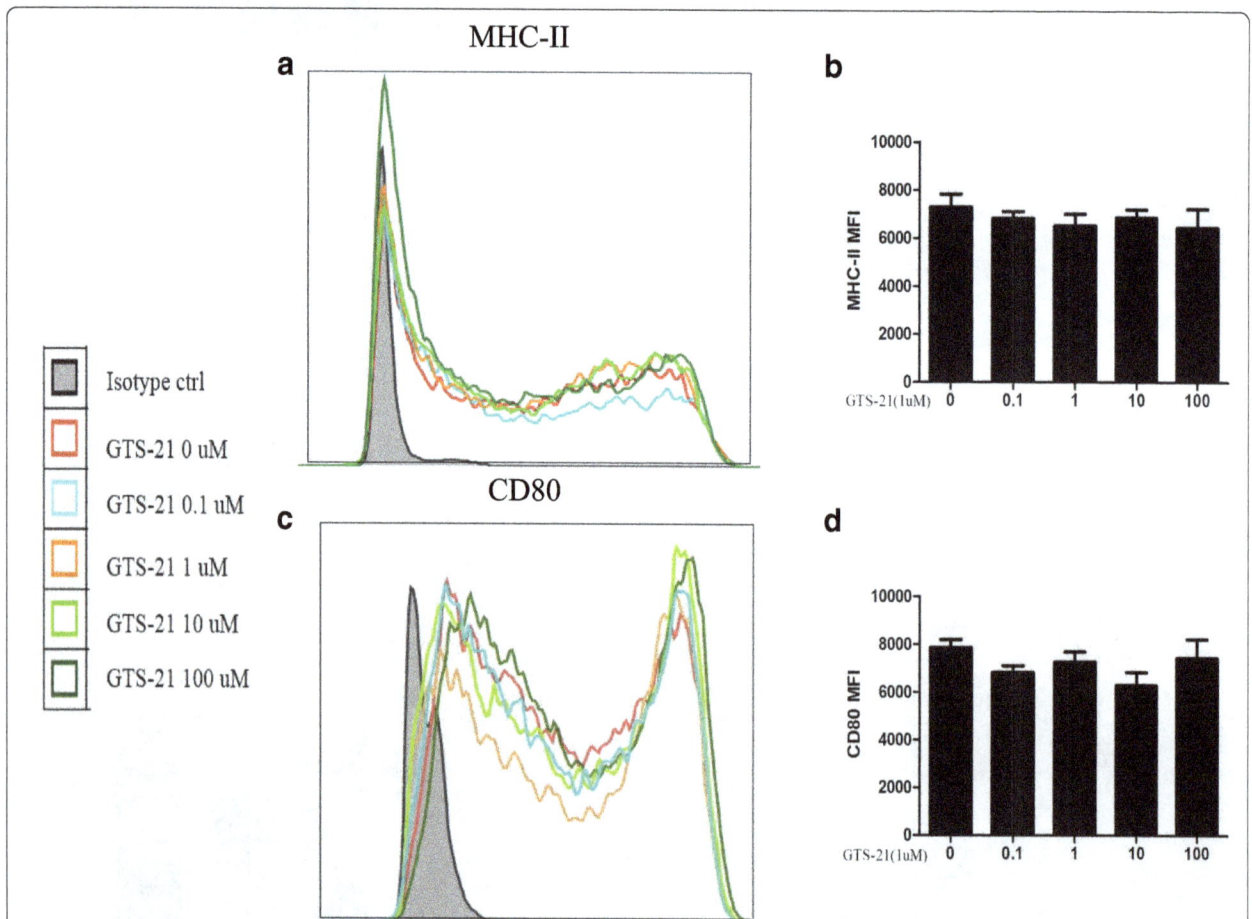

Fig. 6 GTS-21 had no effect on the expression of CD80 and major histocompatibility complex II (MHC II) on the surface of dendritic cells (DCs) during DC maturation. On day 6 of bone marrow–derived dendritic cell culture, immature DCs were stimulated with GTS-21 (0.1, 1, 10, or 100 μmol/L) for 24 h. The expression levels of MHC II and CD80 were detected by using flow cytometry. All data shown were gated on CD11c$^+$ F4/80$^-$ cells. **a**, **c** Histograms of MHC II and CD80 in the CD11c$^+$ F4/80$^-$ cells are shown. **b**, **d** The changes of mean fluorescence intensity (MFI) of MHC II and CD80 were analyzed. Data are expressed as the mean ± standard deviation. All data are representative of three independent experiments. Abbreviation: *ctrl* control

Conclusions

In summary, our research first investigated the anti-inflammatory effect of the cholinergic agonist GTS-21 on DCs in CIA. The present data indicated that GTS-21–mediated activation of the CAP inhibited DC differentiation and ameliorated inflammation in a CIA model. These results may provide new insight into the immune regulatory mechanism underlying the activity of the CAP in RA.

Abbreviations

α7nAChR: α7 subunit of the nicotinic acetylcholine receptor; BMDC: Bone marrow–derived dendritic cell; CAP: Cholinergic anti-inflammatory pathway; CIA: Collagen-induced arthritis; DC: Dendritic cell; GM-CSF: Granulocyte-macrophage colony-stimulating factor; IL: Interleukin; IOD: Integrated optical density; JAK/STAT: Janus kinase/signal transducer and activator of transcription; LPS: Lipopolysaccharide; MAPK: Mitogen-activated protein kinase; MHC II: Major histocompatibility complex II; MLA: Methyllycaconitine; PBS: Phosphate-buffered saline; RA: Rheumatoid arthritis; rmGM-CSF: Recombinant mouse granulocyte-macrophage colony-stimulating factor; TNFα: Tumor necrosis factor-alpha; TRAP: Tartrate-resistant acid phosphatase; VGX: Vagotomy

Acknowledgments

We would like to thank all members of the Department of Rheumatology and Immunology, Xiangya Hospital, Central South University.

Funding

This work was supported by grants from the National Natural Science Foundation of China (81501854, 81571602) and the Fundamental Research Funds for the Central Universitiesof Central South University (2018zzts284).

Authors' contributions

DL contributed to performing experiments, analyzing data, and writing the manuscript. TL, HL, and XZ interpreted data and contributed to writing the manuscript. SL and SW designed the research, interpreted data, and contributed to writing the manuscript. All authors read and approved the final version of the manuscript.

Competing interests

The authors declare that they have no competing interests.

References

1. McInnes IB, Schett G. The pathogenesis of rheumatoid arthritis. N Engl J Med. 2011;365:2205–19.
2. Kubo S, Yamaoka K, Kondo M, Yamagata K, Zhao J, Iwata S, et al. The JAK inhibitor, tofacitinib, reduces the T cell stimulatory capacity of human monocyte-derived dendritic cells. Ann Rheum Dis. 2014;73:2192–8.
3. Stoop JN, Robinson JH, Hilkens CM. Developing tolerogenic dendritic cell therapy for rheumatoid arthritis: what can we learn from mouse models? Ann Rheum Dis. 2011;70:1526–33.
4. Leal Rojas IM, Mok WH, Pearson FE, Minoda Y, Kenna TJ, Barnard RT, et al. Human Blood CD1c(+) Dendritic Cells Promote Th1 and Th17 Effector Function in Memory CD4(+) T Cells. Front Immunol. 2017;8:971.
5. Murphy CA, Langrish CL, Chen Y, Blumenschein W, McClanahan T, Kastelein RA, et al. Divergent pro- and antiinflammatory roles for IL-23 and IL-12 in joint autoimmune inflammation. J Exp Med. 2003;198:1951–7.
6. Miossec P. Dynamic interactions between T cells and dendritic cells and their derived cytokines/chemokines in the rheumatoid synovium. Arthritis Res Ther. 2008;10(Suppl 1):S2.
7. Walsh KP, Mills KH. Dendritic cells and other innate determinants of T helper cell polarisation. Trends Immunol. 2013;34:521–30.
8. Khan S, Greenberg JD, Bhardwaj N. Dendritic cells as targets for therapy in rheumatoid arthritis. Nat Rev Rheumatol. 2009;5:566–71.
9. Ning B, Wei J, Zhang A, Gong W, Fu J, Jia T, et al. Antigen-specific tolerogenic dendritic cells ameliorate the severity of murine collagen-induced arthritis. PLoS One. 2015;10:e0131152.
10. Yang J, Yang Y, Fan H, Zou H. Tolerogenic splenic IDO (+) dendritic cells from the mice treated with induced-Treg cells suppress collagen-induced arthritis. J Immunol Res. 2014;2014:831054.
11. Thome R, Fernandes LG, Mineiro MF, Simioni PU, Joazeiro PP, Tamashiro WM. Oral tolerance and OVA-induced tolerogenic dendritic cells reduce the severity of collagen/ovalbumin-induced arthritis in mice. Cell Immunol. 2012;280:113–23.
12. Schinnerling K, Soto L, Garcia-Gonzalez P, Catalan D, Aguillon JC. Skewing dendritic cell differentiation towards a tolerogenic state for recovery of tolerance in rheumatoid arthritis. Autoimmun Rev. 2015;14:517–27.
13. Hilkens CM, Isaacs JD. Tolerogenic dendritic cell therapy for rheumatoid arthritis: where are we now? Clin Exp Immunol. 2013;172:148–57.
14. Bell GM, Anderson AE, Diboll J, Reece R, Eltherington O, Harry RA, et al. Autologous tolerogenic dendritic cells for rheumatoid and inflammatory arthritis. Ann Rheum Dis. 2017;76:227–34.
15. Inoue T, Tanaka S, Okusa MD. Neuroimmune Interactions in Inflammation and Acute Kidney Injury. Front Immunol. 2017;8:945.
16. Pavlov VA, Wang H, Czura CJ, Friedman SG, Tracey KJ. The cholinergic anti-inflammatory pathway: a missing link in neuroimmunomodulation. Mol Med. 2003;9:125–34.
17. Koopman FA, Vosters JL, Roescher N, Broekstra N, Tak PP, Vervoordeldonk MJ. Cholinergic anti-inflammatory pathway in the non-obese diabetic mouse model. Oral Dis. 2015;21:858–65.
18. Ren C, Tong YL, Li JC, Lu ZQ, Yao YM. The Protective Effect of Alpha 7 Nicotinic Acetylcholine Receptor Activation on Critical Illness and Its Mechanism. Int J Biol Sci. 2017;13:46–56.
19. van Maanen MA, Lebre MC, van der Poll T, LaRosa GJ, Elbaum D, Vervoordeldonk MJ, et al. Stimulation of nicotinic acetylcholine receptors attenuates collagen-induced arthritis in mice. Arthritis Rheum. 2009;60:114–122.
20. Zhou Y, Zuo X, Li Y, Wang Y, Zhao H, Xiao X. Nicotine inhibits tumor necrosis factor-alpha induced IL-6 and IL-8 secretion in fibroblast-like synoviocytes from patients with rheumatoid arthritis. Rheumatol Int. 2012;32:97–104.
21. Li S, Zhou B, Liu B, Zhou Y, Zhang H, Li T, et al. Activation of the cholinergic anti-inflammatory system by nicotine attenuates arthritis via suppression of macrophage migration. Mol Med Rep. 2016;14:5057–64.
22. Wu S, Luo H, Xiao X, Zhang H, Li T, Zuo X. Attenuation of collagen induced arthritis via suppression on Th17 response by activating cholinergic anti-inflammatory pathway with nicotine. Eur J Pharmacol. 2014;735:97–104.
23. Wu S, Zhao H, Luo H, Xiao X, Zhang H, Li T, et al. GTS-21, an alpha7-nicotinic acetylcholine receptor agonist, modulates Th1 differentiation in CD4(+) T cells from patients with rheumatoid arthritis. Exp Ther Med. 2014;8:557–62.
24. Li T, Zuo X, Zhou Y, Wang Y, Zhuang H, Zhang L, et al. The vagus nerve and nicotinic receptors involve inhibition of HMGB1 release and early pro-inflammatory cytokines function in collagen-induced arthritis. J Clin Immunol. 2010;30:213–20.
25. Munyaka P, Rabbi MF, Pavlov VA, Tracey KJ, Khafipour E, Ghia JE. Central muscarinic cholinergic activation alters interaction between splenic dendritic cell and CD4+CD25- T cells in experimental colitis. PLoS One. 2014;9:e109272.
26. Camps M, Ruckle T, Ji H, Ardissone V, Rintelen F, Shaw J, et al. Blockade of PI3Kgamma suppresses joint inflammation and damage in mouse models of rheumatoid arthritis. Nat Med. 2005;11:936–43.
27. Greenhill CJ, Jones GW, Nowell MA, Newton Z, Harvey AK, Moideen AN, et al. Interleukin-10 regulates the inflammasome-driven augmentation of inflammatory arthritis and joint destruction. Arthritis Res Ther. 2014;16:419.
28. Ding HB, Liu KX, Huang JF, Wu DW, Chen JY, Chen QS. Protective effect of exogenous hydrogen sulfide on pulmonary artery endothelial cells by suppressing endoplasmic reticulum stress in a rat model of chronic obstructive pulmonary disease. Biomed Pharmacother. 2018;105:734–41.

29. Tang Y, Cai QH, Wang YJ, Fan SH, Zhang ZF, Xiao MQ, et al. Protective effect of autophagy on endoplasmic reticulum stress induced apoptosis of alveolar epithelial cells in rat models of COPD. Biosci Rep. 2017;37.

30. Miah MA, Yoon CH, Kim J, Jang J, Seong YR, Bae YS. CISH is induced during DC development and regulates DC-mediated CTL activation. Eur J Immunol. 2012;42:58–68.

31. Inaba K, Inaba M, Romani N, Aya H, Deguchi M, Ikehara S, et al. Generation of large numbers of dendritic cells from mouse bone marrow cultures supplemented with granulocyte/macrophage colony-stimulating factor. J Exp Med. 1992;176:1693–702.

32. Chen L, Wang S, Wang Y, Zhang W, Ma K, Hu C, et al. IL-6 influences the polarization of macrophages and the formation and growth of colorectal tumor. Oncotarget. 2018;9:17443–54.

33. Thomas R, Davis LS, Lipsky PE. Rheumatoid synovium is enriched in mature antigen-presenting dendritic cells. J Immunol. 1994;152:2613–23.

34. Thomas R, Quinn C. Functional differentiation of dendritic cells in rheumatoid arthritis: role of CD86 in the synovium. J Immunol. 1996;156:3074–86.

35. Moret FM, Hack CE, van der Wurff-Jacobs KM, de Jager W, Radstake TR, Lafeber FP, et al. Intra-articular CD1c-expressing myeloid dendritic cells from rheumatoid arthritis patients express a unique set of T cell-attracting chemokines and spontaneously induce Th1, Th17 and Th2 cell activity. Arthritis Res Ther. 2013;15:R155.

36. Leung BP, Conacher M, Hunter D, McInnes IB, Liew FY, Brewer JM. A novel dendritic cell-induced model of erosive inflammatory arthritis: distinct roles for dendritic cells in T cell activation and induction of local inflammation. J Immunol. 2002;169:7071–7.

37. Burska A, Boissinot M, Ponchel F. Cytokines as biomarkers in rheumatoid arthritis. Mediat Inflamm. 2014;2014:545493.

38. Myers LK, Rosloniec EF, Cremer MA, Kang AH. Collagen-induced arthritis, an animal model of autoimmunity. Life Sci. 1997;61:1861–78.

39. Stangenberg L, Burzyn D, Binstadt BA, Weissleder R, Mahmood U, Benoist C, et al. Denervation protects limbs from inflammatory arthritis via an impact on the microvasculature. Proc Natl Acad Sci U S A. 2014;111:11419–24.

40. Wu H, Chen J, Song S, Yuan P, Liu L, Zhang Y, et al. beta2-adrenoceptor signaling reduction in dendritic cells is involved in the inflammatory response in adjuvant-induced arthritic rats. Sci Rep. 2016;6:24548.

41. Nanri M, Kasahara N, Yamamoto J, Miyake H, Watanabe H. A comparative study on the effects of nicotine and GTS-21, a new nicotinic agonist, on the locomotor activity and brain monoamine level. Jpn J Pharmacol. 1998;78:385–9.

42. Meyer EM, Kuryatov A, Gerzanich V, Lindstrom J, Papke RL. Analysis of 3-(4-hydroxy, 2-Methoxybenzylidene)anabaseine selectivity and activity at human and rat alpha-7 nicotinic receptors. J Pharmacol Exp Ther. 1998;287:918–25.

43. Pavlov VA, Ochani M, Yang LH, Gallowitsch-Puerta M, Ochani K, Lin X, et al. Selective alpha7-nicotinic acetylcholine receptor agonist GTS-21 improves survival in murine endotoxemia and severe sepsis. Crit Care Med. 2007;35:1139–44.

44. Khan MAS, Khan MF, Kashiwagi S, Kem WR, Yasuhara S, Kaneki M, et al. An ALPHA7 Nicotinic Acetylcholine Receptor Agonist (GTS-21) Promotes C2C12 Myonuclear Accretion in Association with Release of Interleukin-6 (IL-6) and Improves Survival in Burned Mice. Shock. 2017;48:227–35.

45. Ahmed MS, Byeon SE, Jeong Y, Miah MA, Salahuddin M, Lee Y, et al. Dab2, a negative regulator of DC immunogenicity, is an attractive molecular target for DC-based immunotherapy. Oncoimmunology. 2015;4:e984550.

46. Li X, Han Y, Zhou Q, Jie H, He Y, Han J, et al. Apigenin, a potent suppressor of dendritic cell maturation and migration, protects against collagen-induced arthritis. J Cell Mol Med. 2016;20:170–80.

47. Gabrilovich D. Mechanisms and functional significance of tumour-induced dendritic-cell defects. Nat Rev Immunol. 2004;4:941–52.

48. Moretto MM, Lawlor EM, Khan IA. Aging mice exhibit a functional defect in mucosal dendritic cell response against an intracellular pathogen. J Immunol. 2008;181:7977–84.

49. Satpathy AT, Wu X, Albring JC, Murphy KM. Re(de)fining the dendritic cell lineage. Nat Immunol. 2012;13:1145–54.

50. Dumortier H, van Mierlo GJ, Egan D, van Ewijk W, Toes RE, Offringa R, et al. Antigen presentation by an immature myeloid dendritic cell line does not cause CTL deletion in vivo, but generates CD8+ central memory-like T cells that can be rescued for full effector function. J Immunol. 2005;175:855–63.

51. Amigorena S. Fc gamma receptors and cross-presentation in dendritic cells. J Exp Med. 2002;195:F1–3.

52. Kufer P, Zettl F, Borschert K, Lutterbuse R, Kischel R, Riethmuller G. Minimal costimulatory requirements for T cell priming and TH1 differentiation: activation of naive human T lymphocytes by tumor cells armed with bifunctional antibody constructs. Cancer Immun. 2001;1:10.

53. Palucka K, Banchereau J. Dendritic-cell-based therapeutic cancer vaccines. Immunity. 2013;39:38–48.

54. van de Laar L, Coffer PJ, Woltman AM. Regulation of dendritic cell development by GM-CSF: molecular control and implications for immune homeostasis and therapy. Blood. 2012;119:3383–93.

55. Esashi E, Wang YH, Perng O, Qin XF, Liu YJ, Watowich SS. The signal transducer STAT5 inhibits plasmacytoid dendritic cell development by suppressing transcription factor IRF8. Immunity. 2008;28:509–20.

56. van de Laar L, van den Bosch A, Wierenga AT, Janssen HL, Coffer PJ, Woltman AM. Tight control of STAT5 activity determines human CD34-derived interstitial dendritic cell and langerhans cell development. J Immunol. 2011;186:7016–24.

Association between autophagy and inflammation in patients with rheumatoid arthritis receiving biologic therapy

Yi-Ming Chen[1,2,3†], Chun-Yu Chang[4,5†], Hsin-Hua Chen[1,2,3], Chia-Wei Hsieh[2,3], Kuo-Tung Tang[2,3], Meng-Chun Yang[4], Joung-Liang Lan[4,5,6] and Der-Yuan Chen[4,5,6*] (iD)

Abstract

Background: Increasing evidence indicates a pathogenic role of deregulated autophagy in rheumatoid arthritis (RA). We examined the relationship between autophagy and inflammatory parameters in patients with RA receiving biologic therapy.

Methods: In 72 patients with RA and 20 healthy control subjects (HC), autophagosome levels were determined by the mean fluorescence intensity (MFI) of autophagosomotropic dye incorporated into circulating immune cells, and p62 expression levels in immune cells were measured by flow cytometry. We used immunoblotting to examine protein expression of LC3-II and p62 in peripheral blood mononuclear cells.

Results: Patients with RA had significantly higher levels of autophagosome reflected by MFI of Cyto-ID in circulating lymphocytes, monocytes, and granulocytes (median values, 3.6, 11.6, and 64.8, respectively) compared with HC (1.9, 6.0, and 35.8; respectively) (all $p < 0.001$). p62 MFI levels in lymphocytes and granulocytes from patients with RA (17.1 and 8.6, respectively) were significantly lower than those in the corresponding cells from HC (20.2, $p < 0.05$; and 13.1, $p < 0.001$, respectively). Significantly higher levels of LC3-II protein expression in contrast to lower p62 protein levels were observed in patients with RA than in HC. The autophagosome levels in immune cells were significantly correlated with inflammatory parameters in patients with RA, and they were significantly decreased with disease remission after treatment with tumor necrosis factor-α inhibitors or interleukin-6 receptor inhibitor.

Conclusions: Elevated autophagy with significant correlation to inflammation suggests the involvement of autophagy in RA pathogenesis. The effectiveness of biologic therapy might be partly related to the downregulation of autophagy expression.

Keywords: Autophagy, Inflammatory parameters, TNF-α inhibitors, Interleukin-6 receptor inhibitor, Rheumatoid arthritis (RA)

Background

Autophagy is the process of engulfment and degradation of cytoplasmic contents by lysosomes [1, 2]. Autophagy initiation is regulated by the Unc51-like kinase 1 complex [3], and the most critical step in autophagy is autophagosome formation through the conjugation of microtubule-associated protein light chain 3 (LC3) with phosphatidylethanolamine [2]. LC3 consists of a soluble form (LC3-I, 18 kDa) and a lipidated form (LC3-II, 16 kDa). The LC3-binding adaptor p62 (sequestosome 1 [SQSTM1]) binds ubiquitinated substrates, serves as a bridge for the delivery to autophagosome, and then promotes their degradation through a proteasomal pathway [4, 5]. Therefore, decreased p62 levels are associated with autophagy activation. Finally, the autophagosome fuses with a lysosome to form an autolysosome that digests the engulfed cargo [1, 2].

The networks formed by autophagy and inflammation are complex. Autophagy is involved in the induction and suppression of inflammation and vice versa [6–8].

* Correspondence: dychen1957@gmail.com
†Yi-Ming Chen and Chun-Yu Chang contributed equally to this work.
4Rheumatology and Immunology Center, China Medical University Hospital, No. 2, Yude Road, Taichung 40447, Taiwan
5Translational Medicine Laboratory, Rheumatic Diseases Research Center, China Medical University Hospital, Taichung, Taiwan
Full list of author information is available at the end of the article

Proinflammatory cytokines such as tumor necrosis factor (TNF)-α and interleukin (IL)-6 have been shown to stimulate autophagy, and autophagy also contributes to the secretion of these cytokines [9–12]. However, autophagy is tightly regulated in its response to inflammation, such as participating in the clearance of protein complexes (e.g., inflammasomes) through proteasomal degradation [13]. Owing to the multifaceted roles of autophagy in inflammatory responses [6–8], deregulated autophagy has been implicated in the pathogenesis of autoimmune diseases [12, 14, 15].

Rheumatoid arthritis (RA) is an inflammatory disease that leads to chronic synovitis and joint erosion [16]. Proinflammatory cytokines such as TNF-α and IL-6 can promote synovitis, cartilage damage, and bone destruction [16–18]. The importance of TNF-α and IL-6 in RA pathogenesis is supported by the therapeutic effectiveness of biologics targeting cytokines [18–20]. With autophagy tightly regulated to ensure immune homeostasis, its deregulation may serve a pathogenic role in RA [12, 21, 22]. Lin et al. demonstrated that autophagy is activated in RA in a TNF-α-dependent manner in murine model [21], and Connor et al. revealed that TNF-α stimulated autophagy through the induction of endoplasmic reticulum stress response [22]. Recent studies also indicated an increased autophagy in RA fibroblast-like synoviocytes (FLS) but not in osteoarthritis FLS [12, 23, 24], with a dual role of autophagy in regulating the death pathway in RA FLS [25]. In spite of the accumulating evidence supporting the critical role of autophagy in RA [23–25], there were still limited data regarding the association of autophagy with inflammation in human RA.

In this pilot study, we compared the difference in autophagy expression between patients with RA and healthy control subjects (HC). We also examined the correlation between autophagy expression and inflammatory parameters in patients with RA. In addition, we examined the changes of autophagy expression and serum cytokine levels in patients with RA after 6-month therapy with biologics or conventional synthetic disease-modifying antirheumatic drugs (csDMARDs) alone.

Methods
Subjects
In this prospective study, 72 patients with RA who fulfilled the 2010 classification criteria of the American College of Rheumatology/European League Against Rheumatism collaborative initiative [26] were consecutively enrolled. Disease activity was assessed using the 28-joint Disease Activity Score (DAS28) [27], with active status defined as a DAS28 score > 3.2 [28]. Sixty biologic-naïve patients with active RA who had received csDMARDs started therapy with TNF-α inhibitors

(etanercept or adalimumab, $n = 28$) or IL-6R inhibitor (tocilizumab, $n = 32$) in combination with a stable weekly dose of methotrexate 7.5–15 mg according to the guidelines [29], and the other 12 patients continued with csDMARD therapy alone. Twenty age- and sex-matched healthy volunteers served as HC. The Institutional Review Board of Taichung Veterans General Hospital approved this study (CE14307B), and written consent was obtained from each participant according to the Declaration of Helsinki.

Quantitation of autophagosome levels in circulating immune cells by Cyto-ID staining
Cyto-ID, a cationic amphiphilic tracer dye, specifically recognizes autophago(lyso)some and can be quantified using flow cytometry [30]. To determine autophagosome levels in circulating immune cells, the fluorescence of Cyto-ID on the cells was measured by using the Cyto-ID™ Autophagy Detection Kit (Enzo Life Sciences, Farmingdale, NY, USA) according to the manufacturer's protocol and the described technique [31–33]. Briefly, 100 µl of whole blood was stained with 0.25 µl/ml of Cyto-ID Green Autophagy Detection Reagent (Enzo Life Sciences) and 20 µl of phycoerythrin-cyanine 5 (PC5)-conjugated CD45-specific monoclonal antibody (mAb) (Beckman Coulter Life Sciences, Indianapolis IN, USA). Incubation with CD3-, CD14-, CD66b-, and CD45-specific antibodies was done simultaneously with autophagy dye. After incubation for 30 min in the dark at room temperature (RT), cells were reacted with Opti-Lyse Solution (Beckman Coulter Life Sciences) for 10 min to lyse red blood cells. After PBS washing, cells were analyzed by flow cytometry (Beckman Coulter Life Sciences). Monocytes, lymphocytes, and granulocytes were gated on the basis of CD45$^+$ side scatter, and at least 1×10^4 cells from each sample were analyzed. To verify the gated lymphocytes, monocytes, and granulocytes, 100-µl blood samples were stained with 20 µl of fluorescein isothiocyanate (FITC)-conjugated CD3-specific mAb (Beckman Coulter Life Sciences), 20 µl of PC5-conjugated CD14-specific mAb, and 20 µl of FITC-conjugated CD66b-specific mAb, respectively, with 20 µl of PC5-conjugated CD45-specific mAb separately for 15 min at RT. Regarding the subgroups of lymphocytes, 100-µl blood samples were stained with 5 µl of FITC-conjugated CD4-specific mAb (BioLegend, San Diego, CA, USA), 5 µl of PC5-conjugated CD8-specific mAb (Beckman Coulter Life Sciences), and 10 µl of PC5-conjugated CD19-specific mAb (Beckman Coulter Life Sciences) with 5 µl of peridinin chlorophyll protein (PerCP)-conjugated CD3-specific mAb (BD, Franklin Lakes, NJ, USA) separately with autophagy dye for 30 min at RT. Data were expressed as the mean fluorescence intensity (MFI) of Cyto-ID staining. We also

examined autophagosome levels, determined by Cyto-ID staining, in both synovial fluid (SF)-derived and peripheral blood (PB)-derived immune cells from two patients with active RA.

Quantitation of autophagic adaptor p62 levels in immune cells using flow cytometry

Intracellular immunofluorescent staining of p62 molecule was performed following fixation and permeabilization using the modified method of a previous study [33]. Briefly, 50 µl of whole blood was stained with 20 µl of FITC-conjugated CD45-specific mAb for 15 min at RT. Cells were fixed by adding 100 µl of reagent 1 (Beckman Coulter Life Sciences) for 15 min and were centrifuged for 5 min at $300 \times g$. After removal of the supernatant, 100 µl of reagent 2 (Beckman Coulter Life Sciences) was added for permeabilization for 10 min, and cells were subsequently incubated with PerCP-conjugated p62/SQSTM1 mAb (clone 5H7E2; Novus Biologicals, Littleton, CO, USA) for 15 min in the dark at RT. PerCP-conjugated immunoglobulin G1 (R&D Systems, Minneapolis, MN, USA) was used as an isotype control. Cells were immediately analyzed using flow cytometry (Beckman Coulter Life Sciences).

Determination of autophagy expression using Western blot analysis

Total proteins were extracted from peripheral blood mononuclear cell (PBMC) lysates from 25 patients with active RA and 10 HC. The proteins were separated by 10–12% SDS-PAGE and then transferred to polyvinylidene fluoride membranes (Bio-Rad Laboratories, Hercules, CA, USA). Immunoblots were performed using primary antibodies (1:1000 dilution) overnight at 4 °C against LC3-II (Abcam, Cambridge, MA, USA), p62 (Abcam), and glyceraldehyde 3-phosphate dehydrogenase (GAPDH) (Santa Cruz Biotechnology, Dallas, TX, USA), followed by incubation with horseradish peroxidase-conjugated antirabbit secondary antibody (1:5000) for 1 h at 37 °C (Santa Cruz Biotechnology). The luminescent signal was detected by using the Fujifilm LAS-3000 image detection system (Fujifilm, Tokyo, Japan), and image processing and data quantification were performed using Multi Gauge version 2.02 software (Fujifilm). The LC3-II/LC3-I ratio was calculated as LC3-II expression levels divided by LC3-I expression levels, and the p62 expression levels were normalized to GAPDH.

Plasma antioxidant capacity

The measurement of the total antioxidant capacity (TAC) of biological fluids provides an indication of the overall capability to counteract ROS. Plasma levels of TAC were measured using a colorimetric assay kit (BioVision Incorporated, Milpitas, CA, USA). 6-Hydroxy-

2,5,7,8-tetramethylchroman-2-carboxylic acid (Trolox) was used to standardize antioxidants, with all the other antioxidants being measured in Trolox equivalents. The Cu^{2+} was reduced to Cu^+ by the antioxidant factors in the sample coupled with a colorimetric probe. For calibration, 1 mM Trolox in dimethyl sulfoxide-water was used. Each microtiter plate was filled with either 100 µl of calibrators (0, 4, 8, 16, or 20 nmol Trolox) or 100 µl of diluted serum. Then, 100 µl of freshly prepared Cu^{2+} working solution was added, and the mixture was incubated at RT for 1.5 h. The sample absorbance was analyzed at 570 nm as a function of Trolox equivalent concentrations according to the manufacturer's instructions. The antioxidant capacity was presented in nmol/µl.

Determination of serum levels of proinflammatory cytokines

Serum levels of TNF-α and IL-6 were determined using an enzyme-linked immunosorbent assay (PeproTech Inc., Rocky Hill, NJ, USA) according to the manufacturer's instructions.

Statistical analysis

Results are presented as the mean ± SD or median (IQR). The Mann-Whitney U test was used for between-group comparison of autophagy expression, cytokine levels, and oxidative stress status evidenced by TAC levels. The correlation coefficient was obtained by Spearman's rank test. For evaluation of the changes of autophagy expression and serum cytokine levels during the follow-up period in patients with RA, the Wilcoxon signed-rank test was employed. $p < 0.05$ was considered significant.

Results

Clinical characteristics of patients with RA

As illustrated in Table 1, 69.4% of patients with RA were positive for rheumatoid factor (RF), and 61.1% were positive for anticitrullinated peptide antibodies (ACPA). As expected, patients with RA scheduled for biologic therapy had higher disease activity at baseline than those receiving csDMARDs alone. However, there were no significant differences in the positive rates of RF or ACPA, daily dose of corticosteroids, or the proportion of used csDMARDs among patients with RA receiving different therapies. There were no significant differences in demographic data between patients with RA and HC.

MFI of Cyto-ID in circulating immune cells from patients with RA and HC

Representative cytometric histograms of Cyto-ID-staining obtained from one patient with RA and one HC are shown in Fig. 1a and b. Significantly higher values of MFI were observed in circulating lymphocytes,

Table 1 Clinical characteristics, laboratory findings, and autophagy expression at baseline

	TNF-α inhibitors (n = 28)	IL-6R inhibitor (n = 32)	csDMARDs alone (n = 12)	HC (n = 20)
Mean age (years)	56.7 ± 12.1	55.5 ± 14.1	58.1 ± 14.3	53.3 ± 11.4
Female (%)	22 (78.6%)	24 (75.0%)	10 (83.3%)	15 (75.0%)
RF positivity (%)	22 (78.6%)	20 (62.5%)	8 (66.7%)	NA
ACPA positivity (%)	19 (67.9%)	18 (56.3%)	7 (58.3%)	NA
ESR (mm/first hour)	44.4 ± 30.0*	35.8 ± 21.8	30.5 ± 22.6	NA
CRP (mg/dl)	2.3 ± 2.5*	2.0 ± 2.3	1.3 ± 1.4	NA
DAS28 at baseline	5.89 ± 0.59*	5.95 ± 0.70*	4.80 ± 0.71	NA
Daily steroid dose (mg)	6.3 ± 1.6	6.5 ± 1.5	5.6 ± 1.9	NA
Baseline csDMARDs				
MTX + SSZ + HCQ	23 (82.1%)	26 (81.3%)	10 (83.4%)	NA
SSZ + HCQ + Cyc	2 (7.1%)	3 (9.4%)	1 (8.3%)	NA
MTX + SSZ	1 (3.6%)	1 (3.1%)	0 (0.0%)	NA
MTX + SSZ + Cyc	1 (3.6%)	0 (0.0%)	1 (8.3%)	NA
MTX+ SSZ + HCQ + Cyc	1 (3.6%)	2 (6.2%)	0 (0.0%)	NA

Abbreviations: ACPA Anticitrullinated peptide antibodies, *CRP* C-reactive protein, *csDMARDs* Conventional synthetic disease-modifying antirheumatic drugs, *Cyc* Cyclosporine, *DAS28* Disease Activity Score in 28 joints, *ESR* Erythrocyte sedimentation rate, *HCQ* Hydroxychloroquine, *IL-6R* Interleukin-6 receptor, *MTX* Methotrexate, *NA* Not applicable, *RF* Rheumatoid factor, *SSZ* Sulfasalazine, *TNF-α* Tumor necrosis factor-α
Data are presented as mean ± SD, number (percent), or median (25th–75th quartiles)
*$p < 0.05$ vs. HC by Mann-Whitney U test for between-group comparison of numerical variables

monocytes, and granulocytes from patients with RA (median 3.6, IQR 2.9–5.0; 11.6, IQR 8.7–15.5; 64.8, IQR 49.1–78.1; respectively) compared with those from HCs (1.9, IQR 1.1–3.2; 6.0, IQR 3.7–8.1; 35.8, IQR 29.3–42.7; respectively, all $p < 0.001$) (Fig. 1c–e).

MFI of Cyto-ID in circulating CD4⁺ T cells, CD8⁺ T cells, and CD19⁺ B cells from patients with RA and HC

Representative cytometric histograms of MFI of Cyto-ID in circulating CD4⁺ T cells, CD8⁺ T cells, and CD19⁺ B cells obtained from one patient with RA and one HC are shown in Additional file 1: Figure S1A. Significantly higher values of MFI were observed in circulating CD4⁺ and CD8⁺ T cells from patients with RA (median 93.5, IQR 69.4–126.3; 114.0, IQR 87.5–143.0, respectively) than in those from HC (median 46.7, IQR 25.5–71.0; 54.0, IQR 30.5–82.8, both $p < 0.05$) (Fig. 1b, c). However, no significant difference in MFI of CD19⁺ B cells was observed between patients with RA and HC (median 439.5, IQR 205.0–1187.5 versus 500, IQR 135.5–750.7) (Fig. 1d).

MFI of Cyto-ID in synovial fluid immune cells from patients with RA

Given that immune cells barely exist in SF of patients with osteoarthritis or HC, their PB-derived immune cells were used to serve as controls. Our results showed that MFI of Cyto-ID was significantly higher in SF granulocytes (7846 and 8857, respectively) than in PB-derived

granulocytes (2131 and 2364, respectively) from two patients with active RA (Additional file 1: Figure S1E–G).

MFI of p62 in circulating immune cells from patients with RA and HC

Representative examples of cytometric histograms of p62 levels obtained from one patient with active RA and one HC are shown in Fig. 2a and b. Significantly lower MFI values of p62 were observed in circulating lymphocytes and granulocytes from patients with RA (median 17.1, IQR 14.4–20.6; and 8.6, IQR 6.4–10.8, respectively) than in those from HC (20.2, IQR 17.3–23.1, $p < 0.05$; and 13.1, IQR 10.0–18.5, $p < 0.001$; respectively) (Fig. 2c and e). However, there was no difference in the MFI of p62 in circulating monocytes between patients with RA and HC.

Plasma levels of total antioxidant capacity in patients with RA and HC

Significantly lower TAC levels (median 55.1 nmol/μl, IQR 50.3–61.5 nmol/μl) were shown in patients with RA than in HC (59.0 nmol/μl, IQR 56.2–65.8 nmol/μl; $p < 0.05$). Plasma TAC levels were also negatively associated with autophagosome levels reflected by Cyto-ID MFI in circulating granulocytes from patients with RA ($r = -0.313, p < 0.01$).

Serum cytokine levels in patients with RA and HC

Patients with RA had significantly higher levels of TNF-α and IL-6 (median 172 pg/ml, IQR 117–308 pg/ml; and 917 pg/ml, IQR 455–2842 pg/ml, respectively)

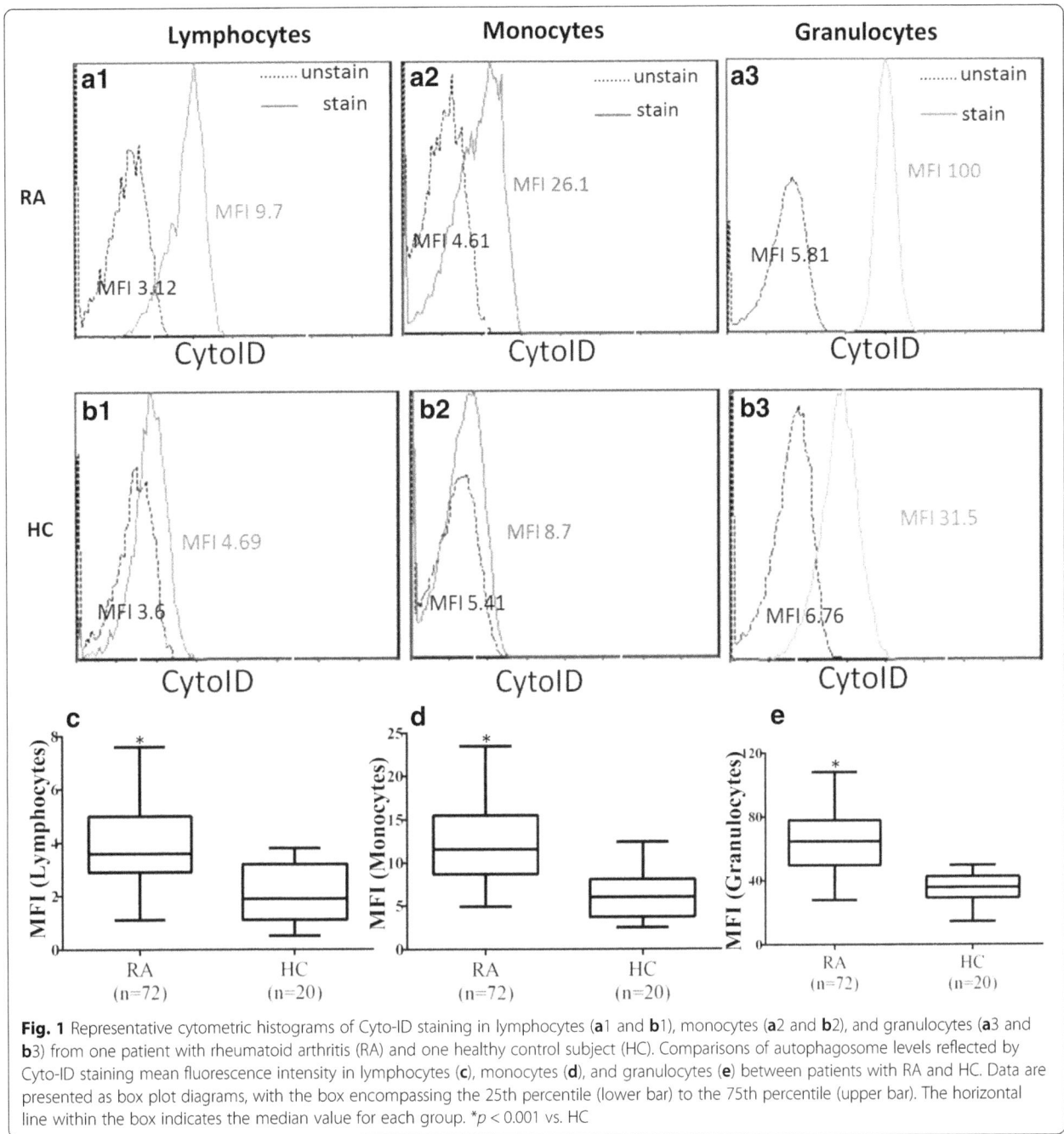

Fig. 1 Representative cytometric histograms of Cyto-ID staining in lymphocytes (**a**1 and **b**1), monocytes (**a**2 and **b**2), and granulocytes (**a**3 and **b**3) from one patient with rheumatoid arthritis (RA) and one healthy control subject (HC). Comparisons of autophagosome levels reflected by Cyto-ID staining mean fluorescence intensity in lymphocytes (**c**), monocytes (**d**), and granulocytes (**e**) between patients with RA and HC. Data are presented as box plot diagrams, with the box encompassing the 25th percentile (lower bar) to the 75th percentile (upper bar). The horizontal line within the box indicates the median value for each group. *$p < 0.001$ vs. HC

compared with HC (82 pg/ml, IQR 50–97 pg/ml; and 231 pg/ml, IQR 159-452 pg/ml, respectively; $p < 0.001$).

Correlations between autophagy expression and inflammatory parameters in RA

As illustrated in Table 2, DAS28 and C-reactive protein (CRP) levels at baseline were significantly and positively correlated with the autophagosome levels in circulating lymphocytes, monocytes, and granulocytes. Serum TNF-α levels were also positively correlated with the autophagosome levels in lymphocytes, monocytes, and granulocytes, and serum IL-6 levels were positively correlated with the autophagosome levels in lymphocytes. On the contrary, DAS28 scores were negatively correlated with p62 levels in the circulating lymphocytes, monocytes, or granulocytes, and CRP levels were negatively with p62 levels in lymphocytes. Serum TNF-α levels were also negatively correlated with p62 levels in lymphocytes, monocytes, and granulocytes. However, there was no significant association between the levels of autophagosome or p62 and ACPA levels in patients with RA (data not shown).

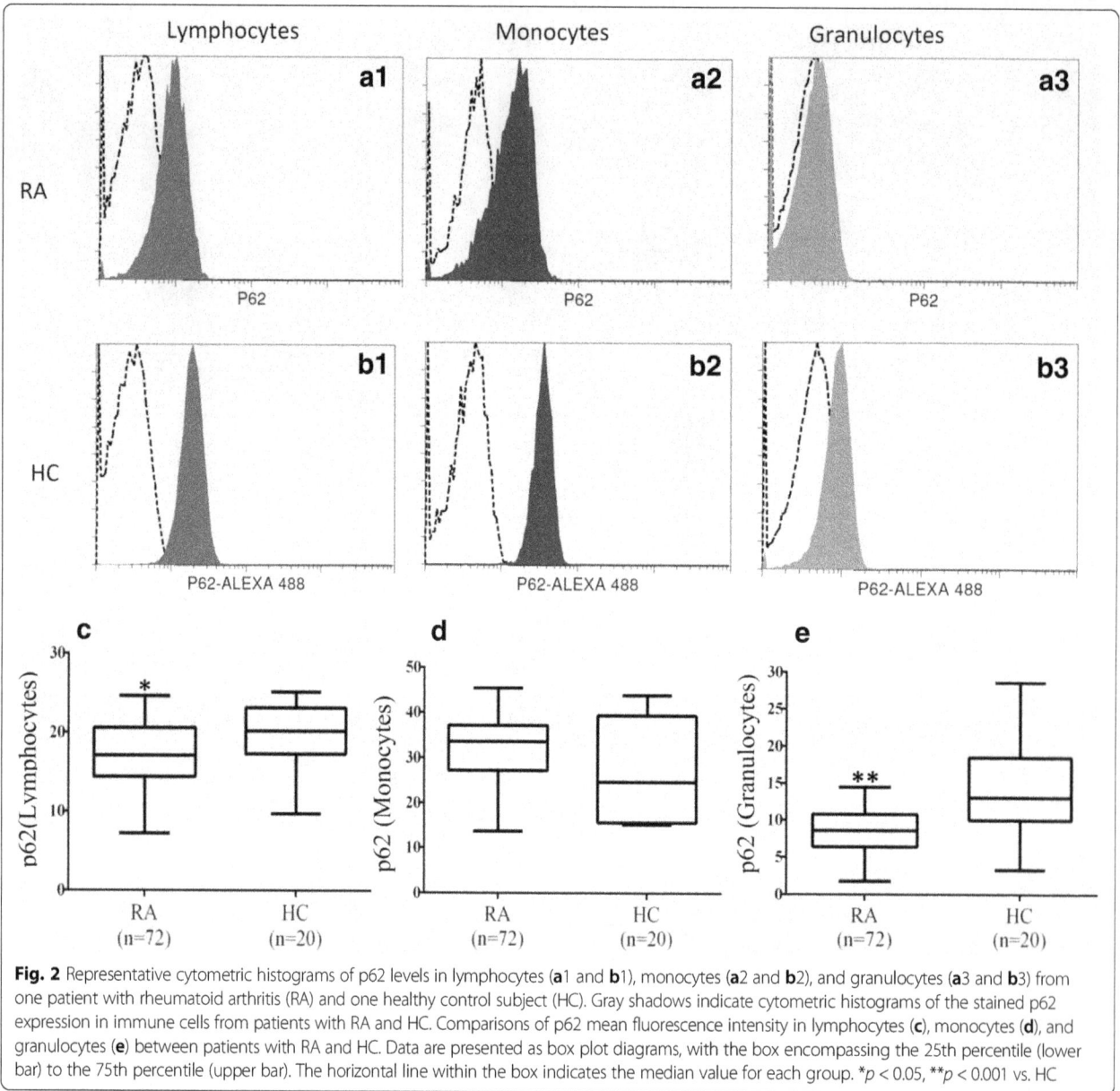

Fig. 2 Representative cytometric histograms of p62 levels in lymphocytes (**a**1 and **b**1), monocytes (**a**2 and **b**2), and granulocytes (**a**3 and **b**3) from one patient with rheumatoid arthritis (RA) and one healthy control subject (HC). Gray shadows indicate cytometric histograms of the stained p62 expression in immune cells from patients with RA and HC. Comparisons of p62 mean fluorescence intensity in lymphocytes (**c**), monocytes (**d**), and granulocytes (**e**) between patients with RA and HC. Data are presented as box plot diagrams, with the box encompassing the 25th percentile (lower bar) to the 75th percentile (upper bar). The horizontal line within the box indicates the median value for each group. $*p < 0.05$, $**p < 0.001$ vs. HC

Table 2 Correlation between autophagy expression and inflammatory parameters in 72 patients with rheumatoid arthritis

Autophagy expression	DAS28	CRP	TNF-α	IL-6
Cyto-ID MFI in lymphocyte	0.522***	0.285*	0.325**	0.252*
Cyto-ID MFI in monocyte	0.478***	0.262*	0.320**	0.200
Cyto-ID MFI in granulocyte	0.486***	0.365**	0.247*	0.141
P62 MFI in lymphocyte	−0.309**	−0.297*	−0.336**	−0.197
P62 MFI in monocyte	−0.325**	−0.221	−0.293*	−0.188
P62 MFI in granulocyte	−0.249*	−0.130	−0.258*	−0.022

Abbreviations: CRP C-reactive protein, DAS28 Disease Activity Score in 28 joints, IL-6 Interleukin 6, MFI Mean fluorescence intensity, TNF-α Tumor necrosis factor-α
$*p < 0.05$, $**p < 0.01$, $***p < 0.001$ were determined by Spearman's rank-correlation test

Autophagy protein expression in PBMCs from patients with RA and HC

Representative immunoblot analyses of autophagy expression in PBMC lysates were obtained from one patient with active RA and one HC (Fig. 3a). The LC3-II expression levels were significantly higher in patients with active RA (median 3.55, IQR 2.05–7.82) than in HC (0.86, IQR 0.52–1.63; $p < 0.005$) (Fig. 3b). In contrast, patients with RA had significantly lower levels of p62 expression (0.47, IQR 0.13–0.67) than HC (1.66, IQR 0.99–3.17; $p < 0.001$) (Fig. 3c).

Given that lymphocytes and monocytes comprise the majority of PBMCs, we estimated autophagosome levels in PBMCs by summing the Cyto-ID MFI in both lymphocytes and monocytes. We examined the correlation between

a

LC3-I (18kDa)
LC3-II (16kDa)

P62 (47 KDa)

GAPDH (37 KDa)

RA   HC

b

LC3II/LC3I (ratio)

RA   HC

c

P62 expression (fold)

RA   HC

Fig. 3 Representative example of LC3-II/LC3-I and p62 protein expression in peripheral blood mononuclear cell lysates from one patient with rheumatoid arthritis (RA) and one healthy control subject (HC) (**a**). Comparisons of protein expression levels of LC3-II/LC3-I (**b**) and p62 (**c**) in patients with RA and HC are shown. Data are presented as box plot diagrams, with the box encompassing the 25th percentile (lower bar) to the 75th percentile (upper bar). The horizontal line within the box indicates median value for each group. *$p < 0.005$, **$p < 0.001$ versus HC, determined by Mann-Whitney U test

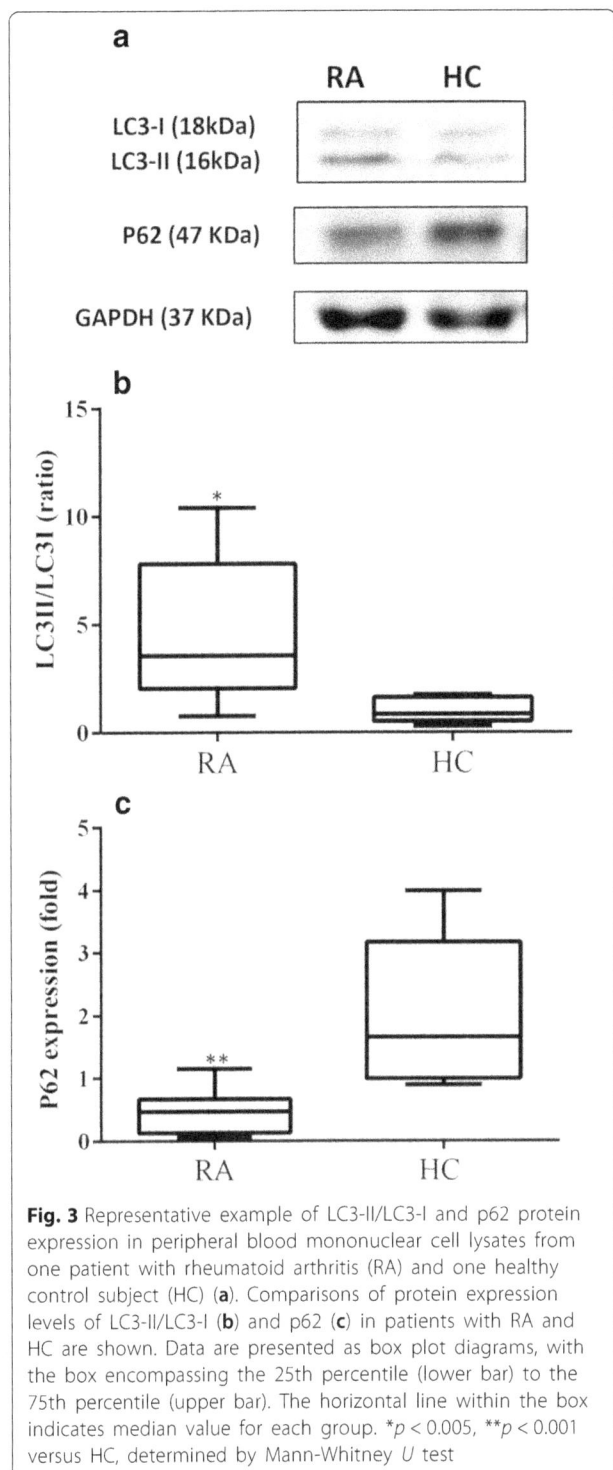

Change of autophagy expression and serum cytokine levels in patients with RA after 6 months of therapy

Sixty patients were available for examining autophagy expression before (at baseline) and after 6-month biologic therapy or csDMARDs alone. As shown in Fig. 4a, the autophagosome levels of circulating lymphocytes, monocytes, and granulocytes significantly declined (median 3.2, IQR 2.8–4.9 vs. 2.7, IQR 1.6–3.8, $p < 0.05$; 12.1, IQR 8.2–15.2 vs. 7.5, IQR 5.8–11.0, $p < 0.005$; 60.0, IQR 44.7–86.0 vs. 48.0, IQR 34.7–61.0, $p < 0.005$; respectively), paralleling the decrease of DAS28 (6.0, IQR 5.4–6.4 vs. 3.9, IQR 3.2–4.5, $p < 0.001$) in patients after 6-month anti-TNF-α therapy. In patients with RA receiving different TNF-α inhibitors, there was no significant difference in the change of autophagy expression between etanercept-treated and adalimumab-treated patients.

In patients after 6-month anti-IL-6R therapy (Fig. 4b), MFI of Cyto-ID in lymphocytes, monocytes, and granulocytes significantly declined (4.2, IQR 3.0–5.3 vs. 2.8, IQR 1.9–3.8; 13.5, IQR 9.3–16.8 vs. 9.5, IQR 5.5–11.9; 71.3, IQR 53.0–86.8 vs. 49.2, IQR 33.3–61.1, all $p < 0.001$), paralleling the decrease of DAS28 (6.0, IQR 5.4–6.5 vs. 3.2, IQR 3.0–3.8, $p < 0.001$). Although DAS28 also significantly decreased (5.2, IQR 4.2–5.9 vs. 3.1, IQR 3.0–3.9, $p < 0.05$) in those receiving csDMARDs alone, there was no significant change in MFI values of Cyto-ID in circulating lymphocytes, monocytes, or granulocytes (Fig. 4c).

Regarding the changes in serum cytokine levels, TNF-α levels significantly declined in patients with RA receiving any of the following medications for 6 months: TNF-α inhibitor, IL-6R inhibitor, or csDMARDs alone (median 165.8 pg/ml, IQR 132.8–265.4 pg/ml vs. 78.5 pg/ml, IQR 38.8–136.0 pg/ml, $p < 0.01$; 175.2 pg/ml, IQR 114.0–324.3 pg/ml vs. 119.2 pg/ml, IQR 39.7–168.6 pg/ml, $p < 0.001$; 183.6 pg/ml, IQR 90.9–276.3 pg/ml vs. 36.1 pg/ml, IQR 25.2–93.1, $p < 0.05$). Although serum IL-6 levels also decreased significantly (873.9 pg/ml, IQR 470.2–2545.1 pg/ml vs. 752.9 pg/ml, IQR 373.9–1163.0 pg/ml, $p < 0.005$) in patients with RA receiving IL-6R inhibitor, serum IL-6 levels did not show significant changes in those receiving TNF-α inhibitors (median 1342.3 pg/ml, IQR 462.5–2869.7 pg/ml vs. 1044.8 pg/ml, IQR 428.4–1801.1 pg/ml, $p = 0.277$) or csDMARDs alone (median 799.9 pg/ml, IQR 449.2–1887.9 pg/ml vs. 223.3 pg/ml, IQR 121.0–1042.3 pg/ml, $p = 0.128$) (Fig. 4d, e).

Discussion

Although autophagy has recently emerged as an important regulator in the induction and maintenance of joint inflammation [8, 21–25, 34], the pathogenic association between autophagy and inflammation in RA has rarely been explored. To our knowledge, the present study is the first to demonstrate significantly higher levels of

autophagy protein expression and autophagosome levels in PBMCs. The results showed a positive correlation between LC3-II expression levels and autophagosome levels ($r = 0.573$, $p < 0.01$) and a negative correlation between p62 levels in immunoblotting and autophagosome levels in Cyto-ID staining ($r = -0.423$, $p < 0.05$).

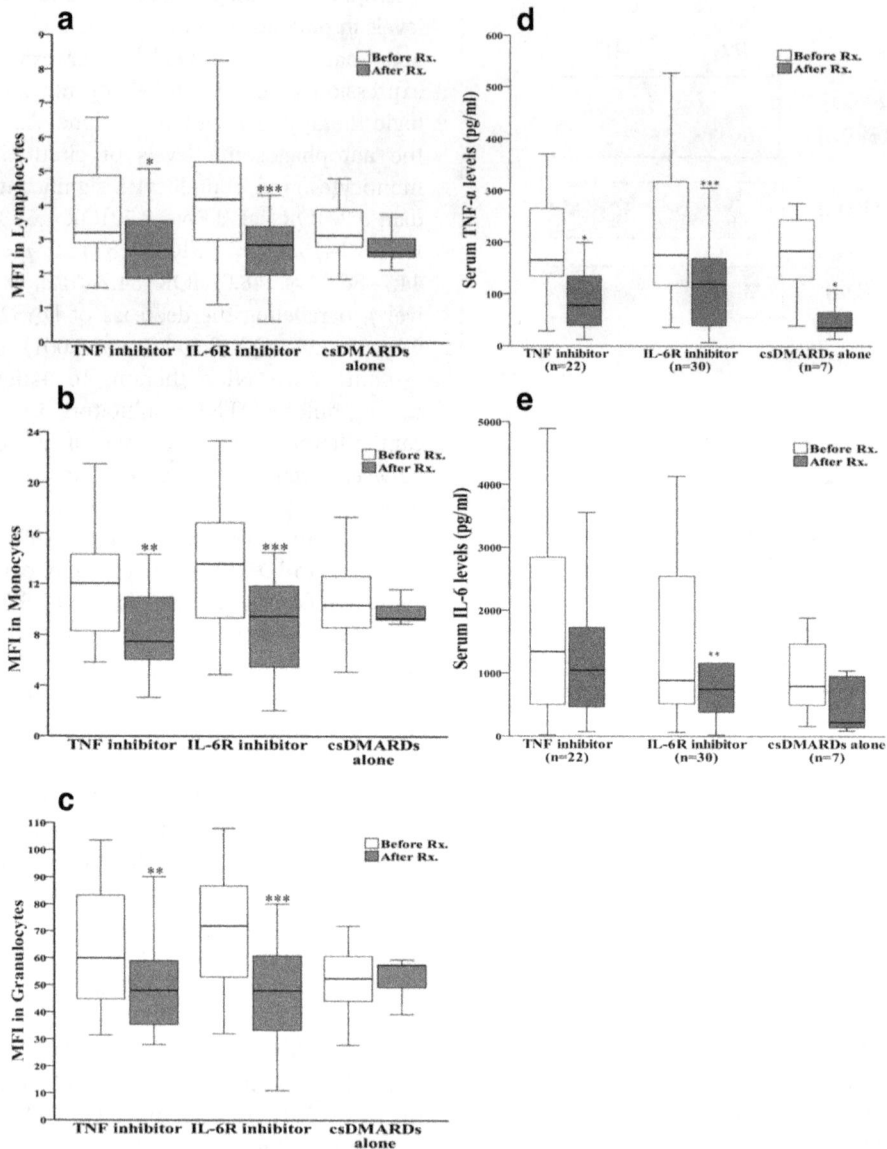

Fig. 4 The changes in autophagosome levels evidenced by Cyto-ID mean fluorescence intensity in circulating (**a**) lymphocytes, **b** monocytes, and (**c**) granulocytes and the change in (**d**) serum tumor necrosis factor-α levels as well as (**e**) interleukin (IL)-6 levels after 6-month therapy in patients with rheumatoid arthritis. Data are presented as the mean ± SEM. *$p < 0.05$, **$p < 0.005$, ***$p < 0.001$ vs. before treatment, as determined by Wilcoxon signed-rank test

autophagosomes, as evidenced by the MFI of Cyto-ID, in circulating immune cells from patients with RA than in HC. The protein expression of LC3-II, an indicator of autophagosome formation, was also elevated in patients with RA. We also revealed significantly lower p62 levels in patients with RA than in HC, as revealed by flow cytometry and immunoblot analyses, indicating increased autophagic activity in patients with RA. In addition, the autophagosome levels in circulating immune cells were significantly correlated with inflammatory parameters in patients with RA. These observations suggest a potential involvement of activated autophagy in RA pathogenesis.

Autophagosome formation, a critical step in the autophagic process [1, 4], was significantly increased in circulating lymphocytes, monocytes, and granulocytes from our patients with RA. Among the circulating lymphocytes, significantly higher levels of autophagosome were observed in circulating CD4[+] T and CD8[+] T cells, but not in CD19[+] B cells, from patients with RA than in HC. Van Loosdregt et al. similarly found an increased autophagy in CD4[+] T cells and CD8[+] T cells of patients with RA compared with HC [34]. We also revealed that the elevated protein expression of LC3-II, an indicator of autophagosome formation [1, 2], was positively associated with Cyto-ID MFI in circulating immune cells from patients with RA. Moreover, autophagosome levels were markedly higher in SF granulocytes than in PB-derived granulocytes in patients with active RA (Additional file 1: Figure S1F–H), in agreement with other recent reports showing that autophagy expression is higher in granulocytes from SF than in those from PB in patients with RA [35]. Previous reports also showed an increased autophagy in RA and persistent activation of the autophagy pathway in FLS from patients with RA or in murine arthritis [23–25]. Therefore, it is reasonable to speculate that increased autophagy in immune cells from patients with RA may result in their persistent activation, particularly at the site of inflammation. In our study, autophagosome levels in immune cells from patients with RA were positively correlated with DAS28, CRP levels, and TNF-α values. Moreover, the autophagosome levels in circulating immune cells declined significantly, paralleling the decrease of serum TNF-α values, in our patients with RA undergoing effective treatment. These observations suggest an association between elevated autophagy and RA-related inflammation, as has been shown in other previous studies [21, 36].

Excessive generation of ROS driven by overproduction of proinflammatory cytokines such as TNF-α participates in an inflammatory process in RA. An efficient antioxidant system catalyzes the inactivation of ROS. Previous studies have revealed increased oxidative stress along with low antioxidant levels and reduced antioxidant capacity in plasma of patients with RA [37]. Plasma TAC levels, as determined in our study, reflect the global combined antioxidant capacity of all individual antioxidants in plasma. We have demonstrated significantly lower TAC levels in patients with RA than in HC, indicating an increased oxidative stress in human RA [37]. Zhang et al. also revealed that excessive ROS cause mitochondrial damage and then induce autophagy in adjuvant-arthritis (AA) rats [38]. In agreement with their findings that resveratrol, an antioxidant, could suppress oxidative stress by reducing autophagy expression in AA rats [38], an inverse correlation between plasma TAC levels and autophagosome levels in circulating granulocytes was observed in our patients with RA.

With p62-bound ubiquitinated substrates incorporated into the autophagosome and then degraded into the autolysosomes, p62 level is selectively degraded by autophagy [39] and serves as a readout of autophagic flux [4, 5]. Thus, the decreases of p62 levels reflect autophagic activation [40]. In the present study, the p62 MFI in circulating immune cells and p62 protein expression in PBMCs from patients with RA were significantly lower than in those from HC, with the p62 MFI in immune cells negatively correlated with RA inflammatory parameters (Table 2). The combination of increased

autophagosome formation and decreased p62 levels suggests autophagic activation in RA. Yang et al. demonstrated the upregulated expression of LC3-II as well as decreased p62 expression in RA FLS [12], also indicating an activated autophagy in RA.

Consistent with previous reports [16–18], significantly higher levels of serum inflammatory cytokines, including TNF-α and IL-6, were found in our patients with RA than in HC. The positive correlation between TNF-α levels and autophagosome levels in circulating immune cells from patients with RA further supports the findings that TNF-α could stimulate the conversion of LC3-I into LC3-II, an indicator of autophagosome formation [21]. In addition, we revealed a significant reduction of autophagosome levels, serum TNF-α levels, and disease activity in patients with RA after 6-month anti-TNF-α therapy (Fig. 4). In an animal model of RA, the inhibition of autophagy could also alleviate synovial inflammation [41]. The inhibitory effect of anti-TNF-α therapy on autophagy may be responsible for its associated increase of infection risk, particularly tuberculosis [10]. Besides, the positive correlation between serum IL-6 levels and autophagosome levels in circulating lymphocytes is in agreement with the previous finding that the knockdown of autophagic initiation ameliorates activated lymphocyte-derived DNA-induced murine lupus through an inhibition of IL-6 [42]. The significant reduction of autophagy expression in our patients with RA after 6-month anti-IL-6R therapy is also similar to previous reports that anti-IL6R therapy was effective in the treatment of glioblastoma by blocking autophagy [43], and the inhibition of autophagy could reduce osteoclastogenesis and prevent structural damage in RA [21]. However, whether the changes in autophagy expression following biologic therapy are related to a cytokine blocking effect needs to be further validated.

In spite of the novel findings in this pilot study, there were still some limitations. We enrolled a limited number of patients with active RA who were followed throughout 6-month therapies. Because the medications used, such as corticosteroids, may influence autophagy through downregulating proinflammatory cytokine secretion [44], their interference should be considered. In contrast to the results of a previous report in an early RA cohort [45], we did not reveal a significant association between autophagy expression and ACPA levels in patients with RA. This discrepancy may be explained by the fact that most of the patients enrolled in our study were not in an early RA stage. Therefore, a long-term study enrolling a larger group of patients, including an early RA population, is required for the validation of our findings.

Last, there is increasing evidence suggesting that autophagy serves a crucial role as a macrophage-intrinsic negative regulator of the inflammasome [46]. The stimulation of macrophages with an autoantigen-autoantibody immunocomplex leads to mitochondrial damage that further activates the inflammasome [46]. Given that autophagy and inflammasome activation are interrelated in autoimmune diseases [46, 47], the insights into the regulation of inflammasome activity by autophagy in RA should be investigated in future studies.

Conclusions

The elevated autophagy expression with positive correlation to disease activity and inflammatory parameters in patients with RA suggests the involvement of activated autophagy in the pathogenesis of this disease. Our preliminary results also indicated that the therapeutic effectiveness of biologics may be related at least in part to their downregulation of autophagy expression. The elucidation of the pathogenic role of autophagy in RA may allow for the development of novel pharmaceutical agents in the future [44, 48].

Additional file

Additional file 1: Figure S1. Representative cytometric histograms of Cyto-ID staining in circulating CD4$^+$ T cells (A1), CD8$^+$ T cells (A2), and CD19$^+$ B cells (A3) from one patient with rheumatoid arthritis (RA) and one healthy control subject (HC). Comparisons of autophagosome levels reflected by Cyto-ID-staining MFI, in CD4$^+$ T cells (B), CD8$^+$ T cells (C) and CD19$^+$ B cells (D) between patients with RA and HC. Data are presented as box plot diagrams, with the box encompassing the 25th percentile (lower bar) to the 75th percentile (upper bar). The horizontal line within the box indicates median value for each group. *$p < 0.05$ versus HC. Representative cytometric histograms of Cyto-ID staining in peripheral blood (PB)-derived granulocytes (E) and synovial fluid (SF)-derived granulocytes (F). Comparisons of autophagosome levels in PB-derived and SF-derived granulocytes in patients with RA (G). (TIF 1427 kb)

Abbreviations

AA: Adjuvant-arthritis; ACPA: Anticitrullinated peptide antibodies; CRP: C-reactive protein; csDMARD: Conventional synthetic disease-modifying anti-rheumatic drug; Cyc: Cyclosporine; DAS28: 28-joint Disease Activity Score; ESR: Erythrocyte sedimentation rate; FITC: Fluorescein isothiocyanate; FLS: Fibroblast-like synoviocytes; HC: Healthy control subjects; HCQ: Hydroxychloroquine; IL-6: Interleukin 6; IL-6R: Interleukin 6 receptor; LC3: Light chain 3; mAb: Monoclonal antibody; MFI: Mean fluorescence intensity; MTX: Methotrexate; PBMC: Peripheral blood mononuclear cell; PC5: Phycoerythrin-cyanine 5; PerCP: Peridinin chlorophyll protein; RA: Rheumatoid arthritis; RF: Rheumatoid factor; RT: Room temperature; SF: Synovial fluid; SQSTM1: Sequestosome 1; SSZ: Sulfasalazine; TAC: Total antioxidant capacity; TNF: Tumor necrosis factor

Acknowledgements

This work was supported by a grant (MOST 104-2314-B-075A-005-MY3) from the National Science Council, Taiwan. The authors thank the Biostatistics Task Force of Taichung Veterans General Hospital, Taichung, Taiwan.

Funding

This work was supported by a grant (MOST 104-2314-B-075A-005-MY3) from the National Science Council, Taiwan.

Authors' contributions

YMC conceived of this study, designed the study, acquired clinical data, analyzed data, and drafted and revised the manuscript. CYC conceived of this study and performed data acquisition and statistical analysis. HHC, CWH, KTT, and JLL performed clinical assessments on study subjects and conducted the analysis of data. MCY performed the flow cytometric analysis and data acquisition. DYC generated the original hypothesis, designed the study, acquired clinical data, analyzed data, and drafted and revised the manuscript. All authors made substantive intellectual contributions to the present study and approved the final manuscript.

Competing interests

The authors declare that they have no competing interests.

Author details

[1]Division of Allergy, Immunology and Rheumatology, Department of Medical Research, Taichung Veterans General Hospital, Taichung City, Taiwan. [2]Faculty of Medicine, National Yang Ming University, Taipei, Taiwan. [3]Institute of Biomedical Science and Rong Hsing Research Center for Translational Medicine, Chung Hsing University, Taichung, Taiwan. [4]Rheumatology and Immunology Center, China Medical University Hospital, No. 2, Yude Road, Taichung 40447, Taiwan. [5]Translational Medicine Laboratory, Rheumatic Diseases Research Center, China Medical University Hospital, Taichung, Taiwan. [6]School of Medicine, China Medical University, Taichung, Taiwan.

References

1. Mizushima N. Autophagy: process and function. Genes Dev. 2007;21:2861–73.
2. Mizushima N, Komatsu M. Autophagy: renovation of cells and tissues. Cell. 2011;147:728–41.
3. Cao Y, Klionsky DJ. Physiological functions of Atg6/Beclin 1: a unique autophagy-related protein. Cell Res. 2007;17:839–49.
4. Seibenhener ML, Babu JR, Geetha T, et al. Sequestosome 1/p62 is a polyubiquitin chain binding protein involved in ubiquitin proteasomal degradation. Mol Cell Biol. 2004;24:8055–68.
5. Bjorkoy G, Lamark T, Brech A, et al. p62/SQSTM1 forms protein aggregates degraded by autophagy and has a protective effect on huntingtin-induced cell death. J Cell Biol. 2005;171:603–14.
6. Levine B, Mizushima N, Virgin HW. Autophagy in immunity and inflammation. Nature. 2011;469:323–35.
7. Saitoh T, Akira S. Regulation of innate immune responses by autophagy-related proteins. J Cell Biol. 2010;189:925–35.
8. Deretic V. Multiple regulatory and effector roles of autophagy in immunity. Curr Opin Immunol. 2009;21:53–62.
9. Harris J. Autophagy and cytokines. Cytokine. 2011;56:140–4.
10. Harris J, Keane J. How tumour necrosis factor blockers interfere with tuberculosis immunity. Clin Exp Immunol. 2010;161:1–9.
11. Roca H, Varsos ZS, Sud S, et al. CCL2 and interleukin-6 promote survival pf human CD11b$^+$ peripheral blood mononuclear cells and induce M2-type macrophage polarization. J Biol Chem. 2009;284:34342–54.
12. Yang R, Zhang Y, Wang L, et al. Increased autophagy in fibroblast-like synoviocytes leads to immune enhancement in rheumatoid arthritis. Oncotarget. 2017;8:15420–30.
13. Shi CS, Shenderov K, Huang NN, et al. Activation of autophagy by inflammatory signals limits IL-1β production by targeting ubiquitinated inflammasomes for destruction. Nat Immunol. 2012;13:255–63.
14. Sridhar S, Botbol Y, Macian F, Cuervo AM. Autophagy and disease: two sides to a problem. J Pathol. 2012;226:255–73.
15. Zhou XJ, Zhang H. Autophagy in immunity: implications in etiology of autoimmune/autoinflammatory diseases. Autophagy. 2012;8:1286–99.
16. Choy EH, Panayi GS. Cytokine pathways and joint inflammation in rheumatoid arthritis. N Engl J Med. 2001;344:907–16.
17. Feldmann M, Maini RN. TNF defined as a therapeutic target for rheumatoid arthritis and other autoimmune diseases. Nat Med. 2003;9:1245–50.
18. Furst DE, Emery P. Rheumatoid arthritis pathophysiology: update on emerging cytokine and cytokine-associated cell targets. Rheumatology (Oxford). 2014;53:1560–9.

19. Breedveld FC, Weisman MH, Kavanaugh AF, et al. The PREMIER study: a multicenter, randomized, double-blind clinical trial of combination therapy with adalimumab plus methotrexate versus methotrexate alone or adalimumab alone in patients with early, aggressive rheumatoid arthritis who had not had previous methotrexate treatment. Arthritis Rheum. 2006; 54:26–37.

20. Yazici Y, Curtis JR, Ince A, et al. Efficacy of tocilizumab in patients with moderate to severe active rheumatoid arthritis and a previous inadequate response to disease-modifying antirheumatic drugs: the ROSE study. Ann Rheum Dis. 2012;71:198–205.

21. Lin NY, Beyer C, Giessl A, et al. Autophagy regulates TNFα-mediated joint destruction in experimental arthritis. Ann Rheum Dis. 2013;72:761–8.

22. Connor AM, Mahomed N, Gandhi R, Keystone EC, Berger SA. TNF-α modulates protein degradation pathway in rheumatoid arthritis synovial fibroblasts. Arthritis Res Ther. 2012;14:R62.

23. Xu K, Xu P, Yao JF, et al. Reduced apoptosis correlates with enhanced autophagy in synovial tissues of rheumatoid arthritis. Inflamm Res. 2013; 62:229–37.

24. Shin YJ, Han SH, Kim DS, et al. Autophagy induction and CHOP under-expression promotes survival of fibroblasts from rheumatoid arthritis patients under endoplasmic reticulum stress. Arthritis Res Ther. 2010;12:R19.

25. Kato M, Ospelt C, Gay RE, Gay S, Klein K. Dual role of autophagy in stress-induced cell death in rheumatoid arthritis synovial fibroblasts. Arthritis Rheumatol. 2014;66:40–8.

26. Aletaha D, Neogi T, Silman AJ, et al. The 2010 rheumatoid arthritis classification criteria: an American College of Rheumatology/European League Against Rheumatism collaborative initiative. Ann Rheum Dis. 2010; 69:1580–8.

27. Prevoo MLL, van 't Hof MA, Kuper HH, et al. Modified disease activity scores that include twenty-eight-joint counts: development and validation in a prospective longitudinal study of patients with rheumatoid arthritis. Arthritis Rheum. 1995;38:44–8.

28. Smolen JS, Aletaha D, Bijlsma JW, et al. Treating rheumatoid arthritis to target: recommendations of an international task force. Ann Rheum Dis. 2011;70:631–7.

29. Ledingham J, Deighton C, British Society for Rheumatology Standards, Guidelines and Audit Working Group. Update on the British Society for Rheumatology guidelines for prescribing TNFα blockers in adults with rheumatoid arthritis (update of previous guidelines of April 2001). Rheumatology (Oxford). 2005;44:157–63.

30. Oeste CL, Seco E, Patton WF, et al. Interactions between autophagic and endo-lysosomal markers in endothelial cells. Histochem Cell Biol. 2013;139:659–70.

31. Shvets E, Fass E, Elazar Z. Utilizing flow cytometry to monitor autophagy in living mammalian cells. Autophagy. 2008;4:621–8.

32. Klionsky DJ, Abdalla FC, Abeliovich H, et al. Guidelines for the use and interpretation of assays for monitoring autophagy. Autophagy. 2012;8: 445–544.

33. Clarke AJ, Ellinghaus U, Cortini A, et al. Autophagy is activated in systemic lupus erythematosus and required for plasmablast development. Ann Rheum Dis. 2015;74:912–20.

34. van Loosdregt J, Rossetti M, Spreafico R, et al. Increased autophagy in CD4+ T cells of rheumatoid arthritis patients results in T-cell hyperactivation and apoptosis resistance. Eur J Immunol. 2016;46:2862–70.

35. An Q, Yan W, Zhao Y, Yu K. Enhanced neutrophil autophagy and increased concentrations of IL-6, IL-8, IL-10, and MCP-1 in rheumatoid arthritis. Int Immunopharmacol. 2018;65:119–28.

36. Zhu L, Wang H, Wu Y, et al. The autophagy level is increased in the synovial tissues of patients with active rheumatoid arthritis and is correlated with disease activity. Mediat Inflamm. 2017;2017:7623145.

37. Hitchon CA, El-Gabalawy HS. Oxidation in rheumatoid arthritis. Arthritis Res Ther. 2004;6:265–78.

38. Zhang J, Song X, Cao W, et al. Autophagy and mitochondrial dysfunction in adjuvant-arthritis rats treatment with resveratrol. Sci Rep. 2016;6:32928.

39. Ichimura Y, Kominami E, Tanaka K, Komatsu M. Selective turnover of p62/A170/SQSTM1 by autophagy. Autophagy. 2008;4:1063–6.

40. Komatsu M, Waguri S, Koike M, et al. Homeostatic levels of p62 control cytoplasmic inclusion body formation in autophagy-deficient mice. Cell. 2007;131:1149–63.

41. Li S, Chen JW, Xie X, et al. Autophagy inhibitor regulates apoptosis and proliferation of synovial fibroblasts through the inhibition of PI3K/AKT pathway in collagen-induced arthritis rat model. Am J Transl Res. 2017;9: 2065–76.

42. Li B, Dong C, Shi Y, Xiong S. Blockade of macrophage autophagy ameliorates activated lymphocytes-derived DNA induced murine lupus possibly via inhibition of proinflammatory cytokine production. Clin Exp Rheumatol. 2014;32:705–14.

43. Xue H, Yuan G, Guo X, et al. A novel tumor-promoting mechanism of IL6 and the therapeutic efficacy of tocilizumab: hypoxia-induced IL6 is a potent autophagy initiator in glioblastoma via the p-STAT3-MIR155-3p-CREBRF pathway. Autophagy. 2016;12:1129–52.

44. Feng Y, Li B, Li XY, Wu ZB. The role of autophagy in rheumatic disease. Curr Drug Targets. 2018;19(9):1009–17.

45. Sorice M, Iannuccelli C, Manganelli V, et al. Autophagy generates citrullinated peptides in human synoviocytes: a possible trigger of anti-citrullinated peptide antibodies. Rheumatology (Oxford). 2016;55:1374–85.

46. Zhong Z, Sanchez-Lopez E, Karin M. Autophagy, NLRP3 inflammasome and auto-inflammatory/immune diseases. Clin Exp Rheumatol. 2016; 34(Suppl 98):S12–6.

47. Spalinger MR, Lang S, Gottier C, et al. PTPN22 regulates NLRP3-mediated IL1B secretion in an autophagy-dependent manner. Autophagy. 2017;13: 1590–601.

48. Dai Y, Hu S. Recent insights into the role of autophagy in the pathogenesis of rheumatoid arthritis. Rheumatology (Oxford). 2016;55:403–10.

16

Effect of high-intensity interval training on muscle remodeling in rheumatoid arthritis compared to prediabetes

Brian J. Andonian[1,2]* ⓘ, David B. Bartlett[1], Janet L. Huebner[1], Leslie Willis[1], Andrew Hoselton[1], Virginia B. Kraus[1,2], William E. Kraus[1] and Kim M. Huffman[1,2]

Abstract

Background: Sarcopenic obesity, associated with greater risk of cardiovascular disease (CVD) and mortality in rheumatoid arthritis (RA), may be related to dysregulated muscle remodeling. To determine whether exercise training could improve remodeling, we measured changes in inter-relationships of plasma galectin-3, skeletal muscle cytokines, and muscle myostatin in patients with RA and prediabetes before and after a high-intensity interval training (HIIT) program.

Methods: Previously sedentary persons with either RA ($n = 12$) or prediabetes ($n = 9$) completed a 10-week supervised HIIT program. At baseline and after training, participants underwent body composition (Bod Pod®) and cardiopulmonary exercise testing, plasma collection, and *vastus lateralis* biopsies. Plasma galectin-3, muscle cytokines, muscle interleukin-1 beta (mIL-1β), mIL-6, mIL-8, muscle tumor necrosis factor-alpha (mTNF-α), mIL-10, and muscle myostatin were measured via enzyme-linked immunosorbent assays. An independent cohort of patients with RA ($n = 47$) and age-, gender-, and body mass index (BMI)-matched non-RA controls ($n = 23$) were used for additional analyses of galectin-3 inter-relationships.

Results: Exercise training did not reduce mean concentration of galectin-3, muscle cytokines, or muscle myostatin in persons with either RA or prediabetes. However, training-induced alterations varied among individuals and were associated with cardiorespiratory fitness and body composition changes. Improved cardiorespiratory fitness (increased absolute peak maximal oxygen consumption, or VO₂) correlated with reductions in galectin-3 ($r = -0.57$, $P = 0.05$ in RA; $r = -0.48$, $P = 0.23$ in prediabetes). Training-induced improvements in body composition were related to reductions in muscle IL-6 and TNF-α ($r < -0.60$ and $P < 0.05$ for all). However, the association between increased lean mass and decreased muscle IL-6 association was stronger in prediabetes compared with RA (Fisher r-to-z $P = 0.0004$); in prediabetes but not RA, lean mass increases occurred in conjunction with reductions in muscle myostatin ($r = -0.92$; $P < 0.05$; Fisher r-to-z $P = 0.026$). Subjects who received TNF inhibitors ($n = 4$) or hydroxychloroquine ($n = 4$) did not improve body composition with exercise training.

Conclusion: Exercise responses in muscle myostatin, cytokines, and body composition were significantly greater in prediabetes than in RA, consistent with impaired muscle remodeling in RA. To maximize physiologic improvements with exercise training in RA, a better understanding is needed of skeletal muscle and physiologic responses to exercise training and their modulation by RA disease–specific features or pharmacologic agents or both.

Keywords: Rheumatoid arthritis, High-intensity interval exercise, Sarcopenic obesity, Galectin-3, Myostatin, Cytokines

* Correspondence: brian.andonian@duke.edu
[1]Duke Molecular Physiology Institute, Duke University School of Medicine, 300 N Duke St, Durham, NC 27701, USA
[2]Division of Rheumatology, Duke University School of Medicine, 40 Duke Medicine Circle Drive, Durham, NC 27710, USA

Introduction

Despite improvements in rheumatoid arthritis (RA) disease management with biologic therapies, patients with RA remain at greater risk than the general population for cardiovascular disease (CVD) and reduced life expectancy [1–3]. RA-associated CVD, disability, and increased mortality are linked to adverse changes in body composition, including decreased skeletal muscle mass and increased fat mass—referred to as sarcopenic obesity [4, 5]. We previously reported that RA sketelal muscle is defined by increased interleukin-6 (IL-6), increased inflammation, increased glycolysis, and a dysregulated remodeling transcriptomic and metabolic signature [6]; these findings overall suggests that RA muscle is deficient in adaptation to physical activity and repair of injuries.

In response to injury, skeletal muscle normally relies on a coordinated activation and deactivation of the inflammatory response to produce myofiber hypertrophy and vascular maturation without excess production of collagen or fibrosis [7]. This process requires immune cells, muscle stem (satellite) cells, and fibroblasts. These cells communicate via well-coordinated systemic and local signaling molecules, including cytokines and myokines [8]. IL-6 and myostatin are critical for muscle hypertrophy and remodeling [9]; myostatin is a member of the transforming growth factor-beta superfamily and a potent negative regulator of muscle hypertrophy [10].

Galectin-3, a beta-galactoside–binding lectin important for muscle repair [11], is implicated in synovial inflammation and acts as a pro-inflammatory mediator of disease activity in RA [12, 13]. A regulatory molecule of chronic inflammation, galectin-3 mediates transitions from acute to chronic inflammation to fibrosis and organ scarring [14, 15]. Galectin-3 may serve as a marker of impaired muscle remodeling; in RA, although responses to chronic exercise training are unknown, serum galectin-3 is unchanged after an acute bout of exercise [16].

The pro-inflammatory, pro-glycolytic, dysregulated muscle phenotype of RA is associated with less physical activity, suggesting that exercise training may counteract the impaired muscle remodeling associated with RA [6]. We hypothesized that (1) a high-intensity interval-based training program would improve skeletal muscle remodeling reflected by reductions in remodeling markers: muscle inflammatory cytokines, myostatin, and plasma galectin-3; (2) changes in remodeling markers would be associated with improvements in clinical measures of body composition (goal to increase lean mass and decrease body fat) and cardiopulmonary fitness; and (3) remodeling markers and clinical associations in subjects with RA would differ from those in subjects with prediabetes. A convenience sample of subjects with prediabetes was chosen as a comparator cohort with a CVD risk similar to that of RA.

Methods

Study design and participants

Previously sedentary volunteers with RA underwent a high-intensity interval walking program. Subjects with RA met the following criteria: (1) RA diagnosis meeting American College of Rheumatology (ACR) 1987 criteria who were either seropositive or with hand radiographic joint erosions [17], (2) no medication changes in the previous 3 months; (3) using doses of prednisone of 5 mg per day or less; and (4) exercising less than 2 days per week at baseline.

To better determine RA-specific changes, this report includes a cohort of persons with prediabetes who underwent an identical exercise training and assessment protocol. Subjects with prediabetes met the following criteria: (1) hemoglobin A1c 5.7–6.5%, (2) stable use of all medications for at least 3 months, and (3) exercising less than 2 days per week at baseline. For both groups, exclusions were diagnoses of diabetes mellitus or CVD and an inability to walk unaided on a treadmill. A previously described cross-sectional cohort of subjects with RA [6] was used to compare plasma galectin-3 between RA and age-, gender-, and body mass index (BMI)-matched controls. This cohort was seropositive or with erosive hand disease, met 1987 ACR criteria for RA, had no medication changes in the last 3 months, and was using prednisone 5 mg a day or less; persons with diabetes or CVD diagnoses were excluded. The Duke University Institutional Review Board approved all research protocols, and all subjects provided written informed consent.

Exercise intervention

Supervised exercise sessions occurred three times per week for 10 weeks using graded treadmills and continuous heart rate monitoring (HRM1G Heart Rate Monitor with the compatible FR60 watch; Garmin, Olathe, KS, USA). Each session consisted of a 5-min warm-up, 10 alternating high-intensity (80–90% heart rate reserve) and low-intensity (50–60% heart rate reserve) intervals (60–90 s each), and a 5-min cool-down.

Outcome measures

Primary outcomes were changes in immune cell function and plasma cytokines, which have been previously reported [18]. Medical history questionnaire and additional assessments—body composition, maximal oxygen consumption (VO_2), and disease activity—were conducted at baseline and between 24 and 48 h after the last exercise-training bout (Table 1). Body composition was assessed via air displacement plethysmography by using a BodPod° (BodPod System; Life Measurement Corporation, Concord, CA, USA). Maximal oxygen consumption during exercise, or peak VO_2, was directly assessed via graded exercise treadmill testing. Disease activity was assessed by the Disease Activity Score in 28 joints (DAS-28) as determined from a patient-completed visual analog scale, physician-determined numbers of tender and swollen joints, and erythrocyte sedimentation rate [19].

Participants underwent fasting phlebotomy and Bergstrom needle *vastus lateralis* biopsies [20]. Plasma and flash-frozen muscle tissue were stored at −80 °C until analyses. Plasma concentrations of inflammatory markers, cytokines, and galectin-3 (R&D cat. no. DGAL30) were determined by immunoassay [6, 21]. Skeletal muscle was homogenized and sample concentrations were normalized to initial masses as previously described [6]. Muscle interleukin 1 beta (mIL-1β), mIL-6, mIL-8, muscle tumor necrosis factor-alpha (mTNF-α) (MSD 4-plex; K15053D-1), mIL-10 (MSD K151QUD-1), and myostatin (R&D cat. no. DGDF80) were measured via enzyme-linked immunosorbent assays (ELISAs). Mean concentrations were above the lower limit of detection for each analyte. For all six analytes, mean intra- and inter-assay coefficients of variation were less than 6.5% and 12%, respectively.

Statistical analysis
As determined by the distribution of the variable, continuous outcome variables were compared by using either Student's t tests or Wilcoxon signed-rank tests. Spearman correlations were used to determine the relationships between the plasma and muscle measures. Strengths of associations for the two groups (RA and prediabetes) were compared with Fisher r-to-z transformations [22]. Except for Fisher transformations, all statistical analyses were performed by using SAS 9.4 (SAS Institute, Cary, NC, USA). P values less than 0.05 were considered statistically significant. All data are available from the corresponding author upon reasonable request.

Results
Remodeling markers in RA at baseline
In a previously described RA cohort [6], plasma galectin-3 was significantly ($n = 47$, P <0.05 for all) and positively correlated with plasma IL-6 ($r = 0.29$), prednisone use ($r = 0.42$), BMI ($r = 0.32$), thigh cross-sectional area ($r = 0.46$), intra-muscular fat (thigh muscle density, $r = -0.44$), and age ($r = 0.39$). Plasma galectin-3 was greater in older (age greater than 55) persons with RA ($n = 24$; 8.80 ± 3.5 (standard deviation) ng/mL) than age-, gender-, and BMI-matched healthy controls ($n = 12$; 6.89 ± 1.9 ng/mL; $P = 0.042$; Fig. 1).

Prior to exercise training, those with RA, compared with those with prediabetes, had similar muscle cytokine concentrations but greater plasma galectin-3 and less skeletal muscle myostatin (P <0.05 for myostatin; Table

2). In RA, muscle cytokines were not significantly associated with previously reported plasma cytokines [18].

Changes in remodeling markers with exercise training
For both groups, training produced robust improvements in peak VO$_2$ and DAS-28 (Table 1) [18]. However, plasma galectin-3, skeletal muscle cytokines, and muscle myostatin concentrations did not respond to training in either group (Table 2).

Associations of remodeling markers with cardiorespiratory fitness and body composition in RA
Responses of remodeling markers (muscle inflammatory cytokines, myostatin, and plasma galectin-3) varied among individuals and were associated with cardiorespiratory fitness and body composition responses in RA. Improved cardiorespiratory fitness (peak VO$_2$) correlated with reductions in galectin-3 (Fig. 2). Training-induced improvements in body composition (increased lean mass) were related to reductions in skeletal muscle IL-6 and TNF-α ($r < -0.60$ and P <0.05 for all; Fig. 3). Changes in lean mass and body fat were not associated with changes in plasma galectin-3.

Associations of remodeling markers with cardiorespiratory fitness and body composition in prediabetes
The inverse relationship of improved cardiorespiratory fitness (peak VO$_2$) with reductions in galectin-3 was similar to RA, but non-significant, in prediabetes (Fisher r-to-z $P = 0.81$; Fig. 2). In prediabetes but not RA, body composition improvements correlated with reductions in muscle myostatin ($r = -0.92$; P <0.05; Fisher r-to-z $P = 0.026$; Fig. 3). The association of increased lean mass with decreased muscle IL-6 was significantly stronger in prediabetes (Fisher r-to-z $P = 0.0004$; Fig. 3).

Associations of RA medication use with body composition
All RA participants who achieved the goal combination of increased lean mass and decreased percentage body fat after exercise training ($n = 4$) were taking methotrexate ($n = 3$), sulfasalazine ($n = 1$), or tofacitinib ($n = 1$). In contrast, no person on TNF inhibitor ($n = 4$) or hydroxychloroquine therapy ($n = 4$) achieved the goal combination of increased lean mass and decreased fat mass after exercise training ($r = -0.50$, $P = 0.098$ for both; Table 3).

Discussion
As a systemic marker and regulator of chronic inflammation leading to tissue fibrogenesis, galectin-3 may reflect increased cardiovascular risk in RA resulting from impaired muscle remodeling. Elevated serum levels of galectin-3 are strongly associated with increased morbidity and mortality

Table 1 Participant characteristics

Variable	Rheumatoid arthritis ($n = 12$)	Prediabetes ($n = 9$)
Age, years	63.9 (7.2)	71.4 (4.9)*
Gender		
Female	11 (91.6%)	5 (55.6%)
Race		
Caucasian	11 (91.6%)	8 (88.9%)
African-American	1 (8.4%)	1 (11.1%)
Absolute peak VO$_2$, mL/min		
Pre-HIIT	1.75 (0.38)	1.71 (0.46)
Post-HIIT	1.90 (0.38)**	1.94 (0.57)**
Relative peak VO$_2$, mL/kg per min		
Pre-HIIT	24.9 (6.6)	19.9 (2.7)
Post-HIIT	27.1 (6.9)**	23.1 (3.6)**
BMI, kg/m^2		
Pre-HIIT	27.4 (9.3)	29.4 (3.0)
Post-HIIT	27.6 (9.8)	29.0 (3.0)
Body fat, %		
Pre-HIIT	36.6 (11.6)	39.6 (8.6)
Post-HIIT	37.2 (11.2)	39.1 (8.1)
Lean mass, kg		
Pre-HIIT	44.9 (8.9)	50.1 (12.2)
Post-HIIT	44.7 (7.8)	50.1 (12.0)
Hemoglobin A1c		
Pre-HIIT	5.46 (0.59)	5.99 (0.19)*
Post-HIIT	5.56 (0.41)	5.87 (0.21)*
Disease duration, years	13.3 (7.2)	NA
DAS-28, mean (SD)		
Pre-HIIT	3.1 (2.3)	NA
Post-HIIT	2.3 (1.5)**	NA
Rheumatoid factor–positive	10/12 (83.3%)	NA
Anti-cyclic citrullinated antibody–positive	5/8 (62.5%)	NA
Erosions on radiographs present	9/12 (75.0%)	NA
Medication use		
Infliximab	2 (16.7%)	NA
Adalimumab	2 (16.7%)	NA
Tofacitinib	1 (8.3%)	NA
Methotrexate	6 (50%)	NA
Leflunomide	1 (8.3%)	NA
Sulfasalazine	2 (16.7%)	NA
Hydroxychloroquine	4 (33.3%)	NA
Nonsteroidal anti-inflammatory agents	8 (66.7%)	NA
Prednisone (<5 mg/day)	3 (25%)	NA

Data are presented as mean (SD) for continuous variables and number (percentage) of participants for dichotomous variables.
Abbreviations: *BMI* body mass index, *HIIT* high-intensity interval training, *NA* not applicable, *NSAID* non-steroidal anti-inflammatory drug, *SD* standard deviation, *VO$_2$* maximal oxygen consumption
*P <0.05 for comparisons between rheumatoid arthritis and prediabetes groups
** P <0.05 for comparisons between pre-and post-HIIT rheumatoid arthritis and prediabetes groups

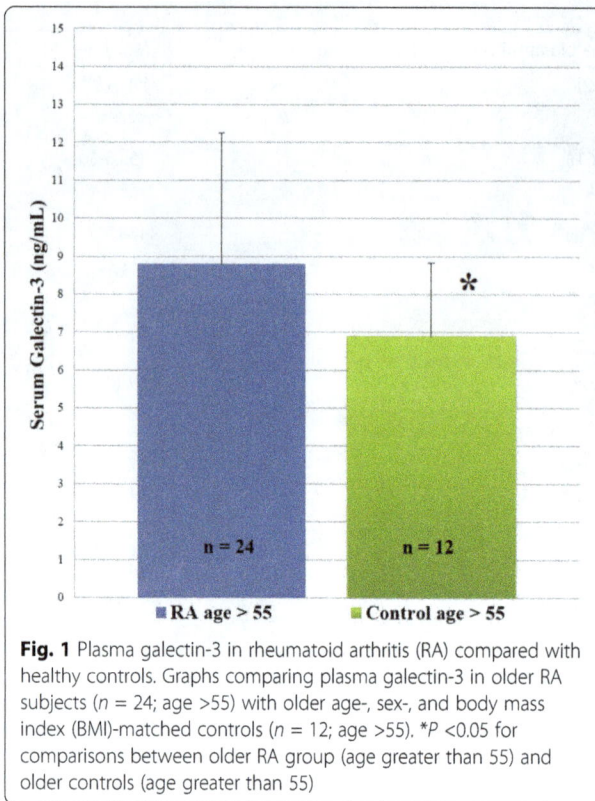

Fig. 1 Plasma galectin-3 in rheumatoid arthritis (RA) compared with healthy controls. Graphs comparing plasma galectin-3 in older RA subjects ($n = 24$; age >55) with older age-, sex-, and body mass index (BMI)-matched controls ($n = 12$; age >55). *P <0.05 for comparisons between older RA group (age greater than 55) and older controls (age greater than 55)

from CVD and heart failure [23, 24]. In the larger, cross-sectional cohort of RA subjects, the strongest associations for galectin-3 were with age and measures of sarcopenic obesity (increased adiposity and reduced muscle mass). In the exercise-training cohort, prediabetes was chosen as a comparator group for having a baseline CVD risk similar to that of RA. Although those with RA were younger than those with prediabetes, RA had greater plasma galectin-3. This finding is aligned with a previous study showing greater levels of galectin-3 in RA sera and synovial fluid

[12]. Thus, galectin-3 may reflect non-traditional CVD risk factors, including sarcopenic obesity, which are present in younger persons with RA [16, 23, 24]. Most important, training-mediated reductions in galectin-3 were associated with improved cardiopulmonary fitness and cardiovascular function, indicative of reduced risk of mortality [25]. These findings suggest that galectin-3 may represent a novel risk factor for CVD and a marker of abnormal muscle remodeling in RA that can be modulated by exercise training.

In contrast to our hypothesis, plasma galectin-3, skeletal muscle cytokines, and muscle myostatin were unaffected by 10 weeks of high-intensity interval training in persons with RA and prediabetes. This is a surprising finding given that RA disease activity, as measured by DAS-28, significantly improved with exercise training, as previously discussed by our group [18]. One explanation for why plasma galectin-3 did not associate with disease activity is that it may more closely represent the chronic inflammatory state leading to CVD and mortality risk in RA as opposed to the acute inflammatory state that likely drives disease activity scores. We hypothesize that a longer duration of exercise training with more robust improvements in cardiorespiratory fitness would likely lead to significant reductions in systemic galectin-3 given the associations discussed above. The mechanisms driving exercise-training effects on acute and chronic systemic and tissue-specific inflammation certainly warrant further investigation.

However, despite insignificant group-level changes, reductions in muscle cytokines mIL-6, mIL-1β, and mTNF-α were associated with the goal body composition changes of increased lean mass and decreased body fat. Perhaps most interestingly, the association of reduced muscle IL-6 with improved body composition was greater in prediabetes than RA. Moreover, in prediabetes but not in RA, myostatin was reduced in association

Table 2 Skeletal muscle remodeling markers

	Rheumatoid arthritis ($n = 12$)		Pre-diabetes mellitus ($n = 9$)	
	Pre-HIIT	Post-HIIT	Pre-HIIT	Post-HIIT
Skeletal muscle concentrations, pg/mL per µg				
IL-1β	0.007 (0.005)	0.009 (0.006)	0.011 (0.010)	0.009 (0.006)
IL-6	0.010 (0.006)	0.013 (0.007)	0.012 (0.006)	0.017 (0.009)
IL-8	0.112 (0.212)	0.121 (0.168)	0.052 (0.024)	0.112 (0.081)
TNF-α	0.008 (0.007)	0.012 (0.006)	0.006 (0.004)	0.009 (0.007)
IL-10	0.009 (0.012)	0.006 (0.004)	0.005 (0.003)	0.005 (0.004)
Myostatin	16.621 (7.463)	20.589 (8.685)	31.884 (14.34)*	34.314 (20.08)*
Plasma concentrations, ng/mL				
Galectin-3	12.21 (6.72)	11.99 (4.22)	8.73 (2.31)	8.71 (2.70)

Sample skeletal muscle concentrations were normalized to initial masses. Continuous variable data are presented as mean (standard deviation). Abbreviations: *HIIT* high-intensity interval training, *IL* interleukin, *TNF-α* tumor necrosis factor-alpha
*P <0.05 for comparisons between rheumatoid arthritis and pre-diabetes mellitus groups

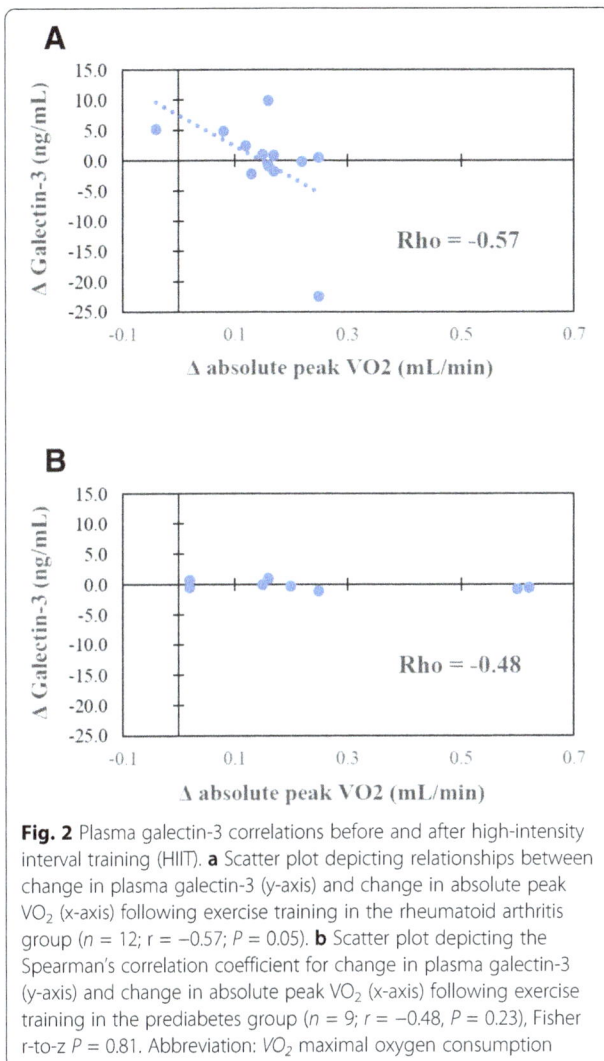

Fig. 2 Plasma galectin-3 correlations before and after high-intensity interval training (HIIT). **a** Scatter plot depicting relationships between change in plasma galectin-3 (y-axis) and change in absolute peak VO$_2$ (x-axis) following exercise training in the rheumatoid arthritis group ($n = 12$; $r = -0.57$; $P = 0.05$). **b** Scatter plot depicting the Spearman's correlation coefficient for change in plasma galectin-3 (y-axis) and change in absolute peak VO$_2$ (x-axis) following exercise training in the prediabetes group ($n = 9$; $r = -0.48$, $P = 0.23$), Fisher r-to-z $P = 0.81$. Abbreviation: VO$_2$ maximal oxygen consumption

with increased muscle mass. These cohort differences signify that skeletal muscle remodeling is impaired in RA even when compared with a group with similar CVD risk; in part, RA disease–specific features or pharmacologic agents (or both) may underlie the impaired adaptations to exercise training.

RA therapeutic agents may prevent or permit improved exercise-mediated muscle remodeling. Intriguingly, of the four patients with improved measures of sarcopenic obesity (combination of a decrease in body fat and an increase in lean body mass) after exercise training, none was concomitantly using TNF inhibitors or hydroxychloroquine. In addition, all four patients on TNF inhibitors had an increase in BMI and body fat at the end of the study. Our findings are supported by others, where tight control of RA disease activity with disease-modifying anti-rheumatic agents (DMARDs) without biologics or exercise training had no overall effect on body composition [26]. Interestingly, as

compared with those who received traditional DMARDs ("triple therapy" with methotrexate, sulfasalazine, and hydroxychloroquine), patients with early RA treated with a TNF inhibitor, infliximab, increased body fat [27]. A randomized trial comparing patients with early RA treated with etanercept compared with methotrexate found no difference in body composition in either group at 24 weeks, but there was a trend toward gaining fat-free mass by those on etanercept [28]. In contrast, patients with RA treated for 24 weeks with tocilizumab, a monoclonal antibody against IL-6 receptor, had no fat mass changes but increased lean mass [29]. Taken together, these results suggest that IL-6 inhibition, as opposed to TNF inhibition, may contribute to beneficial body composition changes in RA.

Obesity, sedentary behavior, and chronic inflammatory diseases such as RA are all associated with a chronic elevation in serum IL-6 [6, 30]. In response to acute exercise and in a TNF-α–independent fashion, skeletal muscle releases IL-6, leading to short-term beneficial metabolic and immunoregulatory effects [31]. With chronic exercise training, basal serum IL-6 is reduced [31]. Although we observed no overall change in skeletal muscle or serum IL-6 with exercise training, reductions in muscle IL-6 were tied to increased muscle mass more closely in subjects with prediabetes compared with RA. One possible explanation is that, in RA, persistently heightened systemic IL-6 contributes to sarcopenic obesity by impairing the normal muscle adaptive responses to exercise training. Specifically, chronic over-expression of systemic IL-6 dampens the skeletal muscle's secretion of, or response to, IL-6 with an acute exercise bout; furthermore, a vicious cycle of chronic inflammation and physical inactivity drives skeletal muscle "IL-6 resistance"—negating of the beneficial effects of IL-6—when released from skeletal muscle as a myokine [9, 32]. Whether IL-6 inhibition is the answer to counteract these maladaptive changes, improve body composition, and in turn decrease risk of CVD in RA merits further study.

In addition to IL-6, impaired myostatin and muscle cytokine signaling may contribute to RA-associated sarcopenic obesity. One would expect lower myostatin, as a potent negative regulator of skeletal muscle growth and hypertrophy, to correspond to greater lean mass [10]. However, despite less myostatin in RA, muscle mass was not greater than an older, prediabetic group. Also, while exercise training did not reduce either group's myostatin concentrations, myostatin responses were related to lean mass changes in prediabetes but not in RA. Thus, reducing myostatin appears insufficient for producing muscle hypertrophy in RA. Similarly, in RA, associations between responses in muscle cytokines and body composition were less pronounced than in prediabetes. Thus,

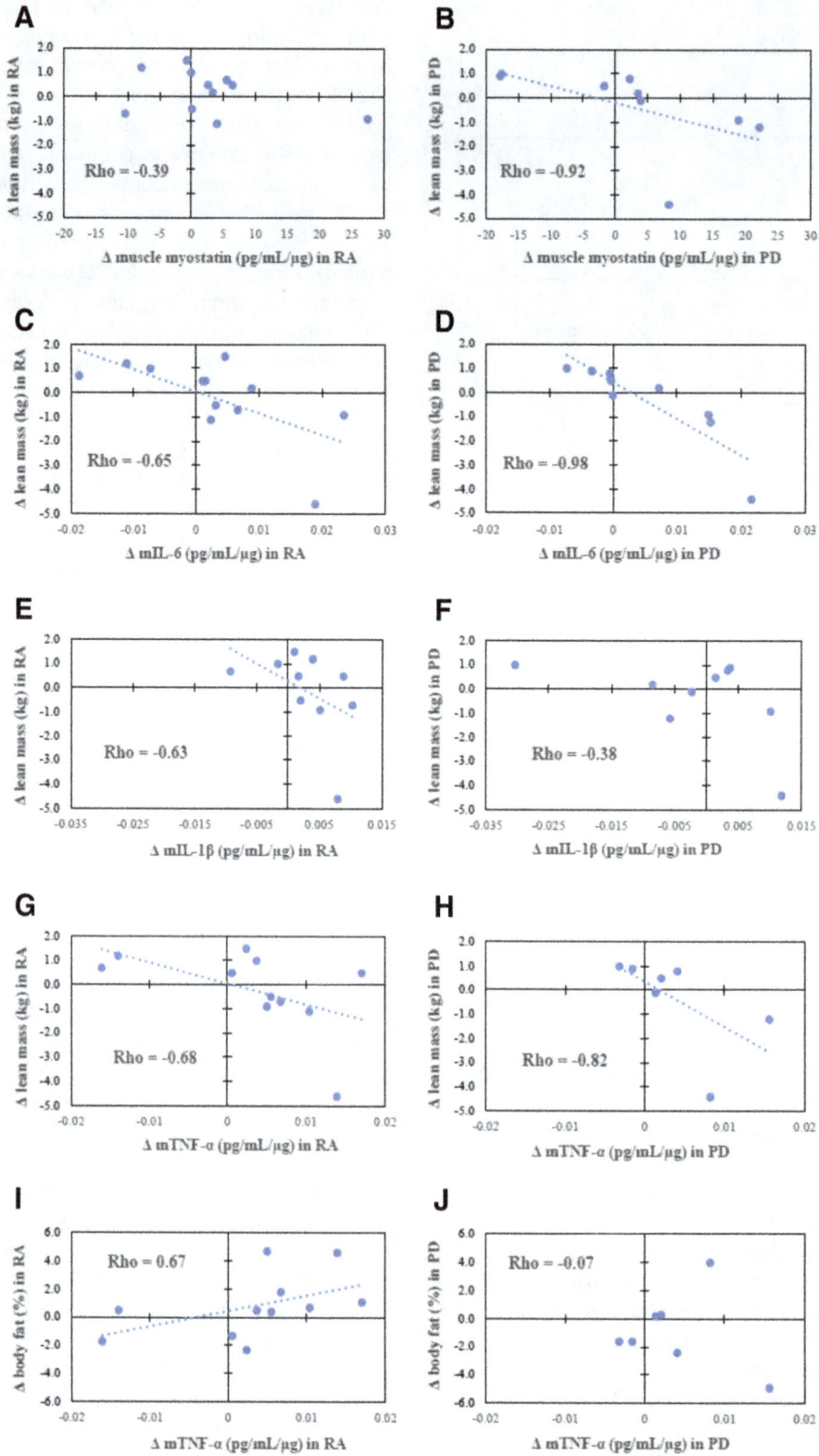

Fig. 3 (See legend on next page.)

(See figure on previous page.)

Fig. 3 Body composition correlations in rheumatoid arthritis (RA) and prediabetes. Scatter plot depicting the relationships between (**a**) change in lean mass (y-axis) and change in muscle myostatin (x-axis) following exercise training in RA ($r = -0.39$, $P = 0.23$); (**b**) change in lean mass and change in muscle myostatin in prediabetes (PD) ($r = -0.92$, $P = 0.0005$), Fisher r-to-z $P = 0.026$; (**c**) change in lean mass and change in muscle interleukin-6 (IL-6) in RA ($r = -0.65$; $P = 0.023$); (**d**) change in lean mass and change in muscle IL-6 in prediabetes ($r = -0.98$, $P <0.0001$), Fisher r-to-z $P = 0.0004$; (**e**) change in lean mass and change in muscle IL-1β in RA ($r = -0.63$; $P = 0.049$); (**f**) change in lean mass and change in muscle IL-1β in prediabetes ($r = -0.38$, $P = 0.31$), Fisher r-to-z $P = 0.516$; (**g**) change in lean mass and change in muscle tumor necrosis factor-alpha (TNF-α) in RA ($r = -0.68$; $P = 0.023$); (**h**) change in lean mass and change in muscle TNF-α in prediabetes ($r = -0.82$, $P = 0.002$), Fisher r-to-z $P = 0.516$; (**i**) change in body fat percentage and change in muscle TNF-α in RA ($r = 0.67$; $P = 0.022$); and (**j**) change in body fat percentage and change in muscle TNF-α in prediabetes ($r = -0.07$, $P = 0.88$), Fisher r-to-z $P = 0.095$

although exercise training may improve coordination of cytokines and myokines critical for skeletal muscle remodeling, in RA, muscle adaptations to exercise training appear disrupted, possibly by external influences such as medication use or systemic immune dysregulation.

As is the nature of a pilot study, this investigation has multiple limitations. With a larger sample size or a longer duration of exercise training, we may have detected significant within- and between-group training-induced changes in skeletal muscle remodeling markers. Additionally, individuals with RA received multiple pharmacologic regimens, complicating analyses to determine effects of individual medications or combinations on muscle remodeling. Despite this, fascinatingly, no patient using a TNF inhibitor or hydroxychloroquine achieved the goal body composition change of a net decrease in body fat and increase in lean mass. Although we did not identify the cellular source of muscle cytokines and myostatin, it is notable that serum cytokines were found to have minimal association with cytokines measured in muscle tissue.

Conclusions

After a 10-week high-intensity interval training program in both RA and prediabetes cohorts, changes in intramuscular cytokine profiles were associated with the goal body composition changes of increased lean muscle mass and decreased body fat percentage. Decreased serum galectin-3 was also associated with decreased intramuscular fat in the cross-sectional RA cohort and with improved cardiorespiratory fitness after exercise training. These findings suggest that exercise-mediated body composition and cardiovascular risk improvements are closely tied to—and likely depend upon—effective muscle remodeling. However, the correlations of muscle remodeling markers (myostatin and cytokines) with favorable body composition outcomes were stronger in prediabetes than in RA. These differences provide further evidence to support the occurrence of abnormal muscle remodeling in RA and offer insights into the etiology of exercise intolerance and disability in RA. Further work should focus on better understanding the complex interplay between disease-modifying pharmacotherapy, exercise, cardiorespiratory fitness, and body composition to better improve disability and decrease the risk of CVD and mortality in RA.

Table 3 Body composition change after high-intensity interval training and rheumatoid arthritis medication use

	Increased lean mass (%)	Decreased fat mass (%)
Medication use		
TNFi	3/4 (75.0%)	0/4 (0.0%)
Tofacitinib	1/1 (100.0%)	1/1 (100.0%)
Methotrexate	4/6 (66.7%)	3/6 (50.0%)
Leflunomide	1/1 (100.0%)	0/1 (0.0%)
Sulfasalazine	1/2 (50.0%)	1/2 (50.0%)
Hydroxychloroquine	1/4 (25.0%)	0/4 (0.0%)
NSAIDs	5/8 (62.5%)	2/8 (25.0%)
Prednisone	3/3 (100.0%)	1/3 (33.3%)

Subjects were identified as achieving increased lean mass if their absolute change in lean mass (kilograms) was greater than zero following exercise training. Subjects were identified as achieving decreased fat mass if their absolute change in fat mass (kilograms) was less than zero following exercise training. Medication use was identified on the basis of whether subjects were taking those medications for the duration of the exercise-training program. Abbreviations: *NSAID* non-steroidal anti-inflammatory agent, *TNFi* tumor necrosis factor inhibitor

Abbreviations
ACR: American College of Rheumatology; BMI: Body mass index; CVD: Cardiovascular disease; DAS-28: Disease Activity Score in 28 joints; DMARD: Disease-modifying anti-rheumatic agent; IL-6: Interleukin-6; RA: Rheumatoid arthritis; TNF: Tumor necrosis factor; VO_2: Maximal oxygen consumption

Acknowledgments
We acknowledge the staff members at the Duke Center for Living for their help with training and with recording of data. We appreciate the support of the Division of Rheumatology and Immunology at Duke University. We acknowledge and greatly appreciate all the participants.

Funding
This work was funded by a Duke Department of Medicine Faculty Resident Research Grant (to BJA) and an EU Marie Curie Outgoing Fellowship Grant (to DBB) (PIOF-GA-2013-629981).

Authors' contributions
BJA, DBB, VBK, WEK, and KMH conceived and designed the study and experimental approach. DBB, LW, and AH performed the physiological and

functional testing and exercise training of participants. KMH performed the skeletal muscle biopsies. JLH completed the plasma galectin-3 and muscle cytokine and myostatin analyses. BJA and KMH performed statistical analyses. BJA wrote the manuscript. All authors contributed to the writing and approval of the final manuscript.

Competing interests
The authors declare that they have no competing interests.

References
1. Svensson AL, Christensen R, Persson F, Løgstrup BB, Giraldi A, Graugaard C, et al. Multifactorial intervention to prevent cardiovascular disease in patients with early rheumatoid arthritis: protocol for a multicentre randomised controlled trial. BMJ Open. 2016;6:e009134.
2. Holmqvist ME, Wedren S, Jacobsson LT, Klareskog L, Nyberg F, Rantapää-Dahlqvist S, et al. Rapid increase in myocardial infarction risk following diagnosis of rheumatoid arthritis amongst patients diagnosed between 1995 and 2006. J Intern Med. 2010;268:578–85.
3. Lindhardsen JO, Ahlehoff O, Gislason GH, Madsen OR, Olesen JB, Torp-Pedersen C, et al. The risk of myocardial infarction in rheumatoid arthritis and diabetes mellitus: a Danish nationwide cohort study. Ann Rheum Dis. 2011;70:929–34.
4. Biolo G, Cederholm T, Muscaritoli M. Muscle contractile and metabolic dysfunction is a common feature of sarcopenia of aging and chronic diseases: from sarcopenic obesity to cachexia. Clin Nutr. 2014;33:737–48.
5. Giles JT, Ling SM, Ferrucci L, Bartlett SJ, Andersen RE, Towns M, et al. Abnormal body composition phenotypes in older rheumatoid arthritis patients: association with disease characteristics and pharmacotherapies. Arthritis Rheum. 2008;59:807–15.
6. Huffman KM, Jessee R, Andonian B, Davis BN, Narowski R, Huebner JL, et al. Molecular alterations in skeletal muscle in rheumatoid arthritis are related to disease activity, physical inactivity, and disability. Arthritis Res Ther. 2017;19:12.
7. Novak ML, Koh TJ. Phenotypic transitions of macrophages orchestrate tissue repair. Am J Pathol. 2013;183:1352–63.
8. Lightfoot AP, Cooper RG. The role of myokines in muscle health and disease. Curr Opin Rheumatol. 2016;28:661–6.
9. Pedersen BK, Febbraio MA. Muscles, exercise and obesity: skeletal muscle as a secretory organ. Nat Rev Endocrinol. 2012;8:457–65.
10. Rodriguez J, Vernus B, Chelh I, Cassar-Malek I, Gabillard JC, Hadj Sassi A, et al. Myostatin and the skeletal muscle atrophy and hypertrophy signaling pathways. Cell Mol Life Sci. 2014;71:4361–71.
11. Rancourt A, Dufresne S, St-Pierre G, Lévesque J, Nakamura H, Kikuchi Y, et al. Galectin-3 and N-acetylglucosamine promote myogenesis and improve skeletal muscle function in the mdx model of Duchenne muscular dystrophy. FASEB J. 2018:fj201701151RRR.
12. Ohshima S, Kuchen S, Seemayer CA, Kyburz D, Hirt A, Klinzing S, et al. Galectin 3 and its binding protein in rheumatoid arthritis. Arthritis Rheum. 2003;48:2788–95.
13. Forsman H, Islander U, Andréasson E, Andersson A, Onnheim K, Karlström A, et al. Galectin 3 aggravates joint inflammation and destruction in antigen-induced arthritis. Arthritis Rheum. 2011;63:445–54.
14. Henderson NC, Sethi T. The regulation of inflammation by galectin-3. Immunol Rev. 2009;230:160–71.
15. Henderson NC, Mackinnon AC, Farnworth SL, Kipari T, Haslett C, Iredale JP, et al. Galectin-3 expression and secretion links macrophages to the promotion of renal fibrosis. Am J Pathol. 2008;172:288–98.
16. Issa SF, Christensen AF, Lottenburger T, Junker K, Lindegaard H, Hørslev-Petersen K, et al. Within-day variation and influence of physical exercise on circulating Galectin-3 in patients with rheumatoid arthritis and healthy individuals. Scand J Immunol. 2015;82:70–5.
17. Arnett FC, Edworthy SM, Bloch DA, McShane DJ, Fries JF, Cooper NS, et al. The American Rheumatism Association 1987 revised criteria for the classification of rheumatoid arthritis. Arthritis Rheum. 1988;31:315–24.
18. Bartlett DB, Willis LH, Slentz CA, Hoselton A, Kelly L, Heubner JL, et al. Ten weeks of high-intensity interval walk training is associated with reduced disease activity and improved innate immune function in older adults with rheumatoid arthritis: a pilot study. Arthritis Res Ther. 2018;20:127.
19. Prevoo ML, van't Hof MA, Kuper HH, van Leeuwen MA, van de Putte LB, van Riel PL. Modified disease activity scores that include twenty eight-joint counts. Development and validation in a prospective longitudinal study of patients with rheumatoid arthritis. Arthritis Rheum. 1995;38:44–8.
20. Bergstrom J. Percutaneous needle biopsy of skeletal muscle in physiological and clinical research. Scand J Clin Lab Invest. 1975;35:609–16.
21. AbouAssi H, Tune KN, Gilmore B, Bateman LA, McDaniel G, Muehlbauer M, et al. Adipose depots, not disease-related factors, account for skeletal muscle insulin sensitivity in established and treated rheumatoid arthritis. J Rheumatol. 2014;41:1974–9.
22. VassarStats: website for statistical computation. Vassar College. 1998–2015. http://vassarstats.net. Accessed May 2017.
23. van der Velde AR, Gullestad L, Ueland T, Aukrust P, Guo Y, Adourian A, et al. Prognostic value of changes in galectin-3 levels over time in patients with heart failure: data from CORONA and COACH. Circ Heart Fail. 2013;6:219–26.
24. Imran TF, Shin HJ, Mathenge N, Wang F, Kim B, Joseph J, et al. Meta-Analysis of the Usefulness of Plasma Galectin-3 to Predict the Risk of Mortality in Patients With Heart Failure and in the General Population. Am J Cardiol. 2017;119:57–64.
25. Harber MP, Kaminsky LA, Arena R, Blair SN, Franklin BA, Myers J, et al. Impact of Cardiorespiratory Fitness on All-Cause and Disease-Specific Mortality: Advances Since 2009. Prog Cardiovasc Dis. 2017;60:11–20.
26. Lemmey AB, Wilkinson TJ, Clayton RJ, Sheikh F, Whale J, Jones HS, et al. Tight control of disease activity fails to improve body composition or physical function in rheumatoid arthritis patients. Rheumatology (Oxford). 2016;55:1736–45.
27. Engvall IL, Tengstrand B, Brismar K, Hafström I. Infliximab therapy increases body fat mass in early rheumatoid arthritis independently of changes in disease activity and levels of leptin and adiponectin: a randomised study over 21 months. Arthritis Res Ther. 2010;12:R197.
28. Marcora SM, Chester KR, Mittal G, Lemmey AB, Maddison PJ. Randomized phase 2 trial of anti-tumor necrosis factor therapy for cachexia in patients with early rheumatoid arthritis. Am J Clin Nutr. 2006;84:1463–72.
29. Tournadre A, Pereira B, Dutheil F, Giraud C, Courteix D, Sapin V, et al. Changes in body composition and metabolic profile during interleukin 6 inhibition in rheumatoid arthritis. J Cachexia Sarcopenia Muscle. 2017;8:639–46.
30. Bastard JP, Jardel C, Bruckert E, Blondy P, Capeau J, Laville M, et al. Elevated levels of interleukin 6 are reduced in serum and subcutaneous adipose tissue of obese women after weight loss. J Clin Endocrinol Metab. 2000;85:3338–42.
31. Fischer CP. Interleukin-6 in acute exercise and training: what is the biological relevance? Exerc Immunol Rev. 2006;12:6–33.
32. Benatti FB, Pedersen BK. Exercise as an anti-inflammatory therapy for rheumatic diseases-myokine regulation. Nat Rev Rheumatol. 2015;11:86–97.

17

Cardiovascular risk factors predate the onset of symptoms of rheumatoid arthritis

Heidi Kokkonen[1]*[iD], Hans Stenlund[2] and Solbritt Rantapää-Dahlqvist[1]

Abstract

Background: Patients with rheumatoid arthritis (RA) are at increased risk of developing cardiovascular disease (CVD). Our aim was to evaluate the impact of factors related to CVD, such as smoking, lipid levels, hypertension, body mass index (BMI) and diabetes, in individuals prior to the onset of symptoms of RA.

Methods: A nested case–control study was performed including data from 547 pre-symptomatic individuals (i.e. individuals who had participated in population surveys in northern Sweden prior to onset of symptoms of RA, median time to symptom onset 5.0 (interquartile range 2.0–9.0) years) and 1641 matched controls. Within the survey, health examinations prior to symptom onset were performed, blood samples were analysed for plasma glucose and lipids, and data on lifestyle factors had been collected with a questionnaire. CVD risk factors were extracted and further analysed with conditional logistic regression models for association with subsequent RA development, including hypertension, apolipoprotein (Apo)B/ApoA1 ratio, BMI, diabetes and smoking habits.

Results: Smoking and BMI $\geq$ 25 (odds ratio (OR) (95% confidence interval (CI)) =1.86 (1.48–2.35) and OR = 1.28 (1.01–1.62) , respectively) were associated with increased risk for future RA development. In women, elevated ApoB/ApoA1 ratio (OR = 1.36 (1.03–1.80)) and smoking (OR = 1.82 (1.37–2.41)) were significantly associated with being pre-symptomatic for RA, whilst in men smoking (OR = 1.92 (1.26–2.92)) and diabetes (OR = 3.62 (95% CI 1.13–11.64)) were significant. In older (>50.19 years) individuals, only smoking (OR = 1.74 (1.24–2.45)) was significantly associated with increased risk of future RA, whereas in younger individuals the significant factors were elevated ApoB/ApoA1 ratio (OR = 1.39 (1.00–1.93)), BMI $\geq$ 25.0 (OR = 1.45 (1.04–2.02)) and smoking (OR = 2.11 (1.51–2.95)). Pre-symptomatic individuals had a higher frequency of risk factors: 41.5% had $\geq$3 compared with 30.4% among matched controls (OR = 2.81 (1.78–4.44)).

Conclusions: Several risk factors for CVD were present in pre-symptomatic individuals and significantly associated with increased risk for future RA. These factors differed in women and men. The CVD risk factors had a greater impact in younger individuals. These results urge an early analysis of cardiovascular risk factors for proposed prevention in patients with early RA.

Keywords: Rheumatoid arthritis, Cardiovascular disease, Body mass index, Apolipoproteins, Diabetes mellitus, Smoking

* Correspondence: heidi.kokkonen@umu.se
[1]Department of Public Health and Clinical Medicine, Rheumatology, Umeå University, Building 6M, 901 87 Umeå, Sweden
Full list of author information is available at the end of the article

Background

Patients with rheumatoid arthritis (RA) have an increased risk of developing several co-morbidities compared with the general population, the commonest co-morbidity being cardiovascular disease (CVD) [1]. Patients with RA also have an increased risk of mortality due to CVD [2–5]. The prevalence of CVD is comparable with that in patients with type 2 diabetes [6]. The aetiology of this increased morbidity and mortality is not fully understood, although traditional risk factors (i.e. cigarette smoking, hypertension, diabetes mellitus and elevated levels of low-density lipoproteins) as well as the inflammatory burden are involved [1, 2, 7, 8].

In a retrospective cohort study, RA patients had a significantly higher risk of hospitalization for either acute or unrecognized myocardial infarction (MI) prior to developing RA [9]. However, in another study no increased risk of ischaemic heart disease, MI or angina pectoris before the onset of RA was reported [10]. The risk of MI was increased, being apparent 1–4 years following diagnosis of RA [11]. In a nested case–control study analysing the presence of risk factors for CVD in individuals prior to development of inflammatory polyarthritis (IP), the only risk factor associated with IP development was smoking [12]. Other CVD risk factors (e.g. total cholesterol, low-density lipoprotein (LDL) cholesterol, systolic and diastolic blood pressure and obesity) were not increased prior to onset of IP [12]. Conversely, a study of individuals prior to onset of symptoms of RA reported a more atherogenic lipid profile with higher levels of total cholesterol, triglycerides and apolipoprotein (Apo)B in addition to lower levels of high-density lipoprotein (HDL) cholesterol compared with control subjects, independent of RF and ACPA, and marginally affected by CRP [13]. A contradictory study reported a significant decrease in levels of total cholesterol as well as LDL-cholesterol and HDL-cholesterol during the 5 years prior to diagnosis of RA compared with non-RA controls [14].

Obesity has been identified as a risk factor for RA [15] and recently we identified that abdominal obesity was associated with an increased risk of subsequent development of RA [16]. After stratification for sex, this association was restricted to men with an early disease onset [16].

The presence of insulin resistance after onset of RA is known, whilst the presence of diabetes before RA onset has been sparsely reported. In one study, the presence of diabetes was associated with increased risk for RA development in women [17].

The aim of this study was to compare lifestyle factors, lipid levels, presence of hypertension and diabetes in individuals prior to onset of symptoms of RA with matched controls in a nested case–control design based on a population-based intervention project from northern Sweden.

Methods

Study cohorts

This study was based on information from the Västerbotten Intervention Programme (VIP) and the Northern Sweden Multinational Monitoring of Trends and Determinants in Cardiovascular Disease (MONICA). The VIP, details of which have been described previously [18], is a population-based study aimed at reducing morbidity and mortality due to CVD and diabetes in northern Sweden. Briefly, since 1991, all individuals aged 40, 50 and 60 years living in the county of Västerbotten are invited to participate in a health assessment at their local primary care centre; the participation rate throughout has been approximately 60% [19]. All participants complete a health questionnaire regarding socioeconomic and demographic status, educational level (analysed as no academic education/university vs academic education/university), self-reported health (including medication) and lifestyle (e.g. exercise and smoking habits). Blood samples were drawn and analysed for total cholesterol, triglycerides, HDL-cholesterol, and LDL-cholesterol according to routine protocols, with excess samples stored at $-80°$ for future analysis. Plasma glucose (baseline) was measured in an overnight fasting sample together with a sample 2 hours after the intake of 75 g anhydrous glucose. Blood pressure was measured twice, the mean value reported. Waist circumference (cm) was measured and the body mass index (BMI; kg/m^2) was calculated.

Details for the registration and survey procedures in the Northern Sweden MONICA project including the two most northern counties have been described previously [20]. Briefly, since 1986, seven population surveys including a physical examination and a questionnaire similar to that used in the VIP have been performed. At examination, blood samples were drawn for analysis, as in the VIP project.

Identification of individuals before onset of symptoms of RA

In 2014, the registers of patients attending the Department of Rheumatology, University Hospital, Umeå, Sweden (the only department within the county) and fulfilling the 1987 ARA criteria for diagnosis of RA since 1995 were co-analysed with those from the VIP and MONICA. This linkage identified 557 individuals having participated in these cohorts prior to the onset of symptoms of joint disease ("pre-symptomatic individual" or case). For each case, three controls were selected randomly, matched for sex, year of birth, participation in the VIP or MONICA and living in a rural or urban area, resulting in 1671 controls without known RA until the end of 2014. In a second evaluation of the cases, 10 of the pre-symptomatic individuals and corresponding controls were excluded due to having experienced symptoms prior to participation in the VIP, resulting in 547 pre-symptomatic individuals (498 (91%) from the

VIP and 49 (9%) from MONICA) and 1641 controls (1494 (91%) from the VIP and 147 (9%) from MONICA) identified for inclusion in this study. The median (Q1–Q3) age of the pre-symptomatic individuals was 50.19 (45.50–59.95) years and for controls was 50.26 (45.94–59.97) years, and the median pre-dating time to symptom onset was 5.0 (2.0–9.0) years. The median (Q1–Q3) duration of follow-up for the controls was 17.0 (14.0–21.0) years.

Analyses of ApoA1 and ApoB
ApoA1 (g/L) and ApoB (g/L) were analysed from stored samples using an immunoturbimetric method (Cobas 8000 instrument; Roche Diagnostics Scandinavia AB).

Statistical analyses
Statistical calculations were performed using SPSS for Windows version 23.0 (IBM Corp., NY, USA). The associations with future RA were analysed in conditional logistic regression models with calculated odds ratios (ORs) and 95% confidence intervals (CIs). All p values are two-sided and $p < 0.05$ was considered statistically significant. Cardiovascular risk factors were selected according to previous studies and scoring systems as risk for CVD, defined as risk if presence of the following are present: hypertension (systolic blood pressure (SBP) ≥ 140 mmHg and/or diastolic blood pressure (DBP) ≥ 90 mmHg, including hypertensive treatment), diabetes (self-reported in questionnaires), BMI ≥ 25.0, elevated ApoB/ApoA1 ratio (women > 0.7, men > 0.8, including lipid lowering therapy) and smoking habits (analysed as current, ex and ever smoker but presented as ever smoker). A risk factor profile was defined as the number of risk factors present (having no risk factor as reference, or having one, two, or three or more) modified from the study by Berry et al. [21]. Results from analyses of HDL-cholesterol and LDL-cholesterol were lacking for approximately two-thirds of the individuals, whereas for the risk factors for CVD chosen to analyse further for associations with future development of RA, data on BMI, blood pressure, diabetes and smoking were available for 98.0–99.5% of the individuals and results of the ApoA1 and ApoB levels were available for 83% of the cases and 85% of the controls. Missing data for the ApoB/ApoA1 ratio was constructed using five imputations modelled by all data on CV risk factors, sex and age using the SPSS 23.0 program (IBM Corp.). Results from the original data are presented.

Results
Smoking, either as current, ex or ever, were all significantly more prevalent among pre-symptomatic individuals compared with controls (OR (95% CI) = 2.74 (2.15–3.51), 1.52 (1.19–1.95) and 2.01 (1.64–2.47), respectively)

(Table 1). This variable was therefore dichotomized into never or ever smokers in subsequent analyses.

The pre-symptomatic individuals had a significantly higher BMI (analysed as a continuous variable) compared with controls in conditional logistic regression models (OR = 1.03 (1.00–1.05)) (Table 1). When stratified for sex, BMI remained significantly higher in the pre-symptomatic women compared with matched controls (OR = 1.03 (1.00–1.06)) (Table 1). The same pattern was observed for waist circumference, with significantly greater circumference for cases compared with controls, remaining significant for women when stratified for sex (Table 1).

A low educational level (no academic/university qualification) was associated with an increased risk for future RA (OR = 1.41 (1.07–1.84)), which was restricted to men (OR = 2.15 (1.23–3.78)) (Table 1).

Lipid levels
Higher levels of ApoA1 were associated with a lower risk for future RA (OR = 0.50 (0.31–0.80)), and this was restricted to women when stratifying for sex (OR = 0.49 (0.28–0.85)) (Table 2). The ApoB/ApoA1 ratio (analysed as a continuous variable) was associated with risk for future RA with a higher ratio among pre-symptomatic women compared with controls (OR = 2.25 (1.25–4.06)) (Table 2). In conditional logistic regression analyses there were no significant differences in the levels of total cholesterol, HDL-cholesterol, LDL-cholesterol or triglycerides in cases compared with controls (Table 2). There were also no differences in these factors after stratification for sex (Table 2).

Plasma glucose and blood pressure
The cases had significantly higher plasma glucose levels at baseline, and after stratification for sex the association with higher risk for future RA was restricted to men (OR = 1.11 (1.00–1.22) and 1.18 (1.01–1.37), respectively) (Table 2). Plasma glucose levels at 2 hours showed no differences in pre-symptomatic individuals compared with controls, and neither did the systolic or diastolic blood pressure (Table 2).

Risk factors for CVD
Results from univariable conditional logistic regression analyses for selected risk factors for CVD (analysed as dichotomous variables), including elevated ApoB/ApoA1 ratio (men ≥0.8 compared with <0.8, women ≥0.7 compared with <0.7), ever smoking (vs never smoking), BMI ≥ 25 (vs BMI < 25.0), diabetes (vs no diabetes) and hypertension (systolic blood pressure (SBP) ≥ 140 mmHg and/or diastolic blood pressure DBP ≥ 90 mmHg including treatment for hypertension compared with SBP < 140 mmHg and DBP < 90 mmHg and no ongoing hypertensive treatment), are presented in Table 3. All factors,

Table 1 Results from conditional logistic regression analyses of pre-symptomatic individuals compared with controls presented for all individuals and stratified for women and men, respectively

	Pre-symptomatic individuals (n = 547)	Controls (n = 1641)	OR (95% CI)	Pre-symptomatic women (n = 372)	Control women (n = 1116)	OR (95% CI)	Pre-symptomatic men (n = 175)	Control men (n = 525)	OR (95% CI)
Smoking ever[a]	366/540 (67.8)	823/1609 (51.1)	2.01 (1.64–2.47)	241/366 (65.8)	548/1096 (50.0)	1.92 (1.50–2.47)	125/174 (71.8)	275/513 (53.6)	2.23 (1.53–3.27)
Current smoker[a]	197/538 (36.6)	326/1603 (20.3)	2.74 (2.15–3.51)	133/365 (36.4)	245/1094 (22.4)	2.01 (1.54–2.61)	64/173 (37.0)	81/509 (15.9)	3.11 (2.09–4.64)
Ex smoker[a]	167/538 (31.0)	491/1603 (30.6)	1.52 (1.19–1.95)	107/365 (29.3)	301/1094 (27.5)	1.56 (1.16–2.10)	60/173 (34.7)	190/509 (37.3)	1.49 (0.97–2.30)
Oral tobacco (snuff)	102/494 (20.6)	278/1491 (18.6)	1.22 (0.91–1.63)	22/329 (6.7)	77/998 (7.7)	0.93 (0.56–1.55)	80/165 (48.5)	201/493 (40.8)	1.40 (0.97–2.00)
BMI (kg/m^2)[b]	25.7 (23.1–28.6) (n = 544)	25.3 (23.1–28.1) (n = 1634)	1.03 (1.00–1.05)	25.5 (22.8–28.6) (n = 369)	25.5 (22.8–28.6) (n = 1111)	1.03 (1.00–1.06)	26.0 (24.0–28.4) (n = 175)	26.0 (24.0–28.4) (n = 523)	1.02 (0.98–1.07)
Waist[c] (cm)	93.0 (82.0–102.0) (n = 103)	89.0 (81.0–97.0) (n = 307)	1.02 (1.00–1.04)	85.5 (78.8–100.0) (n = 70)	85.0 (78.0–93.0) (n = 204)	1.02 (1.00–1.04)	98.0 (93.5–107.0) (n = 33)	96.0 (90.0–102.0) (n = 103)	1.03 (0.99–1.07)
Low education level[b,d]	452/540 (83.7)	1273/1613 (78.9)	1.41 (1.07–1.84)	294/366 (80.3)	854/1101 (77.6)	1.21 (0.88–1.65)	158/174 (90.8)	419/512 (81.8)	2.15 (1.23–3.78)
Hypertensive treatment	76/451 (16.9)	242/1333 (18.2)	0.84 (0.61–1.15)	47/306 (15.4)	168/899 (18.7)	0.70 (0.47–1.04)	29/145 (20.0)	74/434 (17.1)	1.20 (0.70–2.07)
Lipid lowering treatment	14/390 (3.6)	47/1164 (4.0)	0.73 (0.36–1.47)	6/266 (2.3)	24/773 (3.1)	0.46 (0.15–1.42)	8/124 (6.5)	23/391 (5.9)	1.06 (0.42–2.68)

Data presented as n (%) or median (Q1–Q3)

Odds ratio (OR) with 95% confidence interval (CI) in conditional logistic regression

BMI body mass index

[a]Reference group being never smoker

[b]OR per unit of increase

[c]Waist as continuous variable

[d]Low education level = no academic education/university

Table 2 Plasma glucose, blood pressure, total cholesterol, HDL-cholesterol, LDL-cholesterol, ApoA1 and ApoB in pre-symptomatic individuals and controls

	Pre-symptomatic individuals (n = 547)	Controls (n = 1641)	OR (95% CI)	Pre-symptomatic women (n = 372)	Control women (n = 1116)	OR (95% CI)	Pre-symptomatic men (n = 175)	Control men (n = 525)	OR (95% CI)
Plasma glucose, 0 hours (mmol/L)[a]	5.40 (5.05–5.84) (n = 513)	5.40 (5.00–5.80) (n = 1543)	1.11 (1.00–1.22)	5.40 (5.00–5.80) (n = 349)	5.38 (5.00–5.80) (n = 1052)	1.05 (0.92–1.21)	5.50 (5.10–6.00) (n = 164)	5.50 (5.10–5.90) (n = 491)	1.18 (1.01–1.37)
Plasma glucose, 2 hours (mmol/L)[a]	6.60 (5.70–7.30) (n = 470)	6.70 (5.90–7.60) (n = 1473)	0.94 (0.88–1.01)	6.67 (5.80–7.4) (n = 327)	6.80 (6.00–7.70) (n = 1005)	0.92 (0.85–1.00)	6.38 (5.40–7.10) (n = 143)	6.40 (5.40–7.40) (n = 468)	0.98 (0.87–1.10)
Systolic blood pressure (mmHg)[a]	128 (118–140) (n = 542)	129 (118–140) (n = 1637)	1.00 (0.99–1.01)	128 (115–140) (n = 368)	127 (118–140) (n = 1113)	1.00 (0.99–1.01)	128 (120–139) (n = 174)	130 (120–140) (n = 524)	1.00 (0.99–1.01)
Diastolic blood pressure (mmHg)[a]	80 (70–88) (n = 542)	80 (72–86) (n = 1635)	1.00 (0.99–1.01)	79 (70–87) (n = 368)	80 (70–85) (n = 1112)	1.00 (0.98–1.01)	80 (75–90) (n = 174)	80 (75–90) (n = 523)	1.00 (0.99–1.02)
Total cholesterol (mmol/L)[a]	5.74 (5.01–6.49) (n = 535)	5.70 (4.93–6.50) (n = 1619)	1.04 (0.96–1.14)	5.74 (5.01–6.57) (n = 361)	5.71 (4.94–6.57) (n = 1103)	1.04 (0.93–1.16)	5.76 (5.03–6.46) (n = 174)	5.70 (4.90–6.48) (n = 516)	1.06 (0.91–1.23)
Triglycerides (mmol/L)[a]	1.20 (0.89–1.60) (n = 453)	1.18 (0.84–1.70) (n = 1390)	0.95 (0.82–1.10)	1.16 (0.83–1.56) (n = 312)	1.14 (0.80–1.60) (n = 960)	0.95 (0.79–1.15)	1.29 (0.96–1.70) (n = 141)	1.36 (0.95–1.87) (n = 430)	0.94 (0.75–1.18)
HDL-cholesterol (mmol/L)[a]	1.26 (1.04–1.51) (n = 152)	1.32 (1.08–1.60) (n = 517)	0.81 (0.46–1.46)	1.30 (1.10–1.54) (n = 100)	1.40 (1.19–1.66) (n = 341)	0.65 (0.32–1.34)	1.19 (0.92–1.40) (n = 52)	1.14 (0.96–1.39) (n = 176)	1.60 (0.49–5.22)
LDL-cholesterol (mmol/L)[a]	4.13 (3.15–4.76) (n = 143)	4.07 (3.19–4.79) (n = 474)	1.12 (0.90–1.41)	4.08 (3.13–4.61) (n = 96)	4.02 (3.20–4.79) (n = 320)	1.06 (0.80–1.40)	4.28 (3.60–5.06) (n = 47)	4.14 (3.17–4.84) (n = 154)	1.25 (0.85–1.83)
ApoA1 (g/L)[a]	1.39 (1.23–1.57) (n = 453)	1.42 (1.28–1.59) (n = 1389)	0.50 (0.31–0.80)	1.46 (1.28–1.60) (n = 304)	1.47 (1.33–1.63) (n = 943)	0.49 (0.28–0.85)	1.31 (1.15–1.46) (n = 149)	1.32 (1.20–1.47) (n = 446)	0.53 (0.22–1.30)
ApoB (g/L)[a]	1.05 (0.86–1.24) (n = 453)	1.02 (0.86–1.21) (n = 1390)	1.50 (0.96–2.36)	1.02 (0.84–1.22) (n = 304)	1.00 (0.84–1.17) (n = 944)	1.66 (0.95–2.91)	1.11 (0.93–1.28) (n = 149)	1.09 (0.91–1.27) (n = 446)	1.24 (0.58–2.67)
Ratio ApoB/ApoA1	0.75 (0.60–0.93) (n = 453)	0.71 (0.58–0.88) (n = 1389)	2.05 (1.28–3.29)	0.70 (0.57–0.87) (n = 304)	0.67 (0.56–0.82) (n = 943)	2.25 (1.25–4.06)	0.86 (0.69–1.03) (n = 149)	0.82 (0.67–1.00) (n = 446)	1.74 (0.79–3.83)

Data presented as median (Q1–Q3)

Odds ratio (OR) and 95% confidence interval (CI) for future development of rheumatoid arthritis calculated with conditional logistic regression analyses for continuous variables in univariable analyses

Apo apolipoprotein, HDL high-density lipoprotein, LDL low-density lipoprotein

[a]OR per unit of increase

Table 3 Odds ratio (95%) for association of risk factors for cardiovascular disease with future RA from univariable and multivariable conditional logistic regression models

	Elevated ApoB/ApoA1[a]	Smoking, ever[b]	BMI ≥ 25.0[c] (kg/m^2)	Diabetes	Hypertension[d]
Cases	241 (52.9)	366 (67.8)	322 (59.9)	17 (3.1)	78 (14.3)
Controls	667 (47.0)	832 (51.3)	850 (52.7)	27 (1.6)	268 (16.3)
Univariable	1.25 (1.01–1.56)*	2.00 (1.63–2.47)***	1.33 (1.09–1.63)**	1.98 (1.06–3.68)*	0.89 (0.72–1.11)
Multivariable	1.19 (0.95–1.50)	1.86 (1.48–2.35)***	1.28 (1.01–1.62)*	1.75 (0.86–3.58)	0.87 (0.67–1.11)
Univariable, women	1.41 (1.09–1.84)*	1.92 (1.50–2.47)***	1.34 (1.06–1.71)*	1.11 (0.46–2.67)	1.01 (0.77–1.32)
Multivariable, women	1.36 (1.03–1.80)*	1.82 (1.37–2.41)***	1.16 (0.87–1.54)	1.11 (0.41–2.99)	0.99 (0.72–1.34)
Univariable, men	0.99 (0.68–1.43)	2.23 (1.53–3.27)***	1.31 (0.91–1.90)	4.73 (1.71–13.08)**	0.76 (0.52–1.09)
multivariable, men	0.94 (0.63–1.40)	1.92 (1.26–2.92)**	1.56 (1.01–2.39)*	3.62 (1.13–11.64)*	0.67 (0.43–1.03)
Univariable, age ≤ 50.19 years	1.51 (1.11–2.06)**	2.20 (1.62–2.98)***	1.45 (1.09–1.93)*	2.09 (0.56–7.84)	0.88 (0.62–1.26)
Multivariable, age ≤ 50.19 years	1.39 (1.00–1.93)*	2.11 (1.51–2.95)***	1.45 (1.04–2.02)*	1.34 (0.28–6.27)	0.79 (0.53–1.19)
Univariable, age > 50.19 years	1.18 (0.86–1.62)	1.93 (1.43–2.60)***	1.21 (0.91–1.62)	2.10 (1.02–4.36)*	0.91 (0.68–1.20)
Multivariable, age > 50.19 years	0.90 (0.65–1.26)	1.74 (1.24–2.45)**	1.09 (0.77–1.55)	2.07 (0.90–4.81)	0.90 (0.65–1.26)

Data shown for all individuals overall, stratified for sex and age at 50.19 years
Data presented as n (%) or odds ratio (95% confidence interval)
Apo apolipoprotein, *BMI* body mass index, *RA* rheumatoid arthritis
[a]Males > 0.8, females > 0.7 including lipid lowering therapy
[b]Smoking ever compared with never smoking
[c]BMI ≥ 25.0 compared with BMI < 25.0
[d]Systolic blood pressure (SBP) ≥ 140 mmHg and/or diastolic blood pressure (DBP) ≥ 90 mmHg including treatment for hypertension compared with SBP < 140 mmHg and DBP < 90 mmHg and no ongoing hypertensive treatment
*p ≤ 0.05, **p ≤ 0.01, ***p ≤ 0.001, dependent variable case/control

except hypertension, were significantly more frequent among the pre-symptomatic individuals compared with controls (Table 3). In the multivariable model, the factors remaining significantly associated with increased risk for future RA were smoking and BMI ≥ 25.0 (OR = 1.86 (1.48–2.35) and OR = 1.28 (1.01–1.62), respectively) (Table 3), which also remained significant after adjustment for educational level (data not shown).

Stratification based on sex showed that in women the factors significantly associated with increased risk for future RA in the univariable models were smoking (OR = 1.92 (1.50–2.47)), elevated ApoB/ApoA1 ratio (OR = 1.41 (1.09–1.84)) and BMI ≥ 25 (OR = 1.34 (1.06–1.71)). In the multivariable model, smoking and elevated ApoB/ApoA1 ratio remained significantly associated with increased risk for subsequent RA (OR = 1.82 (1.37–2.41) and OR = 1.36 (1.03–1.80), respectively) in women (Table 3), which was unchanged after adjustment for educational level (data not shown). For pre-symptomatic men the significant factors in univariable models were smoking (OR = 2.23 (1.53–3.27)) and diabetes (OR = 4.73 (1.71–13.08)) (Table 3). In the multivariable model the same factors (i.e. smoking and diabetes) were significantly associated with increased risk for future RA in pre-symptomatic men (OR = 1.92 (1.26–2.92) and 3.62 (1.13–11.64), respectively), and additionally BMI ≥ 25.0 (OR = 1.55 (1.01–2.39)) (Table 3), which remained significant after adjustment for education level; furthermore, analyses showed that low educational level was associated with

increased risk for subsequent RA in men (OR = 1.82 (1.02–3.26)) (data not shown).

Inclusion of age as a continuous variable in the conditional logistic regression analyses did not alter the results of the CVD risk factors associated with increased risk for future RA (data not shown). However, age was shown to be a significant factor associated with later RA development. Therefore, analyses were performed where age was stratified according to the median age at 50.19 years to receive two groups similar in size. These analyses showed that most of the risk factors for CVD were only significantly associated with increased risk for subsequent RA among younger pre-symptomatic individuals (Table 3). BMI ≥ 25.0, elevated ApoB/ApoA1 ratio and smoking were all significantly associated with increased risk for development of RA in multivariable conditional logistic regression models in younger individuals (OR = 1.45 (1.04–2.02), OR = 1.39 (1.00–1.93) and OR = 2.11 (1.51–2.95), respectively) (Table 3). In older individuals (>50.19 years), only smoking remained significant in the multivariable model (OR = 1.74 (1.24–2.45)) (Table 3). In older individuals (>50.19 years), only smoking remained significant in the multivariable model (OR = 1.74 (1.24–2.45)) (Table 3).

A variable with combinations of the five selected CVD risk factors was computed. The differences in frequencies between cases and controls of the combinations of no (reference), one, two or ≥ 3 of these risk factors for CVD were significant (χ^2 = 24.26, $p = 2 \times 10^{-5}$). Of the pre-symptomatic individuals, 41.5% had three or more risk factors compared with 30.4% of the controls ($\chi^2 = 19.17$, $p = 1 \times 10^{-5}$). Corresponding numbers for male cases and controls were 47.0% and 39.1% ($\chi^2 = 7.80$, $p = 0.005$) and for female cases and controls were 38.7% and 26.3% ($\chi^2 = 13.05$, $p = 3 \times 10^{-4}$), respectively. Having one, two or ≥ 3 CVD risk factors were all significantly associated with future RA, with the highest OR for three or more risk factors (OR = 2.81 (1.78–4.44)) and significant both for women and men (OR = 2.63 (1.59–4.36) and 5.09 (1.48–17.54), respectively) (Table 4).

Also, the younger pre-symptomatic individuals had significantly higher ORs for combinations of CVD risk factors (OR = 1.80 (1.04–3.14), 2.02 (1.14–3.57) and 4.00 (2.25–7.13) for one, two or ≥ 3 of the factors, respectively, with no risk factor as the reference group), whereas none of the combinations of CVD risk factors were significant among the older individuals (Table 4).

Sensitivity analyses

Sensitivity analyses were performed on pre-symptomatic individuals who had experienced symptoms ≤ 1 year within recruitment into the VIP or MONICA study. This showed that there were no significant differences between them and the rest of the cases regarding age, sex, BMI, ApoB/ApoA1 ratio and systolic or diastolic blood pressure. In the univariable analyses, the association of elevated ApoB/ApoA1 ratio was weakened by exclusion of cases with pre-symptomatic duration ≤ 1 year. However, when stratified for sex the associations were unchanged.

In the multivariable analysis, the association for BMI ≥ 25 for later RA development was altered (OR (95% CI) = 1.24 (0.98–1.58)) and when stratified for sex the significance among male cases was lost (OR (95% CI) = 1.43 (0.92–2.22), $p = 0.11$). Sensitivity analysis after imputation of data for ApoB/ApoA1 did not show any differences for the cardiovascular risk factors, nor for age or sex distributions.

Discussion

In this study we have shown that individuals who subsequently develop RA have increased levels and frequencies of CVD risk factors years before onset of RA. Some of the CVD risk factors prevalent in the pre-symptomatic individuals (e.g. smoking and elevated BMI) have previously been identified as potential risk factors for RA [12, 15, 16].

We have shown that smoking is related to an increased risk of future RA regardless of sex or age with a two-fold increased risk. The other risk factors showed differences when stratified for sex or age. In women the significant risk factor other than smoking was elevated ApoB/ApoA1 ratio, whilst among male cases BMI ≥ 25.0 and diabetes were associated with an increased risk. Diabetes had a four-fold risk, which was the highest of all risk factors studied. In the cohort study by Lahiri et al. [17], being a current smoker was associated with an increased risk of future RA or IP in men, whilst diabetes was associated with an increased risk of RA in women. In the general population, smoking and diabetes have a slightly greater effect in women compared with men for risk of CVD [22], even though male sex is reported to be a risk for developing type 2 diabetes [23].

The relationship between obesity and RA has proved contradictory; a recent meta-analysis of 11 studies concluded that an increased BMI could contribute to higher risk for RA [15]. Recently, we published a study focusing on obesity as a possible risk factor for future RA development based on data from the same cohorts as this study, showing that obesity or abdominal obesity was associated with risk of future RA, mainly in men with an early disease onset [16]. In the present study, a higher BMI was associated with increased risk for future RA, even when adjusting for smoking, ApoB/ApoA1 ratio, diabetes, hypertension and educational level, although, when stratifying for sex, the association of BMI ≥ 25.0 for future RA was restricted to men. The association of being overweight or obese with the risk of RA could potentially be due to both conditions being linked with inflammation,

Table 4 Multivariable conditional logistic regression analyses for subsequent RA stratified for number of risk factors for cardiovascular disease[a] present, stratified for median age (50.19 years) and sex

	No risk factor	One risk factor	Two risk factors	≥ 3 risk factors
All	Reference	1.73 (1.10-2.73)[*]	1.85 (1.17-2.94)[**]	2.81 (1.78-4.44)[***]
Age $\leq$ 50.19 years	Reference	1.80 (1.04-3.14)[*]	2.02 (1.14-3.57)[*]	4.00 (2.25-7.13)[***]
Age > 50.19 years	Reference	1.58 (0.65-3.87)	1.63 (0.69-3.83)	2.08 (0.90-4.85)
Women	Reference	1.47 (0.89-2.42)	1.55 (0.94-2.58)	2.63 (1.59-4.36)[***]
Men	Reference	3.92 (1.10-13.91)[*]	4.12 (1.18-14.36)[*]	5.09 (1.48-17.54)[*]

Data presented as odds ratio (95% confidence interval)

Apo apolipoprotein, *BMI* body mass index, *RA* rheumatoid arthritis

[a]Risk factors for cardiovascular disease: elevated ApoB/ApoA1 ratio (males > 0.8, females > 0.7 including lipid lowering therapy), smoking ever, diabetes (self-reported in questionnaires), hypertension (systolic blood pressure $\geq$ 140 mmHg and/or diastolic blood pressure $\geq$ 90 mmHg including treatment for hypertension), BMI $\geq$ 25

[*]$p \leq 0.05$, [**]$p \leq 0.01$, [***]$p \leq 0.001$, dependent variable case/control. Pre-symptomatic individuals compared with controls (reference being no risk factor present), stratified for age $\leq$ 50.19 years or > 50.19 years and women/men

and consequently with increased levels of inflammatory cytokines. It can be hypothesized that one reason why BMI ≥ 25.0 was not associated with a significant risk for future RA among women in our study was that among these pre-symptomatic individuals a relatively high proportion had yet to reach menopause, when overweight and obesity is known to increase. Additionally, in obese men accumulation of fatty tissue is mainly visceral, with more abundant pro-inflammatory cytokines, whereas in pre-menopausal women it is mainly subcutaneous [24].

Apolipoprotein A1 (ApoA1) is the major apolipoprotein in HDL, and higher levels are associated with a reduced risk for CVD; ApoB is the main apolipoprotein in LDL and therefore atherogenic. Several studies have shown that ApoB and the ratio of ApoB/ApoA1 are a better predictor for CVD and CV events than total cholesterol, LDL-cholesterol and cholesterol/HDL ratio [25–28]. In a study on patients with RA analysing possible predictors for CV events during 18 years, the ratio of ApoB/ApoA1 was predictive for CV events without association with inflammatory markers [29]. In this study we showed that the pre-symptomatic individuals had a significantly higher frequency of elevated ApoB/ApoA1 ratio compared with matched controls, and stratification for sex showed that the association with increased risk for future RA was restricted to women. Consistent with these results, a previous publication reported that blood donors who later developed RA had a more atherogenic lipid profile with higher total cholesterol, triglycerides and ApoB together with decreased HDL-cholesterol, with remaining levels after adjustment for CRP [13]. In a recent study, high serum levels of cholesterol in women were associated with future RA [30].

Hypertension was not more frequent among pre-symptomatic individuals compared with controls. One possible reason for this could be that pre-symptomatic individuals had not yet experienced symptoms of joint disease and, therefore, had no greater usage of NSAIDs, known to increase blood pressure, compared with the controls. The use of glucocorticoids in RA has also been associated with hypertension and could partly explain that there is no difference in the frequency of this condition in pre-symptomatic individuals compared with controls, because the pre-symptomatic individuals had not yet been prescribed any glucocorticoids. Furthermore, it has been suggested that a systemic inflammation with high CRP levels and elevated cytokines can lead to hypertension, as reviewed by Panoulas et al. [31]. Unfortunately, we had no information on CRP levels in the pre-symptomatic individuals but it could be speculated that levels had not reached those observed in newly diagnosed RA patients.

Because age, in addition to the risk factors, had an impact on the association of being pre-symptomatic, individuals were stratified for age. Both elevated ApoB/ApoA1 ratio and BMI ≥ 25.0 are associated with future

development of RA in younger individuals. A recent meta-analysis studying whether the same impact of age and gender on CVD risk was seen in RA as in the general population, with the highest risk among men and older individuals, concluded that the risk of CVD is age dependent [32]. The highest relative risk for CVD was in the youngest RA patients [32]. Interestingly, the results in our study showed that the presence of most of the CVD risk factors was only significantly associated with increased risk among younger pre-symptomatic individuals. The same pattern was observed of having the combination of the CVD risk factors, which were only significantly more prevalent in younger pre-symptomatic individuals compared with matched controls.

One limitation of this study is that approximately 60% of the population participates in the studies at the Medical Biobank. Being male, non-EU country of birth, single living in rural areas, low educational level, low income, being hospitalized more than twice and prior CVD characterized the non-participants [33]. The lack of data from these individuals possibly has an impact on our analyses in several ways, both strengthening and weakening the associations. Additionally, a limitation is that individuals younger than 40 years when affected with RA would be lost from inclusion in our study. Furthermore, for some of the variables, such as information on HDL-cholesterol, LDL-cholesterol and waist circumference, data were lacking and therefore interpretation of these results should be made with caution.

The strengths of this study include the possibility to use data from a well-defined large population-based database incorporating individuals having previously participated by completing questionnaires and donating blood samples to the cohorts in the Medical Biobank prior to onset of symptoms of RA. The blood pressure and anthropometric measurements were assessed by a trained nurse in all individuals. Most of the analyses were undertaken with conditional logistic regression analyses because for each pre-symptomatic individual three controls were selected randomly from the same cohorts and matched for sex, date of birth and year of clinical examination, and rural or urban living area. The subsequent diagnosis of the cases was based on clinical examinations by a rheumatologist. The controls were not clinically examined for presence of joint disease, but until the end of 2014 (when the co-analysis of registers was performed) they were not diagnosed with RA.

We have analysed the associations of the CVD risk factors with the development of future RA, but it is tempting to speculate about the impact of the presence of the CVD risk factors years before onset of symptoms of RA and the known relationship between RA and cardiovascular co-morbidity and mortality [9].

Conclusions

Our results show that several of the known CVD risk factors, of which several are per se related, are present in individuals prior to the onset of symptoms of RA. In pre-symptomatic women both smoking and an elevated ApoB/ApoA1 ratio were significantly more prevalent compared with matched controls, whereas in men smoking, BMI ≥ 25.0 and diabetes were significantly associated with increased risk of future development of RA. Also, the pre-symptomatic individuals had significantly higher frequencies of combinations of the CVD risk factors compared with matched controls, particularly the younger individuals. Together, these results urge a prompt analysis of CVD risk factors for proposed prevention in patients with early RA.

Abbreviations
ACPA: Anti-citrullinated peptide antibodies; Apo: Apolipoprotein; BMI: Body mass index; CVD: Cardiovascular disease; HDL: High-density lipoprotein; LDL: Low-density lipoprotein; MI: Myocardial infarction; MONICA: Northern Sweden Multinational Monitoring of Trends and Determinants in Cardiovascular Disease; OR: Odds ratio; RA: Rheumatoid arthritis; RF: Rheumatoid factor; VIP: Västerbotten Intervention programme

Acknowledgements
The authors would like to thank study participants and the staff involved in the collection of data and blood samples and Professor Göran Hallmans at the Department of Public Health and Clinical Medicine, Nutritional Research, University Hospital, Umeå. Also, they would like to acknowledge Professor Solveig Wållberg Jonsson, Department of Public Health and Clinical Medicine, Rheumatology, University Hospital, Umeå for valuable comments on the manuscript.

Funding
This study was supported by grants from the Swedish Rheumatism Association, the Swedish Research Council (K2013-52X-20307-07-3), King Gustaf V's 80-Year Fund, the Västerbotten county council (ALF) and the Swedish Foundation for Strategic Research, Sweden.

Authors' contributions
SR-D and HK were responsible for study concept and design. SR-D was responsible for acquisition of data. HK was responsible for statistical analysis. HK, HS and SR-D were responsible for analysis and interpretation of data. HK and SR-D were responsible for drafting the manuscript. HK, HS and SR-D were responsible for critical revision of the manuscript. All authors read and approved the final manuscript.

Competing interests
The authors declare that they have no competing interests.

Author details
[1]Department of Public Health and Clinical Medicine, Rheumatology, Umeå University, Building 6M, 901 87 Umeå, Sweden. [2]Department of Public Health and Clinical Medicine, Epidemiology and Global Health, Umeå University, Umeå, Sweden.

References
1. Innala L, Sjöberg C, Möller B, Ljung L, Smedby T, Södergren A, et al. Comorbidity in patients with early rheumatoid arthritis—inflammation matters. Arthritis Res Ther. 2016;18:33.
2. Wållberg-Jonsson S, Johansson H, Ohman ML, Rantapää-Dahlqvist S. Extent of inflammation predicts cardiovascular disease and overall mortality in seropositive rheumatoid arthritis. A retrospective cohort study from disease onset. J Rheumatol. 1999;26:2562–71.
3. Solomon DH, Karlson EW, Rimm EB, Cannuscio CC, Mandl LA, Manson JE, et al. Cardiovascular morbidity and mortality in women diagnosed with rheumatoid arthritis. Circulation. 2003;107:1303–7.
4. Aviña-Zubieta JA, Choi HK, Sadatsafavi M, Etminan M, Esdaile JM, Lacaille D. Risk of cardiovascular mortality in patients with rheumatoid arthritis: a meta-analysis of observational studies. Arthritis Rheum. 2008;59:1690–7.
5. Aviña-Zubieta JA, Thomas J, Sadatsafavi M, Lehman AJ, Lacaille D. Risk of incident cardiovascular events in patients with rheumatoid arthritis: a meta-analysis of observational studies. Ann Rheum Dis. 2012;71:1524–9.
6. van Halm VP, Peters MJ, Voskuyl AE, Boers M, Lems WF, Visser M, et al. Rheumatoid arthritis versus diabetes as a risk factor for cardiovascular disease: a cross-sectional study, the CARRÊ investigation. Ann Rheum Dis. 2009;68:1395–400.
7. Gonzalez A, Maradit Kremers H, Crowson CS, Ballman KV, Roger VL, Jacobsen SJ, et al. Do cardiovascular risk factors confer the same risk for cardiovascular outcomes in rheumatoid arthritis patients as in non-rheumatoid arthritis patients? Ann Rheum Dis. 2008;67:64–9.
8. Innala L, Möller B, Ljung L, Magnusson S, Smedby T, Södergren A, et al. Cardiovascular events in early RA are a result of inflammatory burden and traditional risk factors: a five year prospective study. Arthritis Res Ther. 2011; 13:R131.
9. Maradit-Kremers H, Crowson CS, Nicola PJ, Ballman KV, Roger VL, Jacobsen SJ, et al. Increased unrecognized coronary heart disease and sudden deaths in rheumatoid arthritis. Arthritis Rheum. 2005;52:402–11.
10. Holmqvist ME, Wedrén S, Jacobsson LT, Klareskog L, Nyberg F, Rantapää-Dahlqvist S, et al. No increased occurrence of ischemic heart disease prior to the onset of rheumatoid arthritis. Arthritis Rheum. 2009;60:2861–9.
11. Holmqvist ME, Wedrén S, Jacobsson LT, Klareskog L, Nyberg F, Rantapää-Dahlqvist S, et al. Rapid increase in myocardial infarction risk following diagnosis of rheumatoid arthritis amongst patients diagnosed between 1995 and 2006. J Intern Med. 2010;268:578–85.
12. Goodson NJ, Silman AJ, Pattison DJ, Lunt M, Bunn D, Luben R, et al. Traditional risk factors measured prior to the onset of inflammatory polyarthritis. Rheumatology. 2004;43:731–6.
13. van Halm VP, Nielen MM, Nurmohamed MT, van Schaardenburg D, Reesink HW, Voskuyl AE, et al. Lipids and inflammation: serial measurements of the lipid profile of blood donors who later developed rheumatoid arthritis. Ann Rheum Dis. 2007;66:184–8.
14. Myasoedova E, Crowson CS, Maradit Kremers H, Fitz-Gibbon PD, Therneau TM, Gabriel SE. Total cholesterol and LDL levels decrease before rheumatoid arthritis. Ann Rheum Dis. 2010;69:1310–4.
15. Qin B, Yang M, Fu H, Ma N, Wei T, Tang Q, et al. Body mass index and the risk of rheumatoid arthritis: a systematic review and dose-response meta-analysis. Arthritis Res Ther. 2015;17:86.
16. Ljung L, Rantapää-Dahlqvist S. Abdominal obesity, gender and the risk of rheumatoid arthritis—a nested case-control study. Arthritis Res Ther. 2016;18:277.
17. Lahiri M, Luben RN, Morgan C, Bunn DK, Marshall T, Lunt M, et al. Using lifestyle factors to identify individuals at higher risk of inflammatory polyarthritis (results from the European Prospective Investigation of Cancer-Norfolk and the Norfolk Arthritis Register—the EPIC-2-NOAR Study). Ann Rheum Dis. 2014;73:219–26.
18. Norberg M, Wall S, Boman K, Weinehall L. The Västerbotten Intervention Programme: background, design and implications. Global Health Actions. 2010;3:4643. doi:10.3402/gha.v3i0.4643.
19. Norberg M, Blomstedt Y, Lönnberg G, Nyström L, Stenlund H, Wall S, et al. Community participation and sustainability—evidence over 25 years in the Västerbotten Intervention Programme. Global Health Actions. 2012;5:1–9.
20. Stegmayr B, Lundberg V, Asplund K. The events registration and survey procedures in the Northern Sweden MONICA project. Scand J Public Health. 2003;61:9–17.
21. Berry JD, Dyer A, Cai X, Garside DB, Ning H, Thomas A, et al. Lifetime risks of cardiovascular disease. N Engl J Med. 2012;366(4):321–9.
22. Appelman Y, van Rijn BB, ten Haaf ME, Boersma E, Peters SA. Sex differences in cardiovascular risk factors and disease prevention. Atherosclerosis. 2015; 241:211–8.

23. Wandell PE, Carlsson AC. Gender differences and time trends in incidence and prevalence of type 2 diabetes in Sweden—a model explaining the diabetes epidemic worldwide today? Diabetes Res Clin Pract. 2014;106:e90–2.

24. Palmer BF, Clegg DJ. The sexual dimorphism of obesity. Mol Cell Endocrinol. 2015;402:113–9.

25. Sniderman AD, Furberg CD, Keech A, Roeters van Lennep JE, Frohlich J, Jungner I, et al. Apolipoproteins versus lipids as indices of coronary risk and as targets for statin treatment. Lancet. 2003;361:777–80.

26. Walldius G, Jungner I, Holme I, Aastveit AH, Kolar W, Steiner E. High apolipoprotein B, low apolipoprotein A-I, and improvement in the prediction of fatal myocardial infarction (AMORIS study): a prospective study. Lancet. 2001;358:2026–33.

27. McQueen MJ, Hawken S, Wang X, Ounpuu S, Sniderman A, Probstfield J, et al. Lipids, lipoproteins, and apolipoproteins as risk markers of myocardial infarction in 52 countries (the INTERHEART study): a case-control study. Lancet. 2008;372:224–33.

28. Parish S, Peto R, Palmer A, Clarke R, Lewington S, Offer A, et al. The joint effects of apolipoprotein B, apolipoprotein A_1, LDL cholesterol, and HDL cholesterol on risk: 3510 cases of acute myocardial infarction and 9805 controls. Eur Heart J. 2009;30:2137–46.

29. Öhman M, Öhman ML, Wållberg-Jonsson S. The apoB/apoA1 ratio predict future cardiovascular events in patients with rheumatoid arthritis. Scand J Rheumatol. 2014;43:259–64.

30. Turesson C, Bergström U, Pikwer M, Nilsson JÅ, Jacobsson LT. High serum cholesterol predicts rheumatoid arthritis in women, but not in men: a prospective study. Arthritis Res Ther. 2015;17:284.

31. Panoulas VF, Metsios GS, Pace AV, John H, Treharne GJ, Banks MJ, et al. Hypertension in rheumatoid arthritis. Rheumatology. 2008;47:1286–98.

32. Fransen J, Kazemi-Bajestani SM, Bredie SJ, Popa CD. Rheumatoid arthritis disadvantages younger patients for cardiovascular diseases: a meta-analysis. PLoS One. 2016;11:e0157360.

33. Norberg M, Blomstedt Y, Lönnberg G, Nyström L, Stenlund H, Wall S, et al. Community participation and sustainability—evidence over 25 years in the Västerbotten Intervention Programme. Glob Health Action. 2012;5:19166.

18

Animal models of rheumatoid pain: experimental systems and insights

Bradford D. Fischer, Adeshina Adeyemo, Michael E. O'Leary and Andrea Bottaro[*]

Abstract

Severe chronic pain is one of the hallmarks and most debilitating manifestations of inflammatory arthritis. It represents a significant problem in the clinical management of patients with common chronic inflammatory joint conditions such as rheumatoid arthritis, psoriatic arthritis and spondyloarthropathies. The functional links between peripheral inflammatory signals and the establishment of the neuroadaptive mechanisms acting in nociceptors and in the central nervous system in the establishment of chronic and neuropathic pain are still poorly understood, representing an area of intense study and translational priority. Several well-established inducible and spontaneous animal models are available to study the onset, progression and chronicization of inflammatory joint disease, and have been instrumental in elucidating its immunopathogenesis. However, quantitative assessment of pain in animal models is technically and conceptually challenging, and it is only in recent years that inflammatory arthritis models have begun to be utilized systematically in experimental pain studies using behavioral and neurophysiological approaches to characterize acute and chronic pain stages. This article aims primarily to provide clinical and experimental rheumatologists with an overview of current animal models of arthritis pain, and to summarize emerging findings, challenges and unanswered questions in the field.

Keywords: Arthritis, Inflammation, Pain, Animal models, Nociception

Background

Arthritis pain in human patients

Rheumatoid arthritis (RA) and spondyloarthritis are prevalent inflammatory-erosive joint diseases which affect as many as 2% of the population worldwide, causing severe, debilitating morbidity and major economic costs due to both health care expenditures and lost productivity. Inflammatory arthritides are characterized by progressive joint inflammation and destruction, deformity, loss of mobility, systemic manifestations and severe pain which ultimately hamper basic motility functions, activities of daily living and psychological health in the affected individuals [1, 2].

Therapeutic approaches focused on the underlying inflammatory immunopathology have led to the introduction of targeted biological disease-modifying anti-rheumatic drugs (DMARDs), pioneered by anti-tumor necrosis factor (TNF) agents, which have revolutionized the clinical treatment and dramatically improved long-term outcomes of these diseases [3, 4].

Pain, initially joint localized but often progressing to widespread in advanced stages, is a major component of inflammatory arthritis symptomatology and is typically the primary reason for initial rheumatological referrals [1, 2]. In a subset of patients with advanced disease, chronic pain can also acquire typical neuropathic features [1, 5]. These and other clinical findings support a key role of neurosensitization mechanisms of nociceptive pathways in the central nervous system in the establishment of chronic arthritic pain.

The therapeutic success of biologic DMARDs has provided new insights into the unique qualities of pain manifestations associated with chronic inflammatory arthritis. Notably, patients with a positive response to anti-TNF agents often report rapid initial therapeutic pain suppression which precedes the clinical anti-inflammatory response [1, 6]. This is consistent with a direct role of TNF and other inflammatory cytokines like IL-6 and IL-17 on nociceptor sensitization pathways [7]. Indeed, nociceptors in dorsal root ganglia have been

* Correspondence: bottaro@rowan.edu
Department of Biomedical Sciences, Cooper Medical School of Rowan University, 401 S. Broadway, Camden, NJ 08103, USA

shown to express TNF receptors and to directly respond to TNF stimulation [7].

More problematic for the clinical management of these diseases, however, is that a significant fraction of patients fail to report long-term suppression of pain comparable to their anti-inflammatory clinical response to biologic and other DMARDs [1, 8–10]. Based on these clinical observations and treatment outcomes, therefore, direct inflammatory pain pathways are generally thought to predominate in early-stage arthritis, evolving into chronic-neurogenic pain mechanisms over time [1, 5].

From the patients' perspective, effective management of arthritis-associated pain is a primary therapeutic goal, and a major component of patient-driven disease assessment often underestimated by clinical disease activity scoring tools [2, 10, 11]. A fuller mechanistic understanding of the inflammatory and neuroadaptive mechanisms leading to chronic arthritic pain is therefore required to address a major unmet need in patient care.

This review will first describe existing animal models of arthritis that are commonly utilized for preclinical pain studies, discussing their specific advantages and drawbacks. We will then provide key background on experimental methods for quantitative assessment of pain responses in animal models, highlighting important theoretical and practical challenges, and summarizing recent insights into the mechanisms of arthritic pain.

Animal models of inflammatory joint disease

Animal disease models have proven invaluable to unravel the pathophysiological pathways of inflammatory arthritis, and for investigational testing of therapeutic agents. The most commonly utilized animal species for this purpose are mice and rats, either as strains that spontaneously develop arthritis or as inducible models in which disease can be provoked by administration of arthritogenic stimuli. A number of comprehensive reviews have already covered the range of animal arthritis models, and their features in comparison to human disease pathophysiology and therapeutic responses [12–15]. Here, we will briefly summarize key aspects of a few relevant models, particularly with respect to features such as disease onset, progression and chronicity which may affect their use in pain studies.

Spontaneous arthritis models

Several rodent strains have been reported to be susceptible to development of spontaneous arthritis, but experimental studies have primarily focused on a few genetically modified mouse strains which display full penetrance and reproducible disease progression, especially K/BxN and TNF-transgenic (TNFtg) mice [16, 17].

The K/BxN model K/BxN mice express a T-cell receptor transgene specific for a peptide derived from the ubiquitous enzyme glucose-6-phosphate isomerase (GPI), presented by the I-Ag^7 MHC-II allele [17, 18]. Autoimmunity manifests with onset of joint inflammation around 3–4 weeks of age, progressing over 4–8 weeks to full inflammatory-erosive arthritis. Anti-GPI autoantibodies appear to be the primary drivers of disease, because the transfer of K/BxN serum, or even K/BxN-derived anti-GPI monoclonal antibodies, is sufficient to induce arthritis in other mouse strains (see later) [19]. Histologically, K/BxN disease closely parallels findings in human RA joints, including pannus formation, inflammatory infiltrates and articular erosions. Therefore, K/BxN mice replicate human RA both in the autoimmune pathophysiology and key disease features.

The TNF-transgenic mouse model TNFtg mice, derived in the early 1990s, express a human TNF gene lacking post-transcriptional regulatory elements, and have provided cornerstone evidence for the involvement of TNF in inflammatory arthritis [16]. Commonly used strains range from a single copy (Tg(TNF)3647 strain) to multiple copies (Tg(TNF)197 strain and others) of the TNF transgene [16, 20]. Other TNF-overexpressing strains with similar disease features were later developed, but will not be discussed here.

The 3647-strain TNFtg mice display delayed onset of joint inflammation compared to multicopy transgenics (6–8 weeks of age vs 3–4 weeks), slower disease progression (12–16 weeks from onset to maximal severity) and increased lifespans (over a year with appropriate husbandry) [16, 20]. Because of their late onset and slow progression, single-copy TNFtg mice are particularly suited for the study of processes associated with preclinical disease stages and with progressing chronicity. Although TNFtg disease is not autoimmunity driven, it displays many of the histopathological findings of human RA (synovial hyperplasia, neutrophilic inflammatory infiltrates and joint erosion) and other signs of systemic inflammation. TNFtg mice are therefore an excellent model to investigate TNF-induced inflammatory pathways in human disease.

Inducible arthritis models

Inflammatory arthritis can be induced experimentally in many species, with well-established systems utilizing both rats and mice. Arthritogenic signals in these models can consist of nonspecific inflammatory agents, such as different types of adjuvants; of immunization procedures using specific antigens which cause self-tolerance breakdown; or of passively administered autoreactive antibodies or sera. Compared to spontaneous disease strains, advantages of inducible models include their cost-effectiveness, reduced husbandry needs and reproducibility of existing protocols. Disease typically develops rapidly, limiting the physiological windows for the study of disease onset and progression. Penetrance, persistence and chronicity of arthritis vary depending upon the model.

Adjuvant-induced arthritis and related models Arthritis can be reproducibly induced in susceptible strains of rats (e.g., Lewis or DA rats) by intradermal injection of adjuvants, including complete or incomplete Freund's adjuvant (CFA, IFA), pristane and squalene, or intraarticular administration of streptococcal cell wall products or antigens in presensitized rats or mice [13, 21]. In most applications, disease follows within days of administration, reaches maximal severity within one to a few weeks and is typically followed by remission, which in some protocols is reactivatable by repeated treatments. Disease intensity and course vary depending on the strain and arthritogenic signal. For instance, CFA-induced arthritis is significantly more severe and systemic than that induced by antigen-free adjuvants like IFA or pristane. Pristane-induced arthritis in rats displays a remitting–relapsing "flaring" pattern that resembles human RA. Although the inciting stimulus in adjuvant-induced arthritis is not antigenic, the resulting disease is often associated with MHC-linked susceptibility, production of autoantibodies and/or emergence of autoreactive T-cell clones, reflecting an autoimmune pathophysiology [13].

Collagen-induced arthritis Collagen-induced arthritis (CIA) is the most frequently utilized experimental model of arthritis. Inflammatory arthritis is induced in genetically susceptible rats, mice, rabbits and other species by immunization with type II collagen, typically of bovine origin [22]. In a typical mouse protocol, polyarthritis develops a few weeks post immunization with CFA-emulsified collagen, reaching maximal clinical severity within 2 weeks of onset and persisting in a chronic state thereafter.

Antibody-induced arthritis Evidence that serum from collagen-immunized rats and mice could passively induce arthritis in recipients provided early experimental confirmation of the direct pathogenic role of humoral immunity in arthritis. The same approach is commonly utilized to induce acute, transient arthritis in rats or mice, in models such as collagen-antibody-induced arthritis (CAIA) and K/BxN serum-transfer arthritis [19, 23]. Arthritis in these models is mediated by immune complex deposition in the joints, recruitment of neutrophils and other inflammatory innate components, and is independent of B and T cells [19, 23]. Histologically, bone and cartilage erosions and pannus formation closely resemble human RA. Because the inflammatory response in the joints is rapid, reproducible and intense, the models are best suited for the study of acute mechanisms.

CAIA can be induced in either rats or mice by intravenous transfer of a mixture of anti-collagen II monoclonal antibodies, most often accompanied by intraperitoneal injection of LPS to potentiate the effect. Disease onset follows rapidly after LPS injection, reaching maximal severity in 4–5 days and waning in about an additional week. Repeated injections can exacerbate and extend the response.

Similarly, transfer of serum, antibodies or anti-GPI monoclonals from K/BxN mice (see earlier) can induce rapid (2–3 days) onset of polyarthritis in recipients, with almost complete penetrance and without additional inducers [19].

Experimental systems for analysis of pain-associated responses in animal models

Self-reported pain scores are the primary means for evaluating pain severity in patients. However, objective assessment of pain in animals represents a significant challenge for preclinical research, which has led to the development of several experimental systems which reproducibly mimic pathological pain conditions in humans, including inflammatory and neuropathic pain, and allow assessment of their outcomes. Broadly speaking, animal behavioral models of pain consist of two principal components: experimental manipulation intended to produce a pain-like state; and measurement of behavior presumably indicative of that pain state. These models can be used to experimentally assess pain as well as its relief following the administration of antinociceptive drugs.

Current methods of pain assessment in animals were initially developed in the context of models of induced acute pain from different types of noxious stimuli, or of neuropathic pain following experimental nerve injury, but the same approaches are routinely applied to arthritis pain models. All of these approaches have to overcome the major conceptual hurdle of translating the subjective experience of pain in animal subjects into investigator-observable, quantifiable responses.

Broadly, experimental assessment of pain in animal models relies on the quantification of pain-evoked or pain-suppressed behaviors. Pain-evoked behaviors may occur at very low rates in the absence of pain, and increase in frequency following putative nociceptive stimuli. Examples include footpad withdrawal, jumping, flinching or licking. In contrast, pain-suppressed behaviors are those that occur at high rates in the absence of noxious stimuli and decrease in magnitude or duration after exposure to a noxious stimulus. Some natural behaviors that may be suppressed in this context include locomotor activity, nesting, motor coordination/balance or feeding (e.g., [24]). In each case, measurable changes in behavior may result from pain responses to a normally noxious stimulus, an enhanced response to low-grade painful stimuli (hyperalgesia), or a painful response to a normally non-noxious stimulus (allodynia).

Types of experimental pain models

The basic concept of measuring acute nociceptive pain in animals relies on the input of a normally noxious stimulus followed by the assessment of a withdrawal response. The noxious stimulus can vary in intensity and in modality, such as electrical, mechanical, thermal or chemical [25, 26].

The advantage of these models largely rests in their simplicity, their ability to objectively measure the withdrawal response and their predictive value to assess pharmacological effectiveness of opioid analgesics in humans [25]. However, they have limited clinical relevance and show impaired validity when nonopioid analgesics are tested, such as steroids and nonsteroidal anti-inflammatory drugs (NSAIDs). These and other limitations have led to the development of additional methods to behaviorally assess more clinically relevant pain states, including models of acute and chronic inflammation and neuropathy.

Classic models of acute inflammatory pain include the injection into the hind paw of rodents of chemicals (e.g., formalin or carrageenan), which produce a rapid nociceptive response characterized by paw flinching and licking (formalin), and decreased response thresholds to thermal and mechanical stimuli (i.e., allodynia and hyperalgesia). Neuropathic pain in animals is classically modeled by interventions that cause some degree of nerve injury, such as ligation or chronic constriction. While these systems have good predictive validity in pharmacological studies (e.g., sensitivity to opioids and anticonvulsants), they do not replicate the etiology of most human neuropathic states, nor some of their common clinical manifestations [27, 28].

These experimental systems have been instrumental to unraveling basic neurophysiological pathways of nociception and for pharmacological research, but because of their limited clinical applicability they have been progressively complemented by more pathologically relevant models of chronic and/or neuropathic pain, including the inflammatory arthritis models already described.

Quantifying the perception of pain in animals

The assessment of pain in animals is naturally fraught with conceptual and experimental complexities, and significant research has been carried out in recent years to standardize protocols, identify the impact of critical variables (such as sex, age, behavioral and environmental factors), reduce investigator-associated subjectivity and disruption, and expand the range of testable responses

from strictly sensory to include psychoaffective components [26, 29–31]. A summary of commonly utilized methods is presented in Table 1.

Pain-evoked behaviors The most frequently utilized techniques for assessment of ongoing pain in experimental animals rely on development of hyperalgesia and allodynia, which can be quantitatively measured by assessing withdrawal from non-noxious or subthreshold stimuli. Arguably the most common mechanical stimuli used for this purpose in rodents are von Frey hairs, elastic filaments of varying diameter that buckle at a defined force. Applied to the plantar surface of the paw when the animal is positioned over a wire mesh surface, von Frey hairs of increasing stiffness allow the determination of the mechanical threshold of paw withdrawal. Although less frequently utilized, electrical stimuli can also be applied briefly and quantifiably, and are reproduced easily.

Lowered thresholds of evoked responses to stimuli relative to controls are considered hallmarks of allodynia and hyperalgesia. One limitation of these approaches lies in the subjective measurement of withdrawal responses, which can be obviated by use of automated electronic systems [32, 33]. Assays based on evaluation of weight bearing may be able to more objectively and physiologically identify postural changes in models of joint inflammation [34].

Neurophysiologically, the primary caveat of mechanical and electrical stimuli is that they activate both low-threshold mechanoreceptors and nociceptors, preventing a clear-cut distinction of the pathways involved. Thermal stimulation is thought to be more specific in directly activating nociceptive fibers. Commonly used methods involve applying radiant heat or immersing the distal end of the tail of a restrained animal into a thermostatic water bath. Unrestrained animals can be tested using Hargreaves' method, during which radiant heat is applied to the plantar surface of the footpad via an infrared source to elicit paw withdrawal.

Functional magnetic resonance imaging Functional magnetic resonance imaging (fMRI) measures changes in paramagnetic signals secondary to oxygen extraction from oxyhemoglobin, reflecting metabolic activity in brain tissue. Human fMRI studies have demonstrated activation in specific brain structures following noxious stimuli, including in the lateral thalamus, primary and somatosensory cortex, insular cortex, anterior cingulate cortex, striatum, cerebellum, supplemental motor area and periaqueductal gray matter [35]. Small animal neuroimaging studies have validated the use of fMRI to study pain in animals, showing activation in similar regions [6, 36]. fMRI has the distinct advantage of being

Table 1 Experimental methods of pain assessment in rodent arthritis models

Assessment method [example references]	Response measured	Pain aspect assessed	Advantages	Disadvantages
Von Frey test/mechanical hyperalgesia [6, 32, 33, 48–54, 56, 58, 59, 62]	Pain-evoked behavior: withdrawal threshold from a mechanical stimulus	Mechanical allodynia/ hyperalgesia	Quantitative, well-established protocols	Stimulation of mechanical and nociceptive fibers; possible investigator bias/subjectivity
Hargreaves test/ thermonociception [6, 33, 51, 53, 54, 56–59, 62]	Pain-evoked behavior: withdrawal latency from a thermal stimulus	Thermal allodynia/ hyperalgesia	Quantitative, well-established protocols; primary stimulation of nociceptive fibers	Possible investigator bias/ subjectivity
Ambulatory/locomotor behavior [53, 56, 59, 61–66]	Pain-suppressed behavior: locomotion in an open field	Locomotor activity/ ambulation/exploratory behavior	Automated quantitative measurement; may include affective component	May be affected by nonpain-related outcomes (e.g., motor function)
Grimace scales [38]	Changes in facial expressions associated with pain	Expression of subjective pain perception	Non-interventional; directly linked to individual pain state; may include affective component	Possible investigator bias/ subjectivity; experimenter training needed; further validation in arthritis models required
fMRI [6]	Functional changes in CNS activity associated with pain	Affective CNS responses to pain	Objective measurements; may include affective component	Expensive equipment; high-level investigator training needed; requirement for restraint/ sedation
Gait/dynamic weight bearing analysis [34, 59]	Changes in ambulatory posture or weight distribution	Spontaneous gait changes due to joint pain	Objective, quantitative measurements; automated systems available	Specialized equipment needed.
Operant conditioning [60]	Behavior emitted to receive a reward despite concurrent exposure to a painful stimulus	Affective and/or motivational components of pain perception	Objective, quantitative; automated systems available; may include affective component	Specialized equipment needed
Escape/avoidance [45]	Latency to escape noxious stimulus	Affective and/or motivational components of pain perception	Objective, quantitative; automated systems available; may include affective component	Specialized equipment needed

CNS central nervous system, fMRI functional magnetic resonance imaging

able to assess pain-related effects in brain areas thought to be important in processing both sensory and affective components. However, the approach requires trained personnel and sophisticated equipment, and the use of restraint or sedation to minimize head movement during data acquisition adds obvious confounding variables.

Grimace scales Recent studies have analyzed facial expressions in animals in response to painful stimuli. A 10-point facial expression ("grimace") scale was developed in mice based on orbital tightening (closed eyelid or eye squeeze), nose bulge, cheek bulge, ear position and whisker changes following intraperitoneal administration of acetic acid [37]. Similar scales exist for rats and rabbits, and are being evaluated for other species. Of note, analogous facial expressions are exhibited by humans that verbally report pain, and can be utilized to assess pain responses in nonverbal humans. Grimace scales have shown good reproducibility for trained investigators, especially in acute pain models, and have the distinct advantage of allowing direct assessment of pain in disease models in the absence of additional experimental interventions. However, their applicability to joint inflammation and chronic pain states remains to be fully validated [38].

Pain-suppressed behaviors Although pain-evoked behaviors are most commonly utilized in animal pain studies, pain-suppressed behaviors have also been used to assess pain in animals. These are defined by a decrease of otherwise healthy behaviors that occur at high rates (e.g., feeding, spontaneous ambulatory behavior) following exposure to a noxious stimulus. These have clinical correlates in human chronic pain patients, where suppressed behaviors may include decreased activities of daily living or ambulation, and correlate with signs of clinical depression. Evidence of pain-suppressed behaviors in animals may be quantified by reduced feeding, reduced mating and/or reduced locomotor activity.

Decreased locomotor activity has been associated with pain-like states in animals, including in rodent models of inflammatory and neuropathic pain, although with some discrepancies [39, 40]. As an example, Fig. 1 shows the close quantitative correlation of decreased locomotor activity in TNFtg mice with traditional clinical scores of joint inflammation during disease progression. Models of pain suppressed behaviors such as these can be used to preclinically model the decreased activity observed in patients with RA.

The inclusion of pain-suppressed behaviors in animal testing has several advantages. First, pain-suppressed

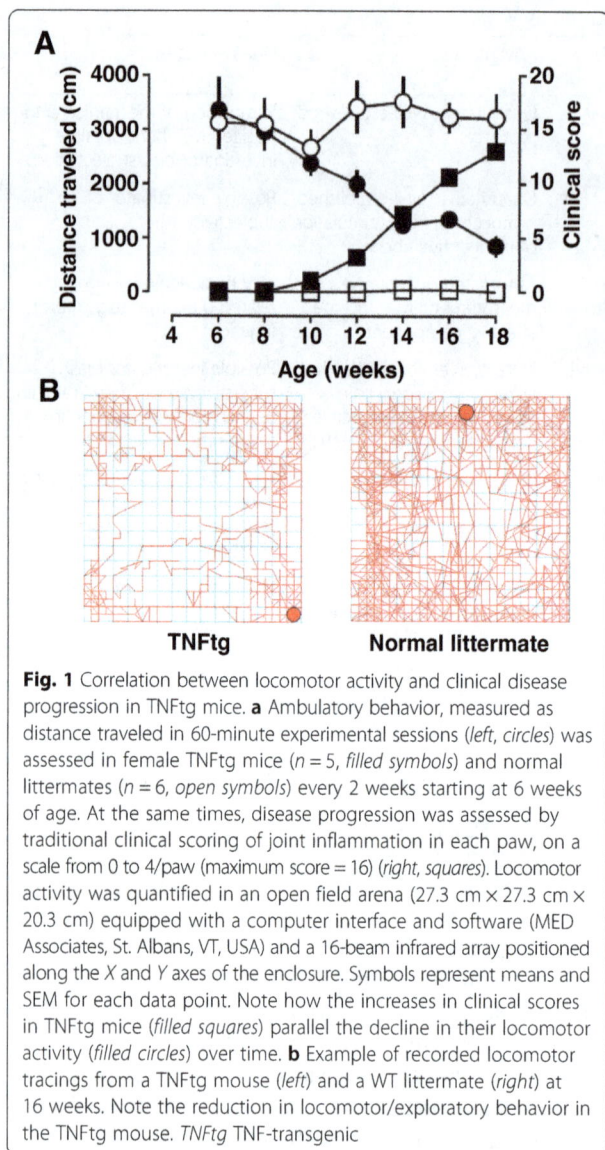

Fig. 1 Correlation between locomotor activity and clinical disease progression in TNFtg mice. **a** Ambulatory behavior, measured as distance traveled in 60-minute experimental sessions (*left, circles*) was assessed in female TNFtg mice (*n* = 5, *filled symbols*) and normal littermates (*n* = 6, *open symbols*) every 2 weeks starting at 6 weeks of age. At the same times, disease progression was assessed by traditional clinical scoring of joint inflammation in each paw, on a scale from 0 to 4/paw (maximum score = 16) (*right, squares*). Locomotor activity was quantified in an open field arena (27.3 cm × 27.3 cm × 20.3 cm) equipped with a computer interface and software (MED Associates, St. Albans, VT, USA) and a 16-beam infrared array positioned along the X and Y axes of the enclosure. Symbols represent means and SEM for each data point. Note how the increases in clinical scores in TNFtg mice (*filled squares*) parallel the decline in their locomotor activity (*filled circles*) over time. **b** Example of recorded locomotor tracings from a TNFtg mouse (*left*) and a WT littermate (*right*) at 16 weeks. Note the reduction in locomotor/exploratory behavior in the TNFtg mouse. *TNFtg* TNF-transgenic

behaviors can be objectively measured using automated equipment (e.g., locomotor activity box, operant response chambers). Second, drugs that produce motor impairment are less likely to produce false positive effects in pain-suppressed assays relative to pain-stimulated behaviors. Third, measures of pain-suppressed behaviors may be used to investigate some of the psychoaffective components of pain and may improve the translational validity of these behaviors toward the clinic. At the same time, the complexities of interpreting animal behavior from a psychoaffective standpoint cannot be understated, and important work needs to be carried out in this area to fully validate these approaches [29, 30].

Operant conditioning and behavioral avoidance Similar to study of pain-suppressed behaviors, behavioral methods can be utilized to explore affective and/or motivational changes that occur in response to pain, bypassing some of the problems associated with pain-evoked responses. Operant procedures may require an animal to predictably emit a defined behavioral response, such as traversing a noxious stimulus (e.g., pass through a heat source), in order to obtain in a positive reinforcer (e.g., food treat) [41, 42]. Place avoidance or preference paradigms are based on the assumption that animals will display aversive behavior toward noxious stimuli (e.g., avoid heated cage areas) or preference for environments associated with reward [43–45]. Changes in avoidance behavior, such as in the presence of persistent pain states or after experimental manipulations (e.g., analgesic drugs), are thought to be related to changes in nociceptive pathways. Assays such as these can be used to study processes that are thought to involve higher brain centers relative to peripheral nociceptors.

Recent advances in animal models of arthritic pain

Although animal models of arthritis have been widely utilized for decades to study not just disease pathogenesis and candidate therapeutics, only in the past 10–15 years have the biological properties of pain in these systems begun to be investigated systematically [46, 47].

Links between inflammation and pain-evoked responses

In all models studied, inflammatory disease is associated with lowered thresholds to mechanical and thermal stimulation, reflecting hyperalgesia and allodynia. However, thermal and mechanical hypersensitivity are not always closely correlated to each other, suggesting that strain-specific and method-specific differences should be considered in evaluating experimental outcomes [33]. In addition, age may be an additional variable, because adjuvant-induced arthritis evoked similar inflammatory responses in young and old mice, but induced higher levels of mechanical hypersensitivity in younger mice using the von Frey test [48]. These discordances aside, sensitization of pain pathways is typically concomitant with the appearance of clinical signs of inflammation, and in some cases it can precede them [46, 49]. This is consistent with pain often being the earliest disease manifestation in human RA patients [1, 50].

Studies focused on the resolution end of the disease spectrum using transient antibody-induced arthritis (e.g., CAIA and K/BxN serum transfer) have shown that pain sensitization can persist for extended periods of time beyond the resolution of inflammation [49, 51, 52]. This also parallels the discordance between the therapeutic control of inflammatory disease and persisting pain experienced by some human RA patients [2, 8–10]. Interestingly, transfer into mice of anti-citrullinated peptide antibodies from human RA patients was recently shown to evoke pain-like induced and suppressed behaviors in the absence of a detectable inflammatory response, suggesting that some pathogenic antibodies may mediate nociceptive signals by distinct, non-inflammatory mechanisms [53].

Neurophysiology of inflammatory pain

Molecular and cellular studies of nociceptors and non-neuronal cell types in dorsal root ganglia (DRG) and spinal cord sensory pathways have begun to elucidate the neurophysiological mechanisms of hyperalgesia in models of arthritis and other inflammatory diseases [32, 52, 54–56]. As in human patients, evidence is accumulating that arthritis chronicity in animal models is associated not just with nociceptor sensitization, but also with bona-fide neuropathic changes, as highlighted by upregulated expression of the neuronal transcription factor ATF3 and other stress markers in DRGs of long-term arthritis models [33, 51, 52, 56, 57]. In the K/BxN serum transfer model, the transition from acute to chronic pain states was shown to be associated with Toll-like receptor 4 function [58], making this molecule and its potential endogenous ligands intriguing therapeutic targets.

Analgesia in chronic arthritis models

Pharmacologically, consistent with a neurogenic mechanism, persistent pain in both CAIA and K/BxN mice appears to be alleviated by gabapentin, but not NSAIDs [49, 51]. A role for leptin-dependent opioid reward mechanisms and analgesia has been identified recently in rat adjuvant-induced arthritis, potentially expanding the usefulness of these models to human addiction studies [45]. TNF antagonists decreased pain responses, as assessed by locomotor/behavioral test and mechanical and thermal hyperalgesia, more rapidly than their anti-inflammatory activity in a model of rat antigen-induced monoarthritis and in TNFtg mice [6, 59]. The latter results correlated with fMRI findings in both animals and human patients, suggesting centrally mediated pain modulation by TNF [6].

Pain-suppressed behavior in arthritis models

Various forms of pain-suppressed spontaneous behaviors, including locomotor activity, as well as operant responses and place avoidance have also been studied in arthritis models, showing strong correlation with clinical disease [45, 60–66]. While the kinetics of clinical disease and suppression of locomotion appear to match closely in rapid-onset models of arthritis [61, 63, 65], the more slowly progressing K/BxN mouse strain displays a significant delay between peak clinical progression and decreased mobility [64]. This finding is suggestive of a psychoaffective component to the pain-suppressed behaviors in this strain. The possibility of depressive-like behavior resulting from chronic inflammatory arthritis was specifically investigated in TNFtg animals; however, the study failed to identify neurobiological or behavioral correlates of depression [66]. Whether these negative results reflect strain-dependent or experimental system differences or can be generalized remains to be established, but this is of course a crucial line of research due to the known psychoaffective component of pain in human RA patients [1, 2].

Conclusions

Although no animal model perfectly recapitulates all aspects of human inflammatory arthritis, the diversity of existing models provides a large armamentarium for elucidating specific pathophysiological mechanisms, including the study of arthritic pain. In this respect, important criteria for model selection include relevant pathophysiology and disease kinetics, especially with regard to chronicity. Similarly, the array of systems currently utilized for the experimental evaluation of pain perception in animals—spanning from traditional quantitation of hyperalgesia and allodynia-linked responses, to behavioral studies, to the more recent neuroimaging and neurobiological approaches—offers important experimental opportunities, while also requiring thoughtful consideration of technical and interpretive caveats. Parallel progress in these two fields will greatly broaden our understanding of pain mechanisms beyond what can be achieved in human studies.

Key priority targets for this research effort include the mechanisms that establish pain chronicity and the emergence of neuropathy in inflammatory arthritis, which are critical for treatment and prevention of symptom progression. Despite the recent pharmacotherapeutic advances, pain remains a major unresolved need in the management of arthritis patients. Animal models have proven instrumental in providing key insights into the inflammatory pathophysiology of arthritis, leading to the biological therapeutics revolution. Application of the same preclinical approaches has great potential for the replication of this success in treating rheumatoid pain.

Acknowledgements
The authors are grateful to Dr Nancy Olsen, Dr Bobby K. Han and Dr Fay Young for critical revision of the manuscript.

Funding
Work on this manuscript was funded in part by the CMSRU Seed Funding Program.

Authors' contributions
AB conceived the review, coordinated the work and wrote the manuscript. BDF and MEO wrote the manuscript. AA contributed Fig. 1 and wrote the manuscript. All authors read and approved the final manuscript.

Competing interests
The authors declare that they have no competing interests.

References

1. Walsh DA, McWilliams DF. Mechanisms, impact and management of pain in rheumatoid arthritis. Nat Rev Rheumatol. 2014;10(10):581–92.

2. Taylor PC, Moore A, Vasilescu R, Alvir J, Tarallo M. A structured literature review of the burden of illness and unmet needs in patients with rheumatoid arthritis: a current perspective. Rheumatol Int. 2016;36(5):685–95.

3. Smolen JS, Aletaha D, Koeller M, Weisman MH, Emery P. New therapies for treatment of rheumatoid arthritis. Lancet. 2007;370(9602):1861–74.

4. Smolen JS, Breedveld FC, Burmester GR, Bykerk V, Dougados M, Emery P, Kvien TK, Navarro-Compan MV, Oliver S, Schoels M, et al. Treating rheumatoid arthritis to target: 2014 update of the recommendations of an international task force. Ann Rheum Dis. 2016;75(1):3–15.

5. Koop SM, ten Klooster PM, Vonkeman HE, Steunebrink LM, van de Laar MA. Neuropathic-like pain features and cross-sectional associations in rheumatoid arthritis. Arthritis Res Ther. 2015;17:237.

6. Hess A, Axmann R, Rech J, Finzel S, Heindl C, Kreitz S, Sergeeva M, Saake M, Garcia M, Kollias G, et al. Blockade of TNF-alpha rapidly inhibits pain responses in the central nervous system. Proc Natl Acad Sci U S A. 2011;108(9):3731–6.

7. Schaible HG. Nociceptive neurons detect cytokines in arthritis. Arthritis Res Ther. 2014;16(5):470.

8. Taylor P, Manger B, Alvaro-Gracia J, Johnstone R, Gomez-Reino J, Eberhardt E, Wolfe F, Schwartzman S, Furfaro N, Kavanaugh A. Patient perceptions concerning pain management in the treatment of rheumatoid arthritis. J Int Med Res. 2010;38(4):1213–24.

9. Lee YC, Cui J, Lu B, Frits ML, Iannaccone CK, Shadick NA, Weinblatt ME, Solomon DH. Pain persists in DAS28 rheumatoid arthritis remission but not in ACR/EULAR remission: a longitudinal observational study. Arthritis Res Ther. 2011;13(3):R83.

10. Smolen JS, Strand V, Koenig AS, Szumski A, Kotak S, Jones TV. Discordance between patient and physician assessments of global disease activity in rheumatoid arthritis and association with work productivity. Arthritis Res Ther. 2016;18(1):114.

11. Nikiphorou E, Radner H, Chatzidionysiou K, Desthieux C, Zabalan C, van Eijk-Hustings Y, Dixon WG, Hyrich KL, Askling J, Gossec L. Patient global assessment in measuring disease activity in rheumatoid arthritis: a review of the literature. Arthritis Res Ther. 2016;18(1):251.

12. Bevaart L, Vervoordeldonk MJ, Tak PP. Evaluation of therapeutic targets in animal models of arthritis: how does it relate to rheumatoid arthritis? Arthritis Rheum. 2010;62(8):2192–205.

13. Bolon B, Stolina M, King C, Middleton S, Gasser J, Zack D, Feige U. Rodent preclinical models for developing novel antiarthritic molecules: comparative biology and preferred methods for evaluating efficacy. J Biomed Biotechnol. 2011;2011:569068.

14. McNamee K, Williams R, Seed M. Animal models of rheumatoid arthritis: how informative are they? Eur J Pharmacol. 2015;759:278–86.

15. Sardar S, Andersson A. Old and new therapeutics for rheumatoid arthritis: in vivo models and drug development. Immunopharmacol Immunotoxicol. 2016;38(1):2–13.

16. Keffer J, Probert L, Cazlaris H, Georgopoulos S, Kaslaris E, Kioussis D, Kollias G. Transgenic mice expressing human tumour necrosis factor: a predictive genetic model of arthritis. EMBO J. 1991;10(13):4025–31.

17. Kouskoff V, Korganow AS, Duchatelle V, Degott C, Benoist C, Mathis D. Organ-specific disease provoked by systemic autoimmunity. Cell. 1996; 87(5):811–22.

18. Monach P, Hattori K, Huang H, Hyatt E, Morse J, Nguyen L, Ortiz-Lopez A, Wu HJ, Mathis D, Benoist C. The K/BxN mouse model of inflammatory arthritis: theory and practice. Methods Mol Med. 2007;136:269–82.

19. Christensen AD, Haase C, Cook AD, Hamilton JA. K/BxN serum-transfer arthritis as a model for human inflammatory arthritis. Front Immunol. 2016;7:213.

20. Li P, Schwarz EM. The TNF-alpha transgenic mouse model of inflammatory arthritis. Springer Semin Immunopathol. 2003;25(1):19–33.

21. Holmdahl R, Lorentzen JC, Lu S, Olofsson P, Wester L, Holmberg J, Pettersson U. Arthritis induced in rats with nonimmunogenic adjuvants as models for rheumatoid arthritis. Immunol Rev. 2001;184:184–202.

22. Brand DD, Kang AH, Rosloniec EF. Immunopathogenesis of collagen arthritis. Springer Semin Immunopathol. 2003;25(1):3–18.

23. Nandakumar KS, Holmdahl R. Collagen antibody induced arthritis. Methods Mol Med. 2007;136:215–23.

24. Zhang Z, Leong DJ, Xu L, He Z, Wang A, Navati M, Kim SJ, Hirsh DM, Hardin JA, Cobelli NJ, et al. Curcumin slows osteoarthritis progression and relieves osteoarthritis-associated pain symptoms in a post-traumatic osteoarthritis mouse model. Arthritis Res Ther. 2016;18(1):128.

25. Le Bars D, Gozariu M, Cadden SW. Animal models of nociception. Pharmacol Rev. 2001;53(4):597–652.

26. Wilson SG, Mogil JS. Measuring pain in the (knockout) mouse: big challenges in a small mammal. Behav Brain Res. 2001;125(1-2):65–73.

27. Bridges D, Thompson SW, Rice AS. Mechanisms of neuropathic pain. Br J Anaesth. 2001;87(1):12–26.

28. Percie du Sert N, Rice AS. Improving the translation of analgesic drugs to the clinic: animal models of neuropathic pain. Br J Pharmacol. 2014;171(12):2951–63.

29. Cobos EJ, Portillo-Salido E. "Bedside-to-Bench" behavioral outcomes in animal models of pain: beyond the evaluation of reflexes. Curr Neuropharmacol. 2013;11(6):560–91.

30. Flecknell P, Leach M, Bateson M. Affective state and quality of life in mice. Pain. 2011;152(5):963–4.

31. Mogil JS, Wilson SG, Wan Y. Chapter 2. Assessing nociception in murine subjects. In: Kruger L, editor. Methods in Pain Research. Boca Raton: CRC Press; 2001. p. 11–39.

32. Clark AK, Grist J, Al-Kashi A, Perretti M, Malcangio M. Spinal cathepsin S and fractalkine contribute to chronic pain in the collagen-induced arthritis model. Arthritis Rheum. 2012;64(6):2038–47.

33. Botz B, Bolcskei K, Kereskai L, Kovacs M, Nemeth T, Szigeti K, Horvath I, Mathe D, Kovacs N, Hashimoto H, et al. Differential regulatory role of pituitary adenylate cyclase-activating polypeptide in the serum-transfer arthritis model. Arthritis Rheumatol. 2014;66(10):2739–50.

34. Quadros AU, Pinto LG, Fonseca MM, Kusuda R, Cunha FQ, Cunha TM. Dynamic weight bearing is an efficient and predictable method for evaluation of arthritic nociception and its pathophysiological mechanisms in mice. Sci Rep. 2015;5:14648.

35. Davis KD. Studies of pain using functional magnetic resonance imaging. In: Casey KL, Bushnell MC, editors. Pain Imaging. Seattle: IASP Press; 2000. p. 195–210.

36. Thompson SJ, Bushnell MC. Rodent functional and anatomical imaging of pain. Neurosci Lett. 2012;520(2):131–9.

37. Langford DJ, Bailey AL, Chanda ML, Clarke SE, Drummond TE, Echols S, Glick S, Ingrao J, Klassen-Ross T, Lacroix-Fralish ML, et al. Coding of facial expressions of pain in the laboratory mouse. Nat Methods. 2010;7(6):447–9.

38. Sotocinal SG, Sorge RE, Zaloum A, Tuttle AH, Martin LJ, Wieskopf JS, Mapplebeck JC, Wei P, Zhan S, Zhang S, et al. The Rat Grimace Scale: a partially automated method for quantifying pain in the laboratory rat via facial expressions. Mol Pain. 2011;7:55.

39. Matson DJ, Broom DC, Cortright DN. Locomotor activity in a novel environment as a test of inflammatory pain in rats. Methods Mol Biol. 2010;617:67–78.

40. Urban R, Scherrer G, Goulding EH, Tecott LH, Basbaum AI. Behavioral indices of ongoing pain are largely unchanged in male mice with tissue or nerve injury-induced mechanical hypersensitivity. Pain. 2011;152(5):990–1000.

41. Neubert JK, Widmer CG, Malphurs W, Rossi HL, Vierck Jr CJ, Caudle RM. Use of a novel thermal operant behavioral assay for characterization of orofacial pain sensitivity. Pain. 2005;116(3):386–95.

42. Nolan TA, Hester J, Bokrand-Donatelli Y, Caudle RM, Neubert JK. Adaptation of a novel operant orofacial testing system to characterize both mechanical and thermal pain. Behav Brain Res. 2011;217(2):477–80.

43. Fuchs PN, McNabb CT. The place escape/avoidance paradigm: a novel method to assess nociceptive processing. J Integr Neurosci. 2012;11(1):61–72.

44. King T, Vera-Portocarrero L, Gutierrez T, Vanderah TW, Dussor G, Lai J, Fields HL, Porreca F. Unmasking the tonic-aversive state in neuropathic pain. Nat Neurosci. 2009;12(11):1364–6.

45. Lim G, Kim H, McCabe MF, Chou CW, Wang S, Chen LL, Marota JJ, Blood A, Breiter HC, Mao J. A leptin-mediated central mechanism in analgesia-enhanced opioid reward in rats. J Neurosci. 2014;34(29):9779–88.

46. Bas DB, Su J, Wigerblad G, Svensson CI. Pain in rheumatoid arthritis: models and mechanisms. Pain Manag. 2016;6(3):265–84.

47. Muley MM, Krustev E, McDougall JJ. Preclinical assessment of inflammatory pain. CNS Neurosci Ther. 2016;22(2):88–101.

48. Weyer AD, Zappia KJ, Garrison SR, O'Hara CL, Dodge AK, Stucky CL. Nociceptor sensitization depends on age and pain chronicity. eNeuro. 2016; 3(1):ENEURO.0115-15.2015.

49. Bas DB, Su J, Sandor K, Agalave NM, Lundberg J, Codeluppi S, Baharpoor A, Nandakumar KS, Holmdahl R, Svensson CI. Collagen antibody-induced arthritis evokes persistent pain with spinal glial involvement and transient prostaglandin dependency. Arthritis Rheum. 2012;64(12):3886–96.

50. Nieto FR, Clark AK, Grist J, Hathway GJ, Chapman V, Malcangio M. Neuron-immune mechanisms contribute to pain in early stages of arthritis. J Neuroinflammation. 2016;13(1):96.

51. Christianson CA, Corr M, Firestein GS, Mobargha A, Yaksh TL, Svensson CI. Characterization of the acute and persistent pain state present in K/BxN serum transfer arthritis. Pain. 2010;151(2):394–403.

52. Su J, Gao T, Shi T, Xiang Q, Xu X, Wiesenfeld-Hallin Z, Hokfelt T, Svensson CI. Phenotypic changes in dorsal root ganglion and spinal cord in the collagen antibody-induced arthritis mouse model. J Comp Neurol. 2015; 523(10):1505–28.

53. Wigerblad G, Bas DB, Fernades-Cerqueira C, Krishnamurthy A, Nandakumar KS, Rogoz K, Kato J, Sandor K, Su J, Jimenez-Andrade JM, et al. Autoantibodies to citrullinated proteins induce joint pain independent of inflammation via a chemokine-dependent mechanism. Ann Rheum Dis. 2016;75(4):730–8.

54. Nieto FR, Clark AK, Grist J, Chapman V, Malcangio M. Calcitonin gene-related peptide-expressing sensory neurons and spinal microglial reactivity contribute to pain states in collagen-induced arthritis. Arthritis Rheumatol. 2015;67(6):1668–77.

55. Pinho-Ribeiro FA, Verri Jr WA, Chiu IM. Nociceptor sensory neuron-immune interactions in pain and inflammation. Trends Immunol. 2017;38(1):5–19.

56. Fischer BD, Ho C, Kuzin I, Bottaro A, O'Leary ME. Chronic exposure to tumor necrosis factor in vivo induces hyperalgesia, upregulates sodium channel gene expression and alters the cellular electrophysiology of dorsal root ganglion neurons. Neurosci Lett. 2017;653:195–201.

57. Segond von Banchet G, Boettger MK, Fischer N, Gajda M, Brauer R, Schaible HG. Experimental arthritis causes tumor necrosis factor-alpha-dependent infiltration of macrophages into rat dorsal root ganglia which correlates with pain-related behavior. Pain. 2009;145(1-2):151–9.

58. Christianson CA, Dumlao DS, Stokes JA, Dennis EA, Svensson CI, Corr M, Yaksh TL. Spinal TLR4 mediates the transition to a persistent mechanical hypersensitivity after the resolution of inflammation in serum-transferred arthritis. Pain. 2011;152(12):2881–91.

59. Boettger MK, Hensellek S, Richter F, Gajda M, Stockigt R, von Banchet GS, Brauer R, Schaible HG. Antinociceptive effects of tumor necrosis factor alpha neutralization in a rat model of antigen-induced arthritis: evidence of a neuronal target. Arthritis Rheum. 2008;58(8):2368–78.

60. Cain CK, Francis JM, Plone MA, Emerich DF, Lindner MD. Pain-related disability and effects of chronic morphine in the adjuvant-induced arthritis model of chronic pain. Physiol Behav. 1997;62(1):199–205.

61. Sasakawa T, Sasakawa Y, Ohkubo Y, Mutoh S. FK506 ameliorates spontaneous locomotor activity in collagen-induced arthritis: implication of distinct effect from suppression of inflammation. Int Immunopharmacol. 2005;5(3):503–10.

62. Inglis JJ, Notley CA, Essex D, Wilson AW, Feldmann M, Anand P, Williams R. Collagen-induced arthritis as a model of hyperalgesia: functional and cellular analysis of the analgesic actions of tumor necrosis factor blockade. Arthritis Rheum. 2007;56(12):4015–23.

63. Hartog A, Hulsman J, Garssen J. Locomotion and muscle mass measures in a murine model of collagen-induced arthritis. BMC Musculoskelet Disord. 2009;10:59.

64. Frommholz D, Illges H. Maximal locomotor depression follows maximal ankle swelling during the progression of arthritis in K/BxN mice. Rheumatol Int. 2012;32(12):3999–4003.

65. Rajasekaran N, Tran R, Pascual C, Xie X, Mellins ED. Reduced locomotor activity correlates with increased severity of arthritis in a mouse model of antibody-induced arthritis. Open J Rheumatol Autoimmune Dis. 2014;4(1):62–8.

66. Suss P, Kalinichenko L, Baum W, Reichel M, Kornhuber J, Loskarn S, Ettle B, Distler JH, Schett G, Winkler J, et al. Hippocampal structure and function are maintained despite severe innate peripheral inflammation. Brain Behav Immun. 2015;49:156–70.

19

Evaluation of newly proposed remission cut-points for disease activity score in 28 joints (DAS28) in rheumatoid arthritis patients upon IL-6 pathway inhibition

M. Schoels[1] (iD), F. Alasti[2], J. S. Smolen[1,2] and D. Aletaha[2*]

Abstract

Background: Stringent remission criteria are crucial in rheumatoid arthritis (RA) assessment. Disease activity score in 28 joints (DAS28)-remission has not been included among American College of Rheumatology/European League Against Rheumatism definitions, because of its association with significant residual disease activity, partly due to high weighting of acute-phase reactants (APR). New, more stringent cut-points for DAS28-remission have recently been proposed that are suggested to reflect remission by clinical and simplified disease activity indices (clinical disease activity index (CDAI), simple disease activity index (SDAI)). However, their stringency in therapies directly influencing APR, like IL-6-blockers, has not been tested. We tested the new cut-points in patients with RA receiving tocilizumab.

Methods: We used data from randomised controlled trials of tocilizumab and evaluated patients in remission according to new DAS28-C-reactive protein (DAS-CRP) and DAS-erythrocyte sedimentation rate (DAS-ESR) cut-points (1.9 and 2.2). We assessed their disease activity state using the CDAI, SDAI and Boolean criteria and analysed their individual residual core set variables, like swollen joint counts (SJC28).

Results: About 50% of patients in DAS28-CRP-remission (<1.9) fell into higher disease activity states when assessed with CDAI, SDAI or Boolean criteria. Also, 15% had three or more (up to eight) SJC. Even higher disease activity was seen in patients classified as being in DAS28-ESR-remission (<2.2).

Conclusions: Even with new, more stringent cut-points, DAS28-remission is frequently associated with considerable residual clinical disease activity, indicating that this limitation of the DAS28 is related to score construction rather than the choice of cut-points.

Keywords: Rheumatoid arthritis, DAS28, Cut-points, Outcomes research, Tocilizumab

Background

Composite measures to define disease activity provide better information than individual variables in the assessment of rheumatoid arthritis (RA) [1]. Among these instruments are dichotomous tools like the American College of Rheumatology (ACR) response criteria, [2] and continuous scores like the simplified and clinical disease activity indices (SDAI and CDAI) [3, 4] and the disease activity score using 28 joint counts (DAS28) in its two versions employing erythrocyte sedimentation rate (ESR) or C-reactive protein (CRP) [5]. The use of continuous measures to assess disease activity states is an important requirement in clinical trials and practice, and achieving a state of low disease activity (LDA) or remission (REM) is a major treatment target in RA [6]. Consequently, stringent remission definitions are crucial for optimising outcomes [7].

DAS28-remission has not been included among the joint remission definitions by the ACR and the European League Against Rheumatism (EULAR), because it is associated with significant residual disease activity in a large proportion of patients [7–9]. Due to the high weight of acute phase reactant (APR) components in the DAS28

* Correspondence: daniel.aletaha@meduniwien.ac.at
[2]Division of Rheumatology, Medical University of Vienna, Waehringer Guertel 18-20, 1090 Vienna, Austria
Full list of author information is available at the end of the article

formula, this impediment becomes particularly prominent when agents that interfere directly with the acute-phase response, like the interleukin-6 (IL-6) pathway inhibitors or Janus kinase (Jak) inhibitors, are used. Recognizing this limitation of the DAS28, which is not seen with the CDAI and SDAI [10], cut-points other than 2.6 have been proposed [11–13]. The most recent approach suggested a DAS28-CRP <1.9 and DAS28-ESR <2.2 to be related best to CDAI-remission [13]. However, survey results show that remission should define a state of at most minimal residual disease activity with no more than two involved joints, swollen and/or tender [7]. As reported previously, upon IL-6 pathway inhibition low APR levels lead to unduly high remission frequencies as assessed by the DAS28 [10] while at the same time allowing for a significant number of residual swollen joints.

Here, we tested the newly proposed cut-points for DAS28-CRP and DAS28-ESR remission in RA patients treated with tocilizumab (TCZ), an approved and widely used antibody to the IL-6 receptor.

Methods

Data

We analysed data from three large, randomized, controlled trials. The LITHE, [14] OPTION, [15] and TOWARD [16] studies evaluated the efficacy of TCZ plus methotrexate/ conventional synthetic disease-modifying anti-rheumatic drugs (csDMARDs) in adult patients with RA with prior non-response to csDMARDs. We were kindly provided with a random 80% data cut by the trial sponsor (Roche). For our analyses, we used data from the TCZ treatment arms, i.e., patients receiving 4 and 8 mg/kg intravenous TCZ in combination with methotrexate or csDMARDs.

Analyses

We examined disease activity parameters in patients who were classified as being in either DAS28-CRP (<1.9) or DAS28-ESR (<2.2) remission after 24 weeks follow up. We analysed levels of core set variables used for calculation of composite scores (formulas compiled in Additional file 1: Table S1), namely SJC/tender joint count (TJC) using 28 joints, patient and evaluator global assessment (PGA, EGA) and CRP and ESR. We contrasted remission according to newly proposed DAS28 cut-points with percentages of REM, LDA, moderate disease activity (MDA) and high disease activity (HDA) using the CDAI [4] or SDAI [3] and also tested Boolean remission criteria [7]. Cut-points for the CDAI (SDAI) were applied as follows: REM ≤2.8 (≤3.3), LDA >2.8 and ≤10 (>3.3 and ≤11), and MDA >10 and ≤22 (>11 and ≤26).

Results

In total, 2423 patients (TCZ: 1613, placebo: 810) were included in the LITHE, OPTION and TOWARD studies

(Additional file 1: Table S2). After 24 weeks of TCZ treatment, 178 patients achieved remission according to the DAS28-CRP <1.9 threshold. Additional file 1: Table S3 shows their baseline characteristics; briefly, mean CRP was 2.6 mg/dl, mean ESR was 46 mm/h, and mean SJC28 was 10.8. Baseline composite scores in DAS28-CRP-remission were: DAS28-CRP 5.6, DAS28-ESR 6.2, SDAI 37.6 and CDAI 35.0. Baseline characteristics of the 235 patients with DAS28-ESR <2.2 at week 24 are also detailed in Additional file 1: Table S3.

Higher remission rates by DAS28 compared to CDAI or SDAI

Among patients in DAS28-CRP-remission, only 47.2% were in remission according to the CDAI while 52.8% were in LDA. SDAI evaluation resulted in 52.8% in REM, 47.2% in LDA and 39.3% in REM according to Boolean criteria (Additional file 1: Table S4). Among the DAS28-ESR remitters, only 30.2% reached CDAI-REM, while 60.9% were in CDAI-LDA, and 8.9% were even in CDAI-MDA (SDAI: 34.5% in REM, 58.3% in LDA, and in 7.2% MDA; Boolean criteria: 24.3% in REM; Additional file 1: Table S4).

Individual disease activity parameters in DAS28-remission

We analysed individual disease activity parameters in patients who reached DAS28-REM at 24 weeks (Table 1). We found that using the SJC in 28 joints (SJC28), up to 8 patients were in DAS28-CRP-REM, and up to 13 were in DAS28-ESR-REM. Figure 1 shows residual numbers of SJC in patients in DAS28-CRP and DAS28-ESR vs. patients in CDAI remission. Almost 15% of remitters had at least three swollen joints; among the 10% of patients with the highest SJC28, the mean SJC was 4.3 (Additional file 1: Table S5), which was made possible by very low APR, i.e., mean CRP of 0.03 mg/dl and mean ESR of 4.2 mm/h. Only 39.3% of patients with DAS28-CRP <1.9 and 24.3% with DAS28-ESR <2.2 fulfilled the Boolean remission definition.

We obtained very similar results for DAS28-ESR-REM regarding number of residual swollen joints (data not shown). Among patients who met DAS28-ESR-remission criteria, but not those for the CDAI, the mean SJC28 was 2.2 (2.8) (Table 1). More than 10% had five or more and >25% had three or more swollen joints. APR in the 10% with the highest number of swollen joints averaged at 0.08 (0.12) mg/dl (CRP) and 2.3 (1.5) mm/h (ESR) (Additional file 1: Table S5).

In addition, DAS28-remission allowed for a patient global assessment of disease activity (PGA) of up to 61 mm (DAS28-CRP-REM), and 89 mm (DAS28-ESR-REM) on the 100 mm visual analogue scale; the evaluator global assessment (EGA) reached up to 63 mm in DAS28-CRP-REM and 75 mm in DAS28-ESR-REM (Table 1). Importantly, this was not the case with the

Table 1 Disease activity parameters of patients in DAS28-CRP or DAS28-ESR remission, but not in SDAI, CDAI or Boolean remission

	DAS28-CRP <1.9 (n = 178)				DAS28-ESR <2.2 (n = 235)			
	No CDAI REM (n = 94)	No SDAI REM (n = 84)	No Boolean REM (n = 108)	All (n = 178)	No CDAI REM (n = 164)	No SDAI REM (n = 154)	No Boolean REM (n = 178)	All (n = 235)
SJC28	1.3 (1.9)	1.5 (1.9)	1.2 (1.8)	0.8 (1.5)	2.2 (2.8)	2.3 (2.9)	2.0(2.8)	1.6 (2.6)
	0 (0.0–8.0)	0 (0.0–8.0)	0.0 (0.0–8.0)	0.0 (0.0–8.0)	1.0 (0.0–13.0)	1.0 (0.0–13.0)	1.0 (0.0–13.0)	0.0 (0.0–13.0)
TJC28	0.1 (0.3)	0.1 (0.2)	0.0 (0.2)	0.1 (0.3)	0.8 (1.3)	0.8 (1.2)	0.7 (1.1)	0.6 (1.0)
	0 (0.0–1.0)	0 (0.0–1.0)	0.0 (0.0–1.0)	0.0 (0.0–1.0)	0.0 (0.0–5.0)	0.0 (0.0–5.0)	0.0 (0.0–5.0)	0.0 (0.0–5.0)
CRP (mg/l)	0.6 (0.8)	0.7 (0.9)	0.7 (0.9)	0.7 (1.0)	1.4 (4.1)	1.4 (4.2)	1.7 (4.8)	1.5 (4.2)
	0.3 (0.2–5.1)	0.3 (0.2–5.1)	0.4 (0.2–5.2)	0.3 (0.2–7.1)	0.4 (0.2–39.7)	0.4 (0.2–39.7)	0.4 (0.2–39.7)	0.4 (0.2–39.7)
ESR (mm/h)	8.4 (10.6)	8.5 (9.8)	8.4 (10.3)	9.3 (12.4)	3.6 (3.1)	3.7 (3.1)	3.9 (3.3)	4.2 (3.5)
	4.0 (0.0–57.0)	5.0 (0.0–45.0)	5.0 (0.0–57.0)	5.0 (.00–91)	3.0 (1.0–16.0)	3.0 (1.0–16.0)	3.0 (1.0–18.0)	3.0 (1.0–18.0)
PGA (mm VAS)	20.4 (14.8)	21.7 (15.2)	20.2 (13.9)	13.7 (13.7)	21.9 (17.8)	22.9 (18.1)	21.4 (17.4)	17.1 (17.0)
	16.0 (0.0–61.0)	19.0 (0–61.0)	16.0 (0.0–61.0)	10.0 (0.0–61.0)	17.5 (0.0–89.0)	19.5 (0.0–89.0)	16.5 (0.0–89.0)	13.0 (0.0–89.0)
EGA (mm VAS)	14.6 (11.4)	15.4 (12.0)	12.2 (11.5)	9.8 (10.4)	14.3 (11.4)	14.7 (11.7)	13.0 (11.5)	11.4 (10.9)
	12.0 (0.0–63.0)	13.0 (0–63.0)	9.0 (0.0–63.0)	7.0 (0.0–63.0)	11.5 (0.0–75.0)	12.0 (0.0–75.0)	10.0 (0.0–75.0)	9.0 (0.0–75.0)
HAQ	0.7 (0.6)	0.7 (0.6)	0.7 (0.6)	0.6 (0.5)	0.7 (0.6)	0.7 (0.6)	0.7 (0.6)	0.6 (0.6)
	0.6 (0.0–2.0)	0.6 (0–2.0)	0.6 (0.0–2.0)	0.4 (0.0–2.0)	0.6 (0.0–2.3)	0.6 (0.0–2.3)	0.6 (0.0–2.3)	0.5 (0.0–2.3)
SDAI	5.0 (1.6)	5.3 (1.5)	4.6 (1.9)	3.3 (2.2)	6.7 (3.3)	7.0 (3.2)	6.3 (3.5)	5.2 (3.7)
	4.7 (2.8–9.5)	4.9 (3.3–9.5)	4.4 (1.3–9.5)	3.1 (0.02–9.5)	5.8 (2.8–19.6)	6.1 (3.4–19.6)	5.6 (1.3–19.6)	4.6 (0.02–19.6)
CDAI	4.9 (1.6)	5.2 (1.5)	4.5 (1.9)	3.2 (2.3)	6.6 (3.3)	6.8 (3.2)	6.2 (3.5)	5.0 (3.7)
	4.6 (2.8–9.5)	4.8 (2.9–9.5)	4.4 (1.2–9.5)	3.0 (0.0–9.5)	5.8 (2.8–19.6)	6.1 (3.2–19.6)	5.5 (0.0–19.6)	4.5 (0.0–19.6)
DAS28–CRP	1.7 (0.2)	1.7 (0.2)	1.6 (0.2)	1.5 (0.3)	2.1 (0.5)	2.1 (0.5)	2.0 (0.5)	1.9 (0.6)
	1.7 (1.1–1.9)	1.7 (1.1–1.9)	1.7 (1.2–1.9)	1.6 (1.0–1.9)	2.0 (1.1–3.7)	2.0 (1.1–3.7)	2.0 (1.2–3.7)	1.8 (1.0–3.7)
DAS28–ESR	1.7 (0.7)	1.7 (0.7)	1.6 (0.7)	1.5 (0.8)	1.6 (0.5)	1.6 (0.5)	1.6 (0.5)	1.5 (0.5)
	1.6 (0.4–3.4)	1.7 (0.5–3.4)	1.6 (0.2–3.4)	1.5 (0.0–3.4)	1.7 (0.4–2.2)	1.8 (0.5–2.2)	1.7 (0.2–2.2)	1.6 (0.0–2.2)

Values are mean (SD) or median (range). *SDAI* simplified disease activity index *CDAI* clinical disease activity index, *REM* remission, *SJC28* swollen joint count using 28 joints, *TJC28* tender joint count using 28 joints, *CRP* C-reactive protein, *ESR* erythrocyte sedimentation rate, *PGA* patient global assessment, *VAS* visual analogue scale, *EGA* evaluator global assessment, *HAQ* health assessment questionnaire, *DAS28-CRP* disease activity score using 28 joint counts and C-reactive protein, *DAS28-ESR* disease activity score using 28 joint counts and erythrocyte sedimentation rate

CDAI and SDAI ratings. Additional file 2: Figure S1 displays individual disease activity parameters that contribute to the calculated composite scores for patients in DAS28-CRP-remission (panel A), and in DAS28-ESR-remission (panel B). As can be seen, in DAS28-remitters, who were in LDA or MDA according to the CDAI, lower APR "compensated" for higher joint counts, allowing maintenance of DAS28-remission despite lower cut-points.

Discussion

In 2011, the ACR and EULAR provided Boolean and index-based remission criteria for trials and clinical practice, implementing survey results and analyses of radiographic and functional outcomes [7]. At that time, the DAS28 remission criteria were not compatible with these important constructs and outcomes. In the meantime, new lower cut-points of 1.9 for DAS28-CRP-remission and 2.2 for DAS28-ESR-remission have been proposed [13].

In the present study, we observed that these cut-points still allow a considerable proportion of patients with RA to be classified as remitters despite the presence of a significant SJC, namely up to 8 in DAS28-CRP remission and 13 in DAS28-ESR remission. These numbers do not represent individual outliers, as approximately 15% and 25%, respectively, of patients in putative remission according to the proposed thresholds had three or more swollen joints.

The SJC is highly related to the progression of joint damage [17], therefore any remission criteria allowing for swollen joints in a substantial number of patients would not pass this important filter of criterion validity, and would not have face validity for most rheumatologists [18]. A majority of patients with DAS28-CRP <1.9 were in LDA according to the CDAI, and about two thirds of patients with DAS28-ESR <2.2 were not in remission as defined by the CDAI, with almost 10% even being in CDAI-MDA. High SJCs were not an isolated finding but rather accompanied by higher PGA score,

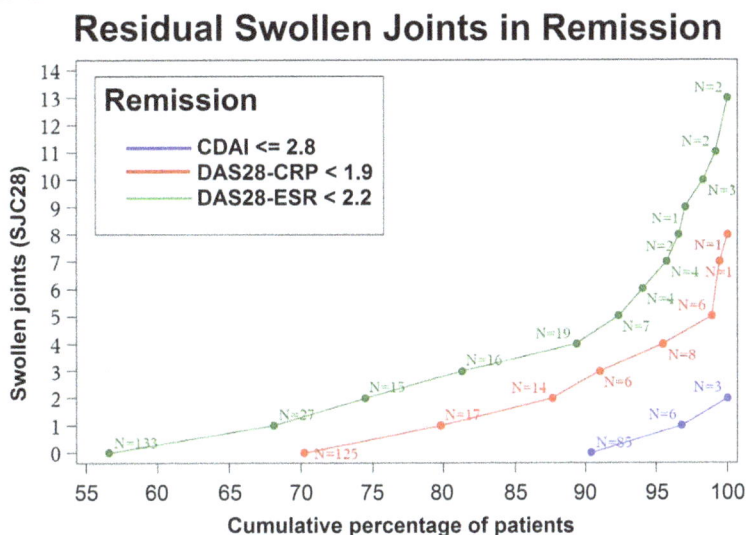

Fig. 1 Residual swollen joints in remission. *X-axis* shows cumulative percent of patients. *Y-axis* shows swollen joint counts (SJC28). *Red line*: counts of patients in remission according to DAS28-CRP (DAS28-CRP <1.9; N = 178); *green line*: remission according to DAS28-ESR (DAS28-ESR <2.2; N = 235); *blue line*: remission according to CDAI (CDAI ≤2.8; N = 94)

pain and EGA ratings and worse function. However, CRP or ESR was lower among DAS28 "remitters" who had CDAI LDA or MDA. Thus, in the formula of DAS28, very low APR within the normal range may compensate for unacceptably high joint counts.

Our results suggest that the problem of DAS28-remission is not related to a specific cut-point, but rather to the construction of the score itself: the complexity, transformations and weighting of the formula will perpetuate the problem, even if the cut-point is dramatically reduced. Indeed, one could have envisaged that lower cut-points would not be the solution as the ACR/EULAR task force had tested a DAS28-ESR threshold of 2.0 and did not find it compatible with optimal outcomes [7]. Also, there was no major difference in sonographic data between cut-points of 2.6 and 2.4 [19]. At the time the DAS28 was introduced, it was a seminal approach to assess disease activity, but remission was only rarely achievable and the weighting of the individual score components was appropriate for higher disease activity states.

When we carried out these analyses for the SDAI, which also includes CRP in its formula, we found remission rates resembling those of the CDAI, a purely clinical score, more closely than those of the DAS28. However, the contribution of CRP to the SDAI only amounts to about 5% [4]. These results emphasise further that not the mere presence but the high weighting of APR in the DAS28 formula may lead to misrepresentation of actual disease activity.

Interestingly, Nishimoto and colleagues conducted correlation analyses between CDAI and DAS28-ESR in 53 patients included in the SATORI study at baseline and follow up [20]. They observed strong correlation between the DAS8 and the CDAI or SDAI and concluded that the DAS28-ESR was a valid tool to assess patients treated with TCZ; nevertheless, this correlation only addressed the relationships between the scores for higher and lower disease activity, which will be found for most scores, and do not provide a comparative answer in the clinical context. In addition, they also reported a threefold difference between rates of DAS28-remission and CDAI-remission after 24 weeks (with the traditional thresholds for DAS28-ESR of <2.6). Finally, patients who were DAS28-ESR remitters but not CDAI/SDAI remitters (*n* = 17) had high residual swollen joints and/or PGA; indeed, among DAS28-remitters, only 44% had no swollen joints, while among SDAI and CDAI remitters almost 90% had no swollen joints. Thus, their data fully support our general assessment.

Also Shaver et al. [21] investigated remission rates using different methods of assessment. In their cross-sectional analysis of data from an outpatient clinic, the authors included RA patients on various therapies, which were partly csDMARDs and partly biological agents, with no further specification. In this cohort, the authors identified a similar if not even greater discrepancy among remission rates: specifically, the prevalence of remission differed dramatically between the scores (28.5% when using the DAS28 compared to 6.5–8.1% when using the CDAI). Thus, these data also support concerns about the high weighting of APRs in the DAS28 formulas, which we have now also shown to affect the DAS28 regardless of the new (lower) thresholds.

Our study has some limitations. First, it focussed on TCZ data only. However, we have previously shown that

DAS28-CRP is also not a reliable instrument for the assessment of remission in tofacitinib therapy [22]. Data on sarilumab, sirukumab and baricitinib need to be obtained to validate the current findings. Second, we did not evaluate radiographic changes. However, when biologic agents are used, we cannot expect joint damage progression even in active disease [23], and the number of placebo-treated patients in remission was very small. Moreover, it has previously been shown that in DAS28 but not in SDAI or CDAI remission, it is mainly the SJC that drives the assessment of joint deterioration, [24] in line with findings that in individual joints swelling is highly related to damage [17].

Conclusions

Lower more stringent remission thresholds for DAS28, as a consequence of the construction of the formula, do not convey sufficient stringency to comply with full clinical remission defined as a state of no or at most minimal disease activity. If one patient in seven to one patient in four who are categorized as being in "remission" has three or more swollen joints, full clinical remission cannot be claimed. Our data further confirm the validity of the ACR/EULAR remission definition, especially when agents interfering directly with APR are employed.

Additional files

Additional file 1: Table S1. Formulas of compound scores for RA assessment. **Table S2.** Baseline characteristics of the LITHE, OPTION and TOWARD trial data provided for the present analyses. **Table S3.** Baseline characteristics of patients achieving DAS28-CRP or DAS28-ESR remission at week 24: investigated cohort. **Table S4.** Comparison of remission rates according to different compound scores (24-week values). **Table S5.** Mean values of core set variables and composite measures in the 10% of patients with the highest swollen joint counts in DAS28-CRP and DAS28-ESR remission (90th percentile of SJC). (DOCX 22 kb)

Additional file 2: Figure S1. Display of individual disease activity parameters among patients with DAS28-CRP<1.9 who attain different states by CDAI after 24 weeks of tocilizumab therapy. Panel a: patients in remission according to DAS28-CRP classification (n=178). Panel b: patients in remission according to DAS28-ESR classification (n=235). X-axis: CDAI disease activity state. Y-axis: Mean values of respective disease activity parameters. (TIF 2475 kb)

Acknowledgements
We thank Roche for the provision of a random sample set of trial data.

Funding
Not applicable.

Authors' contributions
All authors, MS, FA, JS and DA made substantial contributions to conception and design of the study and contributed to analysis and interpretation of data; all authors were involved in drafting the manuscript and revising it; all authors gave final approval of the version to be published.

Competing interests
MS and FA: nothing to disclose; JS: has received grants for his institution from Abbvie, Janssen, Lilly, MSD, Pfizer and Roche and has provided expert advice to and/or had speaking engagements for Abbvie, Amgen, Astra-Zeneca, Astro, Celgene, Celtrion, Glaxo, ILTOO, Janssen, Lilly, Medimmune, MSD, Novartis-Sandoz, Pfizer, Roche, Samsung, Sanofi and UCB; DA: received grants from MSD and BMS, was a speaker for AbbVie, Merck, UCB, Janssen, BMS, Pfizer, Medac and Roche and provided consultancy for Abbvie, Eli Lilly & Co, MSD, Centocor and Janssen.

Author details
[1]Second Department of Internal Medicine, Hietzing Hospital, Vienna, Austria. [2]Division of Rheumatology, Medical University of Vienna, Waehringer Guertel 18-20, 1090 Vienna, Austria.

References

1. van der Heijde DM, van't Hof MA, van Riel PL, et al. Validity of single variables and composite indices for measuring disease activity in rheumatoid arthritis. Ann Rheum Dis. 1992;51(2):177–81.
2. Felson DT, Anderson JJ, Boers M, et al. American College of Rheumatology. Preliminary definition of improvement in rheumatoid arthritis. Arthritis Rheum. 1995;38(6):727–35.
3. Smolen JS, Breedveld FC, Schiff MH, et al. A simplified disease activity index for rheumatoid arthritis for use in clinical practice. Rheumatology (Oxford). 2003;42(2):244–57.
4. Aletaha D, Nell VP, Stamm T, et al. Acute phase reactants add little to composite disease activity indices for rheumatoid arthritis: validation of a clinical activity score. Arthritis Res Ther. 2005;7(4):R796–806.
5. Prevoo ML, van 't Hof MA, Kuper HH, et al. Modified disease activity scores that include twenty-eight joint counts. Development and validation in a prospective longitudinal study of patients with rheumatoid arthritis. Arthritis Rheum. 1995;38:44–8.
6. Smolen JS, Breedveld FC, Burmester GR, et al. Treating rheumatoid arthritis to target: 2014 update of the recommendations of an international task force. Ann Rheum Dis. 2016;75(1):3–15.
7. Felson DT, Smolen JS, Wells G, et al. American College of Rheumatology/ European League Against Rheumatism provisional definition of remission in rheumatoid arthritis for clinical trials. Ann Rheum Dis. 2011;70(3):404–13.
8. Mäkinen H, Kautiainen H, Hannonen P, et al. Is DAS28 an appropriate tool to assess remission in rheumatoid arthritis? Ann Rheum Dis. 2005; 64(10):1410–3.
9. van der Heijde DM, Klareskog L, Boers M, et al. Comparison of different definitions to classify remission and sustained remission: 1 year TEMPO results. Ann Rheum Dis. 2005;64:1582–7.
10. Smolen JS, Aletaha D, Gruben D, et al. Remission Rates with Tofacitinib Treatment in rheumatoid arthritis: a comparison of various remission criteria. Arthritis Rheum. 2016. doi:10.1002/art.39996 [Epub ahead of print].
11. Inoue M, Yamanaka H, Hara M, et al. Comparison of disease activity score (DAS)28-erythrocyte sedimentation rate and DAS28 C-reactive protein threshold values. Ann Rheum Dis. 2007;66(3):407–9.
12. Castrejon I, Ortiz AM, Toledano E, et al. Estimated cutoff points for the 28-joint disease activity score based on C-reactive protein in a longitudinal register of early arthritis. J Rheumatol. 2010;37(7):1439–43.
13. Fleischmann R, van der Heijde D, Koenig AS, et al. How much does Disease Activity Score in 28 joints ESR and CRP calculations underestimate disease activity compared with the Simplified Disease Activity Index? Ann Rheum Dis. 2015;74(6):1132–7.
14. Fleischmann R, Halland AM, Brzosko M, et al. Tocilizumab inhibits structural joint damage and improves physical function in patients with rheumatoid arthritis and inadequate responses to methotrexate: LITHE study 2-year results. J Rheumatol. 2013;40(2):113–26.
15. Smolen JS, Beaulieu A, Rubbert-Roth A, et al. Effect of interleukin-6 receptor inhibition with tocilizumab in patients with rheumatoid arthritis (OPTION study): a double-blind, placebo-controlled, randomised trial. Lancet. 2008; 371(9617):987–97.
16. Genovese MC, McKay JD, Nasonov EL, et al. Interleukin-6 receptor inhibition with tocilizumab reduces disease activity in rheumatoid arthritis with

inadequate response to disease-modifying antirheumatic drugs: the Tocilizumab in Combination With Traditional Disease-Modifying Anti-rheumatic Drug Therapy study. Arthritis Rheum. 2008;58:2968–80.

17. Navarro-Compan MV, Gherghe AM, Smolen JS, et al. Relationship between disease activity indices and their individual components and radiographic progression in RA: a systematic literature review. Rheumatology (Oxford). 2015;54(6):994–1007.

18. Aletaha D, Machold KP, Nell VP, et al. The perception of rheumatoid arthritis core set measures by rheumatologists. Results of a survey. Rheumatology (Oxford). 2006;45(9):1133–9.

19. Balsa A, de Miguel E, Castillo C, et al. Superiority of SDAI over DAS-28 in assessment of remission in rheumatoid arthritis patients using power Doppler ultrasonography as a gold standard. Rheumatology (Oxford). 2010; 49(4):683–90.

20. Nishimoto N, Takagi N. Assessment of the validity of the 28-joint disease activity score using erythrocyte sedimentation rate (DAS28-ESR) as a disease activity index of rheumatoid arthritis in the efficacy evaluation of 24-week treatment with tocilizumab: subanalysis of the SATORI study. Mod Rheumatol. 2010;20(6):539–47.

21. Shaver TS, Anderson JD, Weidensaul DN, et al. The problem of rheumatoid arthritis disease activity and remission in clinical practice. J Rheumatol. 2008; 35:1015–22.

22. Smolen JS, Aletaha D, Gruben D, et al. Remission rates with tofacitinib treatment in rheumatoid arthritis: a comparison of various remission criteria. Arthritis Rheum. 2012;64(Suppl):S334.

23. Smolen JS, Avila JC, Aletaha D. Tocilizumab inhibits progression of joint damage in rheumatoid arthritis irrespective of its anti-inflammatory effects: disassociation of the link between inflammation and destruction. Ann Rheum Dis. 2012;71(5):687–93.

24. Aletaha D, Smolen JS. Joint damage in rheumatoid arthritis progresses in remission according to the Disease Activity Score in 28 joints and is driven by residual swollen joints. Arthritis Rheum. 2011;63(12):3702–11.

20

A phase III, randomized, two-armed, double-blind, parallel, active controlled, and non-inferiority clinical trial to compare efficacy and safety of biosimilar adalimumab (CinnoRA®) to the reference product (Humira®) in patients with active rheumatoid arthritis

Ahmadreza Jamshidi[1]*[iD], Farhad Gharibdoost[1], Mahdi Vojdanian[1], Soosan G. Soroosh[2], Mohsen Soroush[3], Arman Ahmadzadeh[4], Mohammad Ali Nazarinia[5], Mohammad Mousavi[6], Hadi Karimzadeh[7], Mohammad Reza Shakibi[8], Zahra Rezaieyazdi[9], Maryam Sahebari[9], Asghar Hajiabbasi[10], Ali Asghar Ebrahimi[11], Najmeh Mahjourian[12] and Amin Mohammadinejad Rashti[13]

Abstract

Background: This study aimed to compare efficacy and safety of test-adalimumab (CinnoRA®, CinnaGen, Iran) to the innovator product (Humira®, AbbVie, USA) in adult patients with active rheumatoid arthritis (RA).

Methods: In this randomized, double-blind, active-controlled, non-inferiority trial, a total of 136 patients with active RA were randomized to receive 40 mg subcutaneous injections of either CinnoRA® or Humira® every other week, while receiving methotrexate (15 mg/week), folic acid (1 mg/day), and prednisolone (7.5 mg/day) over a period of 24 weeks. Physical examinations, vital sign evaluations, and laboratory tests were conducted in patients at baseline and at 12-week and 24-week visits. The primary endpoint in this study was the proportion of patients achieving moderate and good disease activity score in 28 joints-erythrocyte sedimentation rate (DAS28-ESR)-based European League Against Rheumatism (EULAR) response. The secondary endpoints were the proportion of patients achieving American College of Rheumatology (ACR) criteria for 20% (ACR20), 50% (ACR50), and 70% (ACR70) responses along with the disability index of health assessment questionnaire (HAQ), and safety.

(Continued on next page)

* Correspondence: jamshida@tums.ac.ir
[1]Rheumatology Research Center, Tehran University of Medical Sciences, Tehran, Iran
Full list of author information is available at the end of the article

(Continued from previous page)

Results: Patients who were randomized to CinnoRA® or Humira® arms had comparable demographic information, laboratory results, and disease characteristics at baseline. The proportion of patients achieving good and moderate EULAR responses in the CinnoRA® group was non-inferior to the Humira® group at 12 and 24 weeks based on both intention-to-treat (ITT) and per-protocol (PP) populations (all p values >0.05). No significant difference was noted in the proportion of patients attaining ACR20, ACR50, and ACR70 responses in the CinnoRA® and Humira® groups (all p values >0.05). Further, the difference in HAQ scores and safety outcome measures between treatment arms was not statistically significant.

Conclusion: CinnoRA® was shown to be non-inferior to Humira® in terms of efficacy at week 24 with a comparable safety profile to the reference product.

Keywords: Adalimumab, Biosimilar, CinnoRA®, Rheumatoid arthritis

Background

Rheumatoid arthritis (RA) is a chronic, inflammatory, autoimmune disease of unknown pathophysiology leading to peripheral and symmetrical joint synovitis. The primary systemic manifestations are pain, morning stiffness, fatigue, and weight loss [1–3]. In progressive forms, it may lead to cartilage damage, joint destruction, and joint swelling resulting in impaired physical function and premature morbidity [4–6]. RA mostly develops in the fourth and fifth decades of life, with 80% of the cases occurring between 35 and 50 years of age. The worldwide prevalence of RA is about 0.5–1.0% with a female/male ratio of 2.5:1.0 [7, 8]. Although the presence of chronic inflammation has been proposed as a contributing factor, the exact mechanism of developing RA is still unknown [9].

The management of RA aims primarily at improving patients' quality of life (QoL), achieving low disease activity based on American College of Rheumatology (ACR) and European League Against Rheumatism (EULAR) criteria, and ultimately remission [1, 10]. The treatment options for RA include non-steroidal anti-inflammatory drugs (NSAIDs), glucocorticoids, conventional synthetic disease-modifying antirheumatic drugs (sDMARDs) and biological DMARDs (bDMARDs). RA treatment has developed considerably in recent years, with the early use of methotrexate (MTX) and the addition of targeted bDMARDs in patients with an inadequate response to MTX [10, 11]. In fact, concomitant use of bDMARDs and MTX has been associated with the greatest clinical outcomes in trials and has been approved as the standard of care for patients with moderate-to-severe disease [12]. The stage and severity of the joint condition, the balance between possible adverse effects and expected benefits, and patients' preferences are amongst the influential factors in choosing a DMARD. MTX is the most frequently administered sDMARD and is used either as monotherapy or in combination with other anti-rheumatic drugs. The early onset of action and superior efficacy makes MTX the synthetic agent of choice in the treatment of RA [5, 13]. Similarly, biological agents such as anti-tumor necrosis factor-α (anti-TNF-α) monoclonal antibodies are effective in suppressing disease activity, inhibiting structural deterioration and maintaining physical function. Adalimumab, a fully humanized immunoglobulin (IgG1) monoclonal antibody is produced in genetically modified Chinese hamster ovary cells (CHO). Adalimumab consists of two identical heavy and two identical light chains that bind specifically to the transmembrane TNF, thus blocking the interaction of TNF-α with its receptor [4, 14–16]. Adalimumab was first approved by the US Food and Drug Administration (FDA) in December 2002 for the treatment of RA and is currently approved for the following indications: RA, juvenile idiopathic arthritis (JIA), psoriatic arthritis (PsA), ankylosing spondylitis (AS), Crohn's disease (CD), pediatric CD, ulcerative colitis (UC), psoriasis (PsO), pediatric plaque PsO, hidradenitis suppurativa (HS), and non-infectious uveitis [17, 18].

Biosimilars are biotherapeutic products that are similar to the licensed biological reference products in terms of quality, efficacy, and safety, but often are provided at a lower price [19, 20]. CinnoRA® was developed by CinnaGen Company (Alborz, Iran) as a biosimilar to the innovator adalimumab product (Humira®). This study aimed to evaluate the non-inferiority of test-adalimumab (CinnoRA®) to the reference product in terms of efficacy, tolerability, and safety in patients with active RA.

Methods

Study design

In this randomized, double-blind, non-inferiority trial, a total of 136 patients with active RA were randomized in a 1:1 ratio to receive 40-mg subcutaneous injections of either biosimilar adalimumab (CinnoRA®,

CinnaGen Co., Iran) or the reference product (Humira®, AbbVie Inc., USA) every other week along with methotrexate (15 mg/week), folic acid (1 mg/day), and prednisolone (7.5 mg/day) over a period of 24 weeks. The study was conducted in accordance with the principles of good clinical practice (GCP) and the declaration of Helsinki across 10 referral hospitals in Iran. All the procedures were approved by the Institutional Review Board (IRB) and Ethics committees of each hospital. Patients provided written informed consent forms before initiation of any study-related procedure. The trial is registered in the Iranian registry of clinical trials with the following identification code IRCT2015030321315N1.

Patients' demographic information was recorded at baseline and a thorough medical examination was performed. Vital signs and laboratory examinations were taken from the patients at baseline and at the 12-week and 24-week visits. All the injections were administered by trained nurses at each study site. After initial screening and assessing eligibility, patients were randomized by permuted balanced block randomization with a block size of four. The randomization was implemented using telephone randomization by an independent contract research organization. Allocated treatments were administered to patients based on their enrollment number. Patients, nurses, and physicians were unaware of the size of the blocks and the allocated treatments, and the blinding was maintained till the end of the intervention. Information relating to demographic characteristics, contact history of subjects diagnosed with active tuberculosis (TB), medical history, and prior medications were collected. Body weight and height were measured and a complete physical examination was performed. Also, vital signs including heart rate and blood pressure were measured. Laboratory examinations, including hematological and blood chemistry assessment, measurement of rheumatoid factor, C-reactive protein (CRP), hepatitis B surface antigen, and hepatitis C antibody, urinalysis, and a pregnancy test in women, were performed during a fasting state.

Participants
Adult subjects of each gender who met the following criteria were included in this study: age between 18 and 75 years; active RA diagnosed by EULAR criteria [21]; moderate-to-severe RA for at least 6 months; lack of response to conventional non-biologic anti-rheumatic drugs after at least 12 months of therapy; and the ability to read, understand, and sign the written informed consent form.

Patients with any of the following criteria were excluded from the study: active or latent TB with a purified protein derivative (PPD) tuberculin test more than 5 mm in size or abnormal chest X-ray (CXR); previous treatment with TNF inhibitors; known hypersensitivity to human immunoglobulin proteins or other components of adalimumab formulation; in women, pregnancy, current nursing, or intention to become pregnant during the study; positive serology test for hepatitis B or C or human immunodeficiency virus antibody; ACR functional class IV or wheelchair/bed bound; taking intravenous antibiotics during the 8 weeks prior to screening or receiving oral antibiotic treatment during the 2 weeks before screening; history of serious, relapsing, or chronic infection; hemoglobin less than 8.5 g/dl; platelet count less than 125,000/μl; leukocyte count less than 3500/μl; serum creatinine more than 2 mg/dl; concomitant use of NSAIDs or more than 10 mg/day of prednisolone; receiving intravenous, intramuscular, intra-articular or oral corticosteroids (prednisolone, more than 7.5 mg/day) in the previous 4 weeks; previous treatment with rituximab, azathioprine, or 6-mercaptopurine (6-MP); history of chronic heart failure (CHF); history of myocardial infarction (MI) or unstable angina pectoris within 12 months prior to screening; history of demyelinating diseases or multiple sclerosis; history of malignancy within 5 years prior to screening; and participation in the study judged by the physician to be potentially harmful to the patient.

Efficacy and safety assessment
The percent of patients achieving good and moderate disease activity score (DAS)-based EULAR response was the primary endpoint of this study. The proportion of patients reaching ACR criteria for 20% (ACR20), 50% (ACR50), and 70% (ACR70) improvements after 24 weeks of treatment with adalimumab along with the disability index of the health assessment questionnaire (HAQ), and safety were the secondary endpoints of this study [22, 23]. The incidence of adverse events at each visit was recorded based on patients' reports, vital signs, physical examinations, and laboratory tests.

Statistical analysis
In a study conducted by Broeder et al., 89% of the patients who received adalimumab achieved EULAR response [24]. The sample size of 64 people in each group was estimated by a non-inferiority margin of $\delta = -0.18$ that was based on clinical judgement with 90% power and a 0.025 one-sided significance level. Primary efficacy measures were evaluated using both intention-to-treat (ITT) and per-protocol (PP) populations, while ITT population was used for safety assessment. Data were analyzed using Student's independent samples t test, the Mann-Whitney U test, the normal approximation test, Pearson's chi-square test, and Fisher's exact test. P values <0.05 were considered statistically significant. Data were analyzed using Stata 11.2 software (College Station, TX,

USA) and plotted using GraphPad prism version 6.0 (GraphPad Software, USA).

Results

A total of 216 subjects were screened across 10 hospitals in Iran, of whom 136 patients were considered eligible for participation in this study. Patients were enrolled in the CinnoRA® or Humira® arms (68 subjects in each arm) and 64 patients in each group completed the 24-week study period. Four patients in the CinnoRA® group withdrew from the study for the following reasons: adverse drug reactions (ADR, $n = 2$), positive PPD test ($n = 1$), and poor compliance ($n = 1$). Similarly, four patients in the Humira® group left the trial because of ADR ($n = 3$) and poor compliance ($n = 1$). The study profile is shown in Fig. 1.

Patients who were randomized to the CinnoRA® or Humira® arms had comparable baseline characteristics. The mean age of the participants in the CinnoRA® and Humira® groups was 48.29 ± 12.72 and 47.59 ± 11.48 years, respectively. The mean DAS in 28 joints based on

erythrocyte sedimentation rate (DAS28-ESR) was 5.51 ± 1.24 in the CinnoRA® arm and 5.47 ± 1.28 in the Humira® arm. The baseline characteristics are summarized in Table 1.

At week 12, the DAS28-ESR values were 2.95 ± 1.30, and 2.96 ± 1.41 in the CinnoRA® and Humira® groups, respectively (P value = 0.97); at week 24 the DAS28-ESR values were 2.58 ± 1.06 in the CinnoRA® arm vs. 2.55 ± 1.14 in the Humira® group (p value = 0.88).

According to the PP population, the proportion of patients fulfilling moderate and good EULAR response criteria based on the DAS28-ESR at week 12 was 42.42% and 54.55% in the CinnoRA® arm compared to 37.88% and 51.52% in the Humira® group, respectively (cumulative 12-week good and moderate EULAR response in the PP population 97% in the CinnoRA® vs. 89% in the Humira® arm; p value = 0.08; CI for the difference = –0.9 to 16). At 24 weeks, 28.13% and 70.31% in the CinnoRA® vs. 31.25% and 67.19% in the Humira® arm met the criteria for moderate and good EULAR response, respectively (cumulative 24-week good and moderate EULAR response in the PP

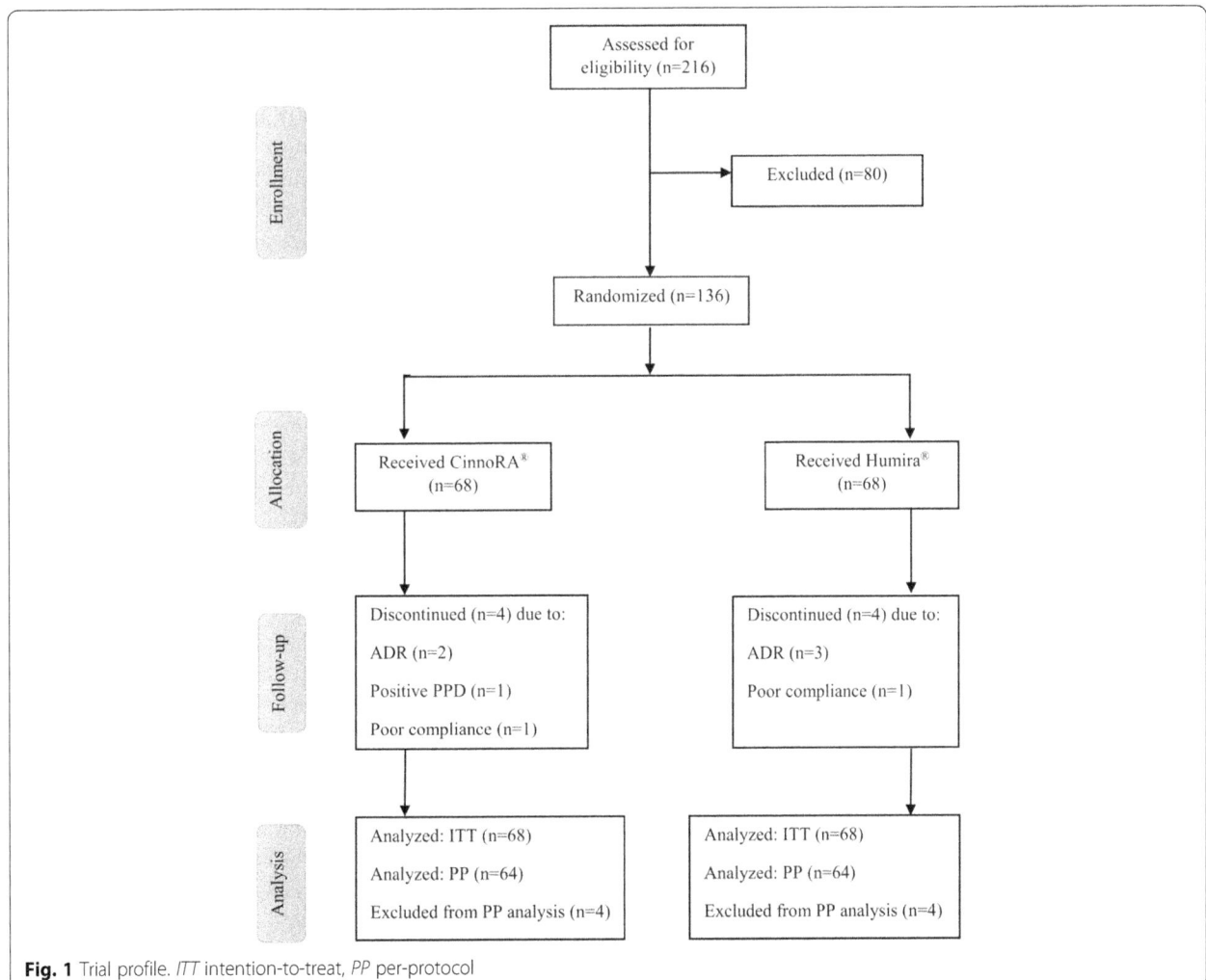

Fig. 1 Trial profile. *ITT* intention-to-treat, *PP* per-protocol

Table 1 Summary of the baseline characteristics of the patients

Variable	CinnoRA®	Humira®	P value
Age	48.29 ± 12.72	47.59 ± 11.48	0.73
Sex, n (%)			
Male	10 (14.71%)	8 (11.76%)	0.85*
Female	58 (85.29%)	60 (88.24%)	
Swollen joint count, 28 joints	9.96 ± 7.39	9.46 ± 6.98	0.69
Tender joint count, 28 joints	9.46 ± 8.23	9.66 ± 7.97	0.88
Patient assessment of pain	67.21 ± 23.51	70.22 ± 21.93	0.44
Patient global assessment of disease activity	70.15 ± 20.35	70.74 ± 22.21	0.87
Physician's global assessment of disease activity	68.97 ± 17.38	70.44 ± 17.68	0.63
CRP (mg/L)	21.40 ± 25.98	18.90 ± 23.90	0.57
ESR (mm/h)	32.65 ± 21.24	31.12 ± 24.01	0.69
HAQ	1.25 (1.38)	1.38 (1.13)	0.56†
DAS28-ESR	5.51 ± 1.24	5.47 ± 1.28	0.87
RF	63.76 ± 57.22	76.95 ± 65.66	0.22

Data are shown as mean ± SD and were analyzed using the independent t test unless stated otherwise. *CRP* C-reactive protein, *DAS28* disease activity score in 28 joints, *ESR* erythrocyte sedimentation rate, *HAQ* health assessment questionnaire, *RF* rheumatoid factor. *Data were analyzed using Pearson's chi-squared test. †Scores are shown as median (interquartile range) and were analyzed using the Mann-Whitney U test

population 98% in the CinnoRA® vs. 98% in the Humira® arm; p value = 1; CI for the difference = −4 to 4). Similarly, in the ITT population, 41.18% and 36.73% achieved moderate EULAR response at 12 weeks in the CinnoRA® and Humira® arms, respectively, and 52.94% in the CinnoRA® arm and 50.00% in the Humira® arm achieved good EULAR response at 12 weeks (cumulative 12-week good and moderate EULAR response in the ITT population 94% in the CinnoRA® vs. 87% in the Humira® arm; p value = 0.14; CI for the difference = −2 to 17). At 24 weeks, moderate EULAR response was attained in 26.47% of patients in the CinnoRA® arm compared to 29.41% in the Humira® arm. However, good EULAR response was achieved in 66.18% of patients in the CinnoRA® arm and 63.24% in the Humira® arm (cumulative 24-week good and moderate EULAR response in the ITT population 93% in the CinnoRA® vs. 93% in the Humira® arm; p value = 1; CI for the difference = −9 to 9). Based on the prespecified margin of 20%, non-inferiority of test-adalimumab to the reference product in terms of the proportion of patients achieving good or moderate EULAR response was confirmed at both the 12-week and 24-week time points (Fig. 2, Table 2).

The median (IQR) HAQ scores at 12 and 24 weeks were 0.25 (0.88) and 0.25 (0.63) in the CinnoRA® arm vs. 0.38 (0.88) and 0.19 (0.63) in the Humira® arm, respectively. The difference between treatment arms was not statistically significant at the respective time points (12 weeks, p value = 0.87; 24 weeks, p value = 0.48).

The proportion of patients achieving ACR20, ACR50, and ACR70 responses at the 12-week time point were 85%, 61%, and 28% in the CinnoRA® arm compared to respective values of 76%, 48%, and 36% in the Humira® arm. At week 24, 92%, 77%, and 47% of the patients in the CinnoRA® arm achieved ACR20, ACR50, and ACR70 responses, respectively, which was similar to those observed in the Humira® arm (89%, 75%, and 53%, respectively). No statistically significant difference was observed between treatment arms at either the 12-week or the 24-week time point (all p values >0.05, Fig. 3).

The incidence of adverse effects was comparable between patients who received test-adalimumab compared to those who took the reference product. Overall, a total of 24 patients (35.29%) in the CinnoRA® arm vs. 30 (44.12%) patients in the Humira® arm reported at least one adverse event. The most prevalent adverse events were local (8.82% with CinnoRA®, 17.65% with Humira®) and respiratory (8.82% with CinnoRA®, 20.59% with Humira®) adverse effects (Table 3).

Discussion

Randomized clinical trials demonstrating comparable efficacy, safety and tolerability of the biosimilar and innovator products are absolutely necessary as well as analytical evidence to establish similar physicochemical and biological actions of the products. Biosimilars improve the availability of more affordable products while offering similar efficacy and safety to the reference product [18, 25–27]. The perception of biosimilarity has been changed over recent years, especially in rheumatology. In September 2016, AMJEVITA™ (Amgen®, Thousand Oaks) was approved by the FDA, as a biosimilar adalimumab for treatment of seven inflammatory diseases. Similarly, Exemptia™, another adalimumab biosimilar, was approved in India. Etanercept and infliximab biosimilars were also authorized in various indications. In May 2016, Inflectra™ was approved by the European Medicines Agency (EMA) and the FDA as an infliximab biosimilar for all indications of the reference infliximab, including RA, AS, PsA, PsO, CD, and UC. In the case of etanercept, the biosimilar HD203 was recently approved in South Korea. In addition, Samsung Bioepis's SB4, known as BRENZYS™ (Samsung Bioepis Co., Ltd., Korea) received regulatory approval from the Korean Ministry of Food and Drug Safety (MFDS), the European Commission (EC), and the Australian Therapeutic Goods Administration (TGA) to be used as a biosimilar alternative to etanercept [18, 28].

In this randomized, double-blind, parallel-group, non-inferiority study, the efficacy and safety of CinnoRA® were compared with those of adalimumab in the

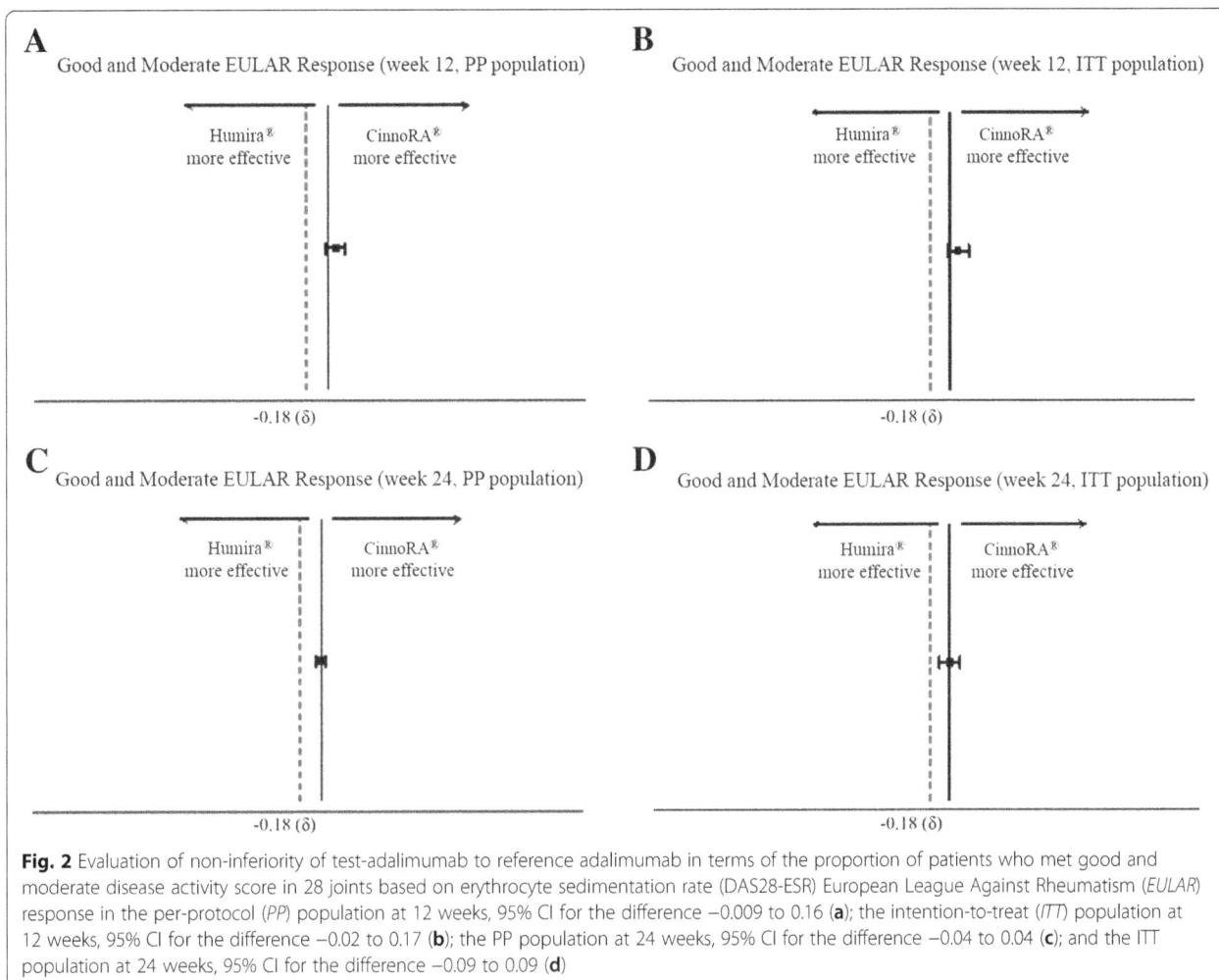

Fig. 2 Evaluation of non-inferiority of test-adalimumab to reference adalimumab in terms of the proportion of patients who met good and moderate disease activity score in 28 joints based on erythrocyte sedimentation rate (DAS28-ESR) European League Against Rheumatism (*EULAR*) response in the per-protocol (*PP*) population at 12 weeks, 95% CI for the difference −0.009 to 0.16 (**a**); the intention-to-treat (*ITT*) population at 12 weeks, 95% CI for the difference −0.02 to 0.17 (**b**); the PP population at 24 weeks, 95% CI for the difference −0.04 to 0.04 (**c**); and the ITT population at 24 weeks, 95% CI for the difference −0.09 to 0.09 (**d**)

treatment of adult patients with active RA. Several studies have assessed the efficacy of 40 mg adalimumab administered subcutaneously every other week, in terms of ACR criteria and DAS-based EULAR response. In the study of Bombardieri et al., the efficacy of adalimumab was evaluated in RA patients for a 12-week period. By the end of week 12, about 60% and 33% of patients achieved ACR20 and ACR50 responses, respectively. Based on EULAR criteria, 76% of patients attained a moderate response and 23% attained a good response. In addition, 12% of patients reached clinical remission, achieving a DAS28 less than 2.6 [29, 30]. In another study, Huang et al. assessed the efficacy and safety of adalimumab in combination with MTX by administrating 40 mg adalimumab every other week for 12 weeks. The results of this multicenter, randomized, double-blind, placebo-controlled clinical trial indicated that 57% of patients achieved ACR20 and 32.2% of them achieved ACR50 responses [31]. In line with previous studies, we evaluated the percentage of patients with moderate-to-good DAS-based EULAR response, which was our

primary outcome measure. Additionally, we compared the number of patients reaching ACR 20, ACR50, and ACR70 responses, along with ESR, CRP, and HAQ status. The percentage of our patients achieving moderate and good EULAR responses increased significantly in both the CinnoRA® and the Humira® arms, and the difference between the two arms was not statistically significant. Further, the percentage of patients reaching ACR20, ACR50, and ACR70 increased significantly during the 6-month period. In the retrospective study of Takeuchi et al. investigating the ability of adalimumab to reduce disease activity in 167 patients with RA, the mean DAS28-ESR score decreased from 5.3 ± 1.3 at baseline to 3.5 ± 1.5 at week 52 ($p < 0.0001$), which is consistent with our findings [32].

Furst et al. conducted a double-blind, placebo-controlled study and assigned patients into groups receiving either adalimumab 40 mg subcutaneously every other week or placebo. The study aimed to evaluate the efficacy of adalimumab when given with standard anti-rheumatic therapy over 24 weeks in patients with active

Table 2 Summary of DAS28-ESR, HAQ, and EULAR response measures

Variable		Week	CinnoRA®	Humira®	P value
DAS28-ESR		12	2.95 ± 1.30	2.96 ± 1.41	0.97*
		24	2.58 ± 1.06	2.55 ± 1.14	0.88*
HAQ		12	0.25 (0.88)	0.38 (0.88)	0.87**
		24	0.25 (0.63)	0.19 (0.63)	0.48**
EULAR response (PP)	No response, n (%)	12	2 (3.03)	7 (10.61)	0.28***
	Moderate response, n (%)		28 (42.42)	25 (37.88)	
	Good response, n (%)		36 (54.55)	34 (51.52)	
	No response, n (%)	24	1 (1.56)	1 (1.56)	0.92***
	Moderate response, n (%)		18 (28.13)	20 (31.25)	
	Good response, n (%)		45 (70.31)	43 (67.19)	
EULAR response (ITT)	No response, n (%)	12	4 (5.88)	9 (13.24)	0.37***
	Moderate response, n (%)		28 (41.18)	25 (36.76)	
	Good response, n (%)		36 (52.94)	34 (50.00)	
	No response, n (%)	24	5 (7.35)	5 (7.35)	0.96***
	Moderate response, n (%)		18 (26.47)	20 (29.41)	
	Good response, n (%)		45 (66.18)	43 (63.24)	

DAS28-ESR disease activity score in 28 joints based on erythrocyte sedimentation rate, *HAQ* health assessment questionnaire, *EULAR* European League Against Rheumatism, *PP* per-protocol, *ITT* intention-to-treat. *Data are shown as mean ± SD and were analyzed using the independent samples t test. **Scores are shown as median (interquartile range) and were analyzed using the Mann-Whitney U test. ***Data were analyzed using Fisher's exact test

RA, who were not adequately responding to such therapies. Similarly, a 24-week follow-up period was considered to evaluate the efficacy and safety of test-adalimumab in rheumatic patients [33].

Aletaha et al. chose the 3-month time point as a critical decision point in the treatment of patients with RA. It seems that patients who have significantly improved by 3 months are more likely to reach their treatment target by 6 months. In fact, achieving responses at 3 months is a good indicator of remission at 12 months, whereas patients with poor responses at 3 months will probably benefit from changing the treatment [34]. In agreement with previous studies, patients in our study who had noticeable improvements at 3 months also had better remission status. Patients in the CinnoRA® arm responded to treatment within a shorter period of time; however, this difference was not statistically significant. In the study of Burmester et al. in rheumatic patients receiving adalimumab for approximately 5 years, the mean HAQ-disability index score decreased in the first 6 months and then remained steady till the end of the study [35]. Similarly, in our study the mean HAQ score decreased significantly in both treatment arms and the difference between the groups was not statistically significant. In fact, as an important therapeutic goal, adalimumab improved social and physical functions in rheumatic patients.

In the safety analyses of the study of Takeuchi et al., the most frequently noted adverse events during one year of treatment with adalimumab were reactions at the drug administration site, with a frequency of 11.40/100 patient-years [32]. Safety was evaluated based on the adverse events reported by patients. All the adverse events were summarized according to the *Medical Dictionary for Regulatory Activities system organ class* (MedDRA SOC). We did not notice any significant difference in the incidence of injection site reactions as the most prevalent adverse events between treatment arms, and our findings were consistent with previous studies.

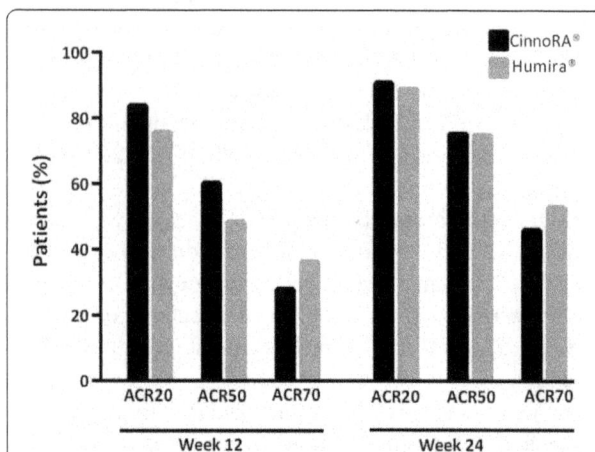

Fig. 3 The proportion of patients achieving American College of Rheumatology 20%, 50% or 70% response (*ACR20, ACR50,* or *ACR70*) following treatment with test or reference adalimumab at 12 and 24 weeks

Table 3 Summary of information relating to the adverse effects in the treatment arms

Adverse effects (AE)		Number (%)	
Organ systems	Type	CinnoRA®	Humira®
Patients with at least one AE, total*		24 (35.29)	30 (44.12)
Dermatologic	Hives	2 (2.94)	5 (7.35)
	Swelling		
	Rash		
Local	Inject site react., erythema	6 (8.82)	12 (17.65)
	Inject site react., itching		
	Inject site react., hemorrhage		
	Inject site react., swelling		
	Inject site react., pain		
Respiratory	Sinusitis	6 (8.82)	14 (20.59)
	Flu-like syndrome		
	Difficulty breathing		
	Respiratory infection		
Gastrointestinal	Nausea	5 (7.35)	2 (2.94)
	Abdominal pain		
Central nervous system	Headache	4 (5.88)	4 (5.88)
Renal	Urinary tract infection	1 (1.47)	1 (1.47)
Neuromuscular	Back pain	1 (1.47)	2 (2.94)
Other	Other	11 (16.18)	6 (8.82)

*Data were analyzed using the Pearson chi-squared test (p value = 0.29). *react.* reaction

Despite having a negative PPD test at the beginning of the study, one of the patients had a positive PPD test 8 weeks later that was probably due to close contact with a patient infected with TB close to the time of study enrollment.

Conclusion

Based on our findings, CinnoRA®, as a biosimilar adalimumab, was shown to be non-inferior to Humira® in the treatment of adult patients with active RA.

Abbreviations

6-MP: 6-Mercaptopurine; ACR: American College of Rheumatology; ADR: Adverse drug reaction; AS: Ankylosing spondylitis; BDMARDs: Biological disease-modifying antirheumatic drugs; CD: Crohn's disease; CHF: Chronic heart failure; CHO: Chinese hamster ovary cells; CI: Confidence interval; CRP: C-reactive protein; CXR: Chest X-ray; DAS28: Disease activity score in 28 joints; EC: European Commission; EMA: European Medicines Agency; ESR: Erythrocyte sedimentation rate; EULAR: European League Against Rheumatism; FDA: Food and Drug Administration; GCP: Good clinical practice; HAQ: Health assessment questionnaire; HAQ DI: Health assessment questionnaire disability index; HS: Hidradenitis suppurativa; IgG1: Immunoglobulin-G1; ITT: Intention-to-treat; JIA: Juvenile idiopathic arthritis; MedDRA SOC: Medical Dictionary for Regulatory Activities system organ class; MFDS: Food and drug safety; MI: Myocardial infarction; MTX: Methotrexate; NSAIDs: Non-steroidal anti-inflammatory drugs; PP: Per-protocol; PPD: Purified protein derivative; PsA: Psoriatic arthritis; PsO: Psoriasis; RA: Rheumatoid arthritis; sDMARDs: Synthetic disease-modifying antirheumatic drugs; TB: Tuberculosis; TGA: Australia's therapeutic goods administration; TNF-α: Tumor necrosis factor-α; UC: Ulcerative colitis

Acknowledgements

The authors thank all the participants in this study.

Funding

This study was completely funded by CinnaGen Co., Iran.

Authors' contributions

AJ participated in the design of the study and drafted the manuscript. FG conceived of the study, participated in its design and coordination, and helped to draft the manuscript. MV participated in the sequence alignment and drafted the manuscript. SS participated in the sequence alignment and drafted the manuscript. MS participated in the design of the study and helped to revise the manuscript. AA participated in the sequence alignment and drafted the manuscript. MN participated in the sequence alignment and drafted the manuscript. MM participated in the design of the study. HK participated in the design of the study. MSH participated in the sequence alignment. ZR participated in the sequence alignment. MS participated in the sequence alignment. AH participated in the sequence alignment. AE participated in the sequence alignment. NM was Clinical Research Coordinator and helped to draft the manuscript. AMwas Clinical Research Coordinator and helped to draft the manuscript. All authors read and approved the final manuscript.

Ethics approval and consent to participate

The study was conducted in accordance with the ethical principles that have their origins in the guidelines of the Iranian Food and Drug Administration (IFDA) and also the Declaration of Helsinki. The project has been approved (Code: 26826 in Tehran and Code: IR.KMU.REC.1394.126 in Kerman) by the Ethics Committee of Tehran university of medical sciences. The Clinical Trial Agreement (CTA) of this trial with the number 665/110693 in on 27 October 2015 was issued by the IFDA by Dr. Mehdi Pirsalehi, the general manager of the Drug and Poison Information Center. The ethics approval of the trial with the number 132091 on 5 January 2015 was issued by the Ethics Committee of Tehran University of Medical Sciences; it was also issued by the Ethics Committee of Kerman University of Medical Sciences with the number IR.KMU.REC.1394.126 on 7 September 2015.

Competing interests

The authors of the study declare no competing interests.

Author details

[1]Rheumatology Research Center, Tehran University of Medical Sciences, Tehran, Iran. [2]AJA university of Medical Sciences Rheumatology research center, Tehran, Iran. [3]AJA university of Medical Sciences Internal medicine, Rheumatology Section, Tehran, Iran. [4]Department of Rheumatology, Loghman e Hakim Hospital, Shahid Beheshti University of Medical Sciences, Tehran, Iran. [5]Shiraz Geriatric Research Center, Shiraz University of Medical Sciences, Shiraz, IR, Iran. [6]Department of Rheumatology, School of Medicine, Shahrekord University of Medical Sciences, Shahrekord AND Behcet's Unit, Rheumatology Research Center, Tehran University of Medical Sciences, Tehran, Iran. [7]Department of Rheumatology, Al-Zahra Hospital, Isfahan, Iran. [8]Endocrinology and Metabolism Research Center, Institute of Basic and Clinical Physiology Sciences, Kerman University of Medical Sciences, Kerman, Iran. [9]Rheumatic Diseases Research Center, Faculty of Medicine, Mashhad University of medical Sciences, Mashhad, Iran. [10]Guilan Rheumatology Research Center, Department of Rheumatology, Razi Hospital, School of Medicine, Guilan University of Medical Sciences, Rasht, IR, Iran. [11]Tabriz University of Medical Sciences, Connective Tissue Reserch Center, Tabriz, Iran. [12]Tehran University of Medical Sciences, Tehran, Iran. [13]Tehran University of Medical Sciences, Faculty of Pharmacy, Tehran, Iran.

References

1. Bértolo MB, Brenol CV, Schainberg CG, Neubarth F, Lima FAC, Laurindo IM, et al. Atualização do consenso brasileiro no diagnóstico e tratamento da artrite reumatóide. Rev Bras Reumatol. 2007;47:151–9.
2. McInnes IB, Schett G. Cytokines in the pathogenesis of rheumatoid arthritis. Nat Rev Immunol. 2007;7(6):429–42.

3. Tugwell P. Pharmacoeconomics of drug therapy for rheumatoid arthritis. Rheumatology (Oxford). 2000;39:43–7.

4. Lee DM, Weinblatt ME. Rheumatoid arthritis. Lancet. 2001;358(9285):903.

5. Kwoh CK, Anderson LG, Greene JM, Johnson DA, O'Dell JR, Robbins ML, Roberts WN, Simms RW, Yood RA. Guidelines for the management of rheumatoid arthritis: 2002 update-American College ofRheumatology Subcommittee on Rheumatoid Arthritis Guidelines. Arthritis Rheum. 2002;46(2):328-46.

6. Alamanos Y, Voulgari PV, Drosos AA, editors. Incidence and prevalence of rheumatoid arthritis, based on the 1987 American College of Rheumatology criteria: a systematic review. Seminars in arthritis and rheumatism. 2006; 36(3):182-8). WB Saunders.

7. Kvien TK. Epidemiology and burden of illness of rheumatoid arthritis. Pharmacoeconomics. 2004;22(1):1–12.

8. Khan MOA, et al. Clinical evaluation of herbal medicines for the treatment of rheumatoid arthritis. Pak J Nutr. 2011;10(1):51-3.

9. Felson DT, Smolen JS, Wells G, Zhang B, Van Tuyl LH, Funovits J, et al. American College of Rheumatology/European League Against Rheumatism provisional definition of remission in rheumatoid arthritis for clinical trials. Arthritis Rheum. 2011;63(3):573–86.

10. Mota LMH, Cruz BA, Brenol CV, Pereira IA, Rezende-Fronza LS, Bertolo MB, et al. 2012 Brazilian Society of Rheumatology Consensus for the treatment of rheumatoid arthritis. Rev Bras Reumatol. 2012;52(2):152–74.

11. Smolen JS, Landewé R, Breedveld FC, Dougados M, Emery P, Gaujoux-Viala C, et al. EULAR recommendations for the management of rheumatoid arthritis with synthetic and biological disease-modifying antirheumatic drugs. Ann Rheum Dis. 2010;69(6):964–75.

12. Singh JA, Furst DE, Bharat A, Curtis JR, Kavanaugh AF, Kremer JM, et al. 2012 Update of the 2008 American College of Rheumatology recommendations for the use of disease-modifying antirheumatic drugs and biologic agents in the treatment of rheumatoid arthritis. Arthritis Care Res. 2012;64(5):625–39.

13. Weinblatt ME, Schiff M, Valente R, Van Der Heijde D, Citera G, Zhao C, et al. Head-to-head comparison of subcutaneous abatacept versus adalimumab for rheumatoid arthritis: findings of a phase IIIb, multinational, prospective, randomized study. Arthritis Rheum. 2013;65(1):28–38.

14. Menninger H, Herborn G, Sander O, Blechschmidt J, Rau R. A 36 month comparative trial of methotrexate and gold sodium thiomalate in the treatment of early active and erosive rheumatoid arthritis. Rheumatology. 1998;37(10):1060–8.

15. Choy EH, Panayi GS. Cytokine pathways and joint inflammation in rheumatoid arthritis. N Engl J Med. 2001;344(12):907–16.

16. Van de Putte L, Atkins C, Malaise M, Sany J, Russell A, Van Riel P, et al. Efficacy and safety of adalimumab as monotherapy in patients with rheumatoid arthritis for whom previous disease modifying antirheumatic drug treatment has failed. Ann Rheum Dis. 2004;63(5):508–16.

17. Food U. Drug Administration Guidance for industry: scientific considerations in demonstrating biosimilarity to a reference product. Rockville: FDA; 2012. 2015.

18. Castañeda-Hernández G, González-Ramírez R, Kay J, Scheinberg MA. Biosimilars in rheumatology: what the clinician should know. RMD open. 2015;1(1):e000010.

19. Medicare Cf, Services M. National health expenditures 2012 highlights. Online verfügbar unter http://www.cms.gov/Research-Statistics-Data-and-Systems/Statistics-Trends-and-Reports/National-HealthExpendData/Downloads/highlights.pdf. 2014.

20. Castaneda-Hernández G, Szekanecz Z, Mysler E, Azevedo VF, Guzman R, Gutierrez M, et al. Biopharmaceuticals for rheumatic diseases in Latin America, Europe, Russia, and India: innovators, biosimilars, and intended copies. Joint Bone Spine. 2014;81(6):471–7.

21. Aletaha D, Neogi T, Silman AJ, Funovits J, Felson DT, Bingham CO, et al. 2010 rheumatoid arthritis classification criteria: an American College of Rheumatology/European League Against Rheumatism collaborative initiative. Arthritis Rheum. 2010;62(9):2569–81.

22. Felson DT, Anderson JJ, Boers M, Bombardier C, Furst D, Goldsmith C, et al. American College of Rheumatology preliminary definition of improvement in rheumatoid arthritis. Arthritis Rheum. 1995;38(6):727–35.

23. Fries JF, Spitz P, Kraines RG, Holman HR. Measurement of patient outcome in arthritis. Arthritis Rheum. 1980;23(2):137–45.

24. den Broeder A, van de Putte L, Rau R, Schattenkirchner M, Van Riel P, Sander O, et al. A single dose, placebo controlled study of the fully human anti-tumor necrosis factor-alpha antibody adalimumab (D2E7) in patients with rheumatoid arthritis. J Rheumatol. 2002;29(11):2288–98.

25. Kaur P, Chow V, Zhang N, Markus R. A randomized, single-blind, single-dose, three-arm, parallel group study in healthy subjects demonstrating pharmacokinetic equivalence of proposed biosimilar ABP 501 with adalimumab. United European Gastroenterol J. 2015;3(5S):A606.

26. Njue C. Statistical considerations for confirmatory clinical trials for similar biotherapeutic products. Biologicals. 2011;39(5):266–9.

27. Fletcher MP. Biosimilars clinical development program: confirmatory clinical trials: a virtual/simulated case study comparing equivalence and non-inferiority approaches. Biologicals. 2011;39(5):270–7.

28. Dörner T, Strand V, Castañeda-Hernández G, Ferraccioli G, Isaacs JD, Kvien TK, et al. The role of biosimilars in the treatment of rheumatic diseases. Ann Rheum Dis. 2012:annrheumdis-2012-202715.

29. Bombardieri S, Ruiz A, Fardellone P, Geusens P, McKenna F, Unnebrink K, et al. Effectiveness of adalimumab for rheumatoid arthritis in patients with a history of TNF-antagonist therapy in clinical practice. Rheumatology. 2007;46(7):1191–9.

30. Hochberg M, Tracy J, Hawkins-Holt M, Flores R. Comparison of the efficacy of the tumour necrosis factor α blocking agents adalimumab, etanercept, and infliximab when added to methotrexate in patients with active rheumatoid arthritis. Ann Rheum Dis. 2003;62 suppl 2:ii13–ii6.

31. Aaltonen KJ, Virkki LM, Malmivaara A, Konttinen YT, Nordström DC, Blom M. Systematic review and meta-analysis of the efficacy and safety of existing TNF blocking agents in treatment of rheumatoid arthritis. PLoS One. 2012;7(1):e30275.

32. Takeuchi T, Tanaka Y, Kaneko Y, Tanaka E, Hirata S, Kurasawa T, et al. Effectiveness and safety of adalimumab in Japanese patients with rheumatoid arthritis: retrospective analyses of data collected during the first year of adalimumab treatment in routine clinical practice (HARMONY study). Mod Rheumatol. 2012;22(3):327–38.

33. Furst DE, Schiff MH, Fleischmann RM, Strand V, Birbara CA, Compagnone D, et al. Adalimumab, a fully human anti tumor necrosis factor-alpha monoclonal antibody, and concomitant standard antirheumatic therapy for the treatment of rheumatoid arthritis: results of STAR (Safety Trial of Adalimumab in Rheumatoid Arthritis). J Rheumatol. 2003;30(12):2563–71.

34. Aletaha D, Alasti F, Smolen JS. Optimisation of a treat-to-target approach in rheumatoid arthritis: strategies for the 3-month time point. Ann Rheum Dis. 2016;75(8):1479-85.

35. Burmester GR, Matucci-Cerinic M, Mariette X, Navarro-Blasco F, Kary S, Unnebrink K, et al. Safety and effectiveness of adalimumab in patients with rheumatoid arthritis over 5 years of therapy in a phase 3b and subsequent postmarketing observational study. Arthritis Res Ther. 2014;16(1):1.

Permissions

List of Contributors

Soshi Takahashi, Sho Sendo, Takaichi Okano, Kengo Akashi and Akio Morinobu
Department of Rheumatology and Clinical Immunology, Kobe University Graduate School of Medicine, 7-5-1, Kusunoki-Cho, Chuo-Ku, Kobe 650-0017, Japan

Jun Saegusa
Department of Rheumatology and Clinical Immunology, Kobe University Graduate School of Medicine, 7-5-1, Kusunoki-Cho, Chuo-Ku, Kobe 650-0017, Japan
Department of Clinical Laboratory, Kobe University Hospital, 7-5-1, Kusunoki-Cho, Chuo-Ku, Kobe 650-0017, Japan

Yasuhiro Irino
Division of Evidence-Based Laboratory Medicine, Kobe University Graduate School of Medicine, 7-5-1, Kusunoki-Cho, Chuo-Ku, Kobe 650-0017, Japan

Pawel A. Kabala and Chiara Angiolilli
Department of Rheumatology and Clinical Immunology, University Medical Center Utrecht, Utrecht, The Netherlands
Department of Clinical Immunology and Rheumatology, Academic Medical Centre/University of Amsterdam, Amsterdam, The Netherlands
Amsterdam Rheumatology and Immunology Center, Amsterdam, The Netherlands
Department of Experimental Immunology, Academic Medical Centre/University of Amsterdam, Amsterdam, The Netherlands
Laboratory of Translational Immunology, University Medical Center Utrecht, Utrecht, The Netherlands

Timothy R. Radstake and Kris A. Reedquist
Department of Rheumatology and Clinical Immunology, University Medical Center Utrecht, Utrecht, The Netherlands
Laboratory of Translational Immunology, University Medical Center Utrecht, Utrecht, The Netherlands

Nataliya Yeremenko, Desiree Pots and Dominique Baeten
Department of Clinical Immunology and Rheumatology, Academic Medical Centre/University of Amsterdam, Amsterdam, The Netherlands
Amsterdam Rheumatology and Immunology Center, Amsterdam, The Netherlands
Department of Experimental Immunology, Academic Medical Centre/University of Amsterdam, Amsterdam, The Netherlands

Aleksander M. Grabiec
Department of Clinical Immunology and Rheumatology, Academic Medical Centre/University of Amsterdam, Amsterdam, The Netherlands
Amsterdam Rheumatology and Immunology Center, Amsterdam, The Netherlands
Department of Experimental Immunology, Academic Medical Centre/University of Amsterdam, Amsterdam, The Netherlands
Department of Microbiology, Faculty of Biochemistry, Biophysics and Biotechnology, Jagiellonian University, Krakow, Poland

Barbara Giovannone
Laboratory of Translational Immunology, University Medical Center Utrecht, Utrecht, The Netherlands
Division of Internal Medicine and Dermatology, Department of Dermatology/Allergology, University Medical Center Utrecht, Utrecht, The Netherlands

Young Bin Joo
Department of Rheumatology, St. Vincent's Hospital, The Catholic University of Korea, Suwon, Republic of Korea

Yul Kim and Gwan-Su Yi
Department of Bio and Brain Engineering, Korea Advanced Institute of Science and Technology, Daejeon, Republic of Korea

Youngho Park, So-Young Bang, Hye-Soon Lee and Sang-Cheol Bae
Department of Rheumatology, Hanyang University Hospital for Rheumatic Diseases, Seoul, Republic of Korea

Kwangwoo Kim
Department of Biology, Kyung Hee University, Seoul, Republic of Korea

Jeong Ah Ryu and Seunghun Lee
Department of Radiology, Hanyang University Hospital, Seoul, Republic of Korea

Divya N. Challa, Zoran Kvrgic, Thomas G. Mason II, Eric L. Matteson, Clement J. Michet Jr, Scott T. Persellin, Daniel E. Schaffer, Theresa L. Wampler Muskardin, Kerry Wright and John M. Davis III
Division of Rheumatology, Mayo Clinic, 200 First St. SW, Rochester, MN 55905, USA

Andrea L. Cheville
Department of Physical Medicine and Rehabilitation, Mayo Clinic, 200 First St. SW, Rochester, MN 55905, USA

Cynthia S. Crowson
Division of Biostatistics Challa et al. Arthritis Research & Therapy (2017) 19:212 Page 12 of 14 and Informatics, Mayo Clinic, 200 First St. SW, Rochester, MN 55905, USA

Tim Bongartz
Department of Emergency Medicine, Vanderbilt University Medical Center, Nashville, TN, USA

Hilde Berner Hammer and Tore K. Kvien
Department of Rheumatology, Diakonhjemmet Hospital, Vinderen, 0319 Oslo, Norway

Lene Terslev
Centre for Rheumatology and Spinal Diseases, Copenhagen University Hospital Rigshospitalet, Copenhagen, Denmark

Vidyanand Anaparti and Xiaobo Meng
Department of Internal Medicine, Rady Faculty of Health Sciences, University of Manitoba, Room 799, 715 McDermot Avenue, Winnipeg, MB R3E 3P4, Canada
Manitoba Centre for Proteomics and Systems Biology, University of Manitoba, Winnipeg, MB, Canada
Rheumatic Diseases Unit, University of Manitoba, Winnipeg, MB, Canada

Hani El-Gabalawy
Department of Internal Medicine, Rady Faculty of Health Sciences, University of Manitoba, Room 799, 715 McDermot Avenue, Winnipeg, MB R3E 3P4, Canada
Manitoba Centre for Proteomics and Systems Biology, University of Manitoba, Winnipeg, MB, Canada

Rheumatic Diseases Unit, University of Manitoba, Winnipeg, MB, Canada
Division of Rheumatology, Faculty of Health Sciences, University of Manitoba, Winnipeg, MB, Canada
Department of Immunology, Rady Faculty of Health Sciences, University of Manitoba, Winnipeg, MB, Canada

Neeloffer Mookherjee
Department of Internal Medicine, Rady Faculty of Health Sciences, University of Manitoba, Room 799, 715 McDermot Avenue, Winnipeg, MB R3E 3P4, Canada
Manitoba Centre for Proteomics and Systems Biology, University of Manitoba, Winnipeg, MB, Canada
Department of Immunology, Rady Faculty of Health Sciences, University of Manitoba, Winnipeg, MB, Canada

Irene Smolik
Department of Internal Medicine, Rady Faculty of Health Sciences, University of Manitoba, Room 799, 715 McDermot Avenue, Winnipeg, MB R3E 3P4, Canada
Rheumatic Diseases Unit, University of Manitoba, Winnipeg, MB, Canada
Division of Rheumatology, Faculty of Health Sciences, University of Manitoba, Winnipeg, MB, Canada

Victor Spicer
Manitoba Centre for Proteomics and Systems Biology, University of Manitoba, Winnipeg, MB, Canada

Hiroshi Sato, Shotaro Masuoka, Soichi Yamada and Toshihiro Nanki
Department of Internal Medicine, Graduate School of Medicine, Toho University, Tokyo, Japan
Division of Rheumatology, Department of Internal Medicine, Toho University School of Medicine, 6-11-1 Omori-Nishi, Ota-ku, Tokyo 143-8541, Japan

Sei Muraoka and Natsuko Kusunoki
Division of Rheumatology, Department of Internal Medicine, Toho University School of Medicine, 6-11-1 Omori-Nishi, Ota-ku, Tokyo 143-8541, Japan

Hideaki Ogasawara and Toshio Imai
KAN Research Institute Inc, 6-8-2 Minatojima-minamimachi, Chuo-Ku, Kobe 650-0047, Japan

Yoshikiyo Akasaka
Unit of Regenerative Diseases Research, Division of Research Promotion and Development, Advanced Medical Research Center, Toho University Graduate School of Medicine, Tokyo, Japan

Naobumi Tochigi
Department of Surgical Pathology, Toho University School of Medicine, Tokyo, Japan

Hiroshi Takahashi and Kazuaki Tsuchiya
Department of Orthopedic Surgery, Toho University School of Medicine, Tokyo, Japan

Shinichi Kawai
Department of Inflammation and Pain Control Research, Toho University School of Medicine, Tokyo, Japan

Ewa Kuca-Warnawin, Weronika Kurowska, Anna Radzikowska, Tomasz Burakowski, Urszula Skalska, Magdalena Massalska, Magdalena Plebańczyk and Włodzimierz Maśliński
Department of Pathophysiology and Immunology, National Institute of Geriatrics, Rheumatology and Rehabilitation (NIGRR), Spartanska 1, 02-637 Warsaw, Poland

Monika Prochorec-Sobieszek
Department of Pathology, National Institute of Geriatrics, Rheumatology, and Rehabilitation (NIGRR), Warsaw, Poland
Department of Diagnostic Hematology, Institute of Hematology and Transfusion Medicine, Warsaw, Poland

Barbara Małdyk-Nowakowska, Iwona Słowińska and Robert Gasik
Department of Rheumoorthopaedic Surgery, National Institute of Geriatrics, Rheumatology and Rehabilitation (NIGRR), Warsaw, Poland

Marina Amaral de Ávila Machado, Cristiano Soares de Moura and Steve Ferreira Guerra
Division of Clinical Epidemiology, Research Institute of McGill University Health Centre, 5252 de Maisonneuve West, Montreal, QC, Canada

Michal Abrahamowicz and Sasha Bernatsky
Division of Clinical Epidemiology, Research Institute of McGill University Health Centre, 5252 de Maisonneuve West, Montreal, QC, Canada

Department of Epidemiology, Biostatistics and Occupational Health, Research Institute of McGill University Health Centre, 5252 de Maisonneuve West, Montreal, QC, Canada

Jeffrey R.Curtis
Division of Clinical Immunology and Rheumatology, University of Alabama at Birmingham, 619 19th Street South, Birmingham, AL SRC 076, USA

Emil Rydell, Jan-Åke Nilsson and Carl Turesson
Rheumatology, Department of Clinical Sciences, Malmö, Lund University, Jan Waldenströms gata 35, SE-202 13 Malmö, Sweden
Department of Rheumatology, Skåne University Hospital, Inga Marie Nilssons gata 32, SE-214 28 Malmö, Sweden

Lennart T. H. Jacobsson
Rheumatology, Department of Clinical Sciences, Malmö, Lund University, Jan Waldenströms gata 35, SE-202 13 Malmö, Sweden
Department of Rheumatology and Inflammation Research, Sahlgrenska Academy at Gothenburg University, Guldhedsgatan 10 A, SE-405 30 Göteborg, Sweden

Kristina Forslind
Department of Research and Education, Helsingborg Hospital, Charlotte Yhlens gata 10, SE-251 87 Helsingborg, Sweden
Rheumatology, Department of Clinical Sciences, Helsingborg, Lund University, Svartbrödragränden 3–5, SE-251 87 Helsingborg, Sweden

Hong J. Kan, Hadi Kharrazi and David Bodycombe
Center for Population Health IT, Department of Health Policy and Management, Johns Hopkins Bloomberg School of Public Health, Hampton House HH502, 624 N. Broadway, Baltimore, MD 21205, USA

Kirill Dyagilev
Cortica US, 425 Broadway, New York, NY 10013, USA

Peter Schulam and Suchi Saria
Computer Science Department, Johns Hopkins University, 3400 N Charles Sreett, Baltimore, MD 21218, USA

Charles T. Molta
Main Line Rheumatology, Lankenau Medical Center, 100 Lancaster Avenue, Wynnewood, PA 19096, USA

Jeffrey R. Curtis
Division of Clinical Immunology and Rheumatology, University of Alabama at Birmingham, 510 20th Street South, Birmingham, AL 35294, USA

Yu-Lan Chen, Jun Jing, Ying-Qian Mo, Jian-Da Ma, Li-Juan Yang, Le-Feng Chen, Dong-Hui Zheng and Lie Dai
Department of Rheumatology, Sun Yat-Sen Memorial Hospital, Sun Yat-Sen University, Guangzhou, People's Republic of China

Xiang Zhang
Department of Radiology, Sun Yat-Sen Memorial Hospital, Sun Yat-Sen University, Guangzhou, People's Republic of China

Tao Yan
Zhongshan School of Medicine, Sun Yat-sen University, Guangzhou, People's Republic of China

Frank Pessler
TWINCORE Center for Experimental and Clinical Infection Research, Hannover, Germany
Helmholtz Center for Infection Research, Braunschweig, Germany

Stanley B. Cohen
Metroplex Clinical Research Center, 8144 Walnut Hill Lane, Suite 810, Dallas, TX 75231, USA

Rieke Alten
Schlosspark-Klinik University Medicine, Heubnerweg 2, 14059 Berlin, Germany

Hideto Kameda
Toho University Ohashi Medical Center, 2-17-6, Ohashi Muguro-ku, Tokyo 153-8515, Japan

Tomas Hala
Center for Clinical and Basic Research, Trida Miru 2800, 530 02 Pardubice, Czech Republic

Sebastiao C. Radominski
Universidade Federal do Paraná, Rua General Carneiro, 181 - Alto da Glória, Curitiba, PR 80.060-900, Brazil

Muhammad I. Rehman
Pfizer Inc., 1 Burtt Road, Andover, MA 01810, USA

Ramesh Palaparthy and Steven Y. Hua
Pfizer Inc., 10777 Science Center Drive, CB1/2103, San Diego, CA 92121, USA

Karl Schumacher and Susanne Schmitt
Hexal AG, Industriestraße 25, D-83607 Holzkirchen, Germany

Claudia Ianos
Pfizer UK, Discovery Park, Ramsgate Road, Sandwich CT13 9ND, UK

K. Lea Sewell
Pfizer Inc., 300 Technology Square, Cambridge, MA 02139, USA

Di Liu, Tong Li, Hui Luo, Xiaoxia Zuo, Sijia Liu and Shiyao Wu
Department of Rheumatology and Immunology, Xiangya Hospital, Central South University, Hunan Province, Changsha 410008, People's Republic of China

Hsin-Hua Chen and Yi-Ming Chen
Division of Allergy, Immunology and Rheumatology, Department of Medical Research, Taichung Veterans General Hospital, Taichung City, Taiwan
Faculty of Medicine, National Yang Ming University, Taipei, Taiwan
Institute of Biomedical Science and Rong Hsing Research Center for Translational Medicine, Chung Hsing University, Taichung, Taiwan

Chia-Wei Hsieh and Kuo-Tung Tang
Faculty of Medicine, National Yang Ming University, Taipei, Taiwan
Institute of Biomedical Science and Rong Hsing Research Center for Translational Medicine, Chung Hsing University, Taichung, Taiwan

Meng-Chun Yang
Rheumatology and Immunology Center, China Medical University Hospital, No. 2, Yude Road, Taichung 40447, Taiwan

Chun-Yu Chang
Rheumatology and Immunology Center, China Medical University Hospital, No. 2, Yude Road, Taichung 40447, Taiwan
Translational Medicine Laboratory, Rheumatic Diseases Research Center, China Medical University Hospital, Taichung, Taiwan

Joung-Liang Lan and Der-Yuan Chen
Rheumatology and Immunology Center, China Medical University Hospital, No. 2, Yude Road, Taichung 40447, Taiwan
Translational Medicine Laboratory, Rheumatic Diseases Research Center, China Medical University Hospital, Taichung, Taiwan
School of Medicine, China Medical University, Taichung, Taiwan

David B. Bartlett, Janet L. Huebner, Leslie Willis, Andrew Hoselton and William E. Kraus
Duke Molecular Physiology Institute, Duke University School of Medicine, 300 N Duke St, Durham, NC 27701, USA

Brian J. Andonian, Virginia B. Kraus and Kim M. Huffman
Duke Molecular Physiology Institute, Duke University School of Medicine, 300 N Duke St, Durham, NC 27701, USA
Division of Rheumatology, Duke University School of Medicine, 40 Duke Medicine Circle Drive, Durham, NC 27710, USA

Heidi Kokkonen and Solbritt Rantapää-Dahlqvist
Department of Public Health and Clinical Medicine, Rheumatology, Umeå University, Building 6M, 901 87 Umeå, Sweden

Hans Stenlund
Department of Public Health and Clinical Medicine, Epidemiology and Global Health, Umeå University, Umeå, Sweden

Bradford D. Fischer, Adeshina Adeyemo, Michael E. O'Leary and Andrea Bottaro
Department of Biomedical Sciences, Cooper Medical School of Rowan University, 401 S. Broadway, Camden, NJ 08103, USA

M. Schoels
Second Department of Internal Medicine, Hietzing Hospital, Vienna, Austria

J. S. Smolen
Second Department of Internal Medicine, Hietzing Hospital, Vienna, Austria
Division of Rheumatology, Medical University of Vienna, Waehringer Guertel 18-20, 1090 Vienna, Austria

F. Alasti and D. Aletaha
Division of Rheumatology, Medical University of Vienna, Waehringer Guertel 18-20, 1090 Vienna, Austria

Ahmadreza Jamshidi
Rheumatology Research Center, Tehran University of Medical Sciences, Tehran, Iran

Soosan G. Soroosh
AJA university of Medical Sciences Rheumatology research center, Tehran, Iran

Mohsen Soroush
AJA university of Medical Sciences Internal medicine, Rheumatology Section, Tehran, Iran

Arman Ahmadzadeh
Department of Rheumatology, Loghman e Hakim Hospital, Shahid Beheshti University of Medical Sciences, Tehran, Iran

Mohammad Reza Shakibi
Endocrinology and Metabolism Research Center, Institute of Basic and Clinical Physiology Sciences, Kerman University of Medical Sciences, Kerman, Iran

Index

* 9 7 8 1 6 3 9 2 7 4 7 6 5 *